Ethnic Validity, Ecology, and Psychotherapy

A Psychosocial Competence Model

APPLIED CLINICAL PSYCHOLOGY

Series Editors:
Alan S. Bellack, *Medical College of Pennsylvania at EPPI, Philadelphia, Pennsylvania,* and Michel Hersen, *University of Pittsburgh, Pittsburgh, Pennsylvania*

Current Volumes in this Series

ACTIVITY MEASUREMENT IN PSYCHOLOGY AND MEDICINE
Warren W. Tryon

BEHAVIORAL CONSULTATION AND THERAPY
John R. Bergan and Thomas R. Kratochwill

BEHAVIORAL CONSULTATION IN APPLIED SETTINGS
An Individual Guide
Thomas R. Kratochwill and John R. Bergan

THE CHALLENGE OF COGNITIVE THERAPY
Applications to Nontraditional Populations
Edited by T. Michael Vallis, Janice L. Howes, and Philip C. Miller

CLINICAL PSYCHOLOGY
Historical and Research Foundations
Edited by C. Eugene Walker

ETHNIC VALIDITY, ECOLOGY, AND PSYCHOTHERAPY
A Psychosocial Competence Model
Forrest B. Tyler, Deborah Ridley Brome, and Janice E. Williams

HANDBOOK OF BEHAVIOR MODIFICATION WITH THE MENTALLY RETARDED
Second Edition
Edited by Johnny L. Matson

HANDBOOK OF CLINICAL BEHAVIOR THERAPY WITH THE ELDERLY CLIENT
Edited by Patricia A. Wisocki

PSYCHOLOGY
A Behavioral Overview
Alan Poling, Henry Schlinger, Stephen Starin, and Elbert Blakely

USING RATIONAL-EMOTIVE THERAPY EFFECTIVELY
A Practitioner's Guide
Edited by Michael E. Bernard

A Continuation Order Plan is available for this series. A continuation order will bring delivery of each new volume immediately upon publication. Volumes are billed only upon actual shipment. For further information please contact the publisher.

Ethnic Validity, Ecology, and Psychotherapy

A Psychosocial Competence Model

APPLIED CLINICAL PSYCHOLOGY

Current Volumes in this Series

ACTIVITY MEASUREMENT IN PSYCHOLOGY AND MEDICINE
Warren W. Tryon

BEHAVIORAL CONSULTATION AND THERAPY
John R. Bergan and Thomas R. Kratochwill

BEHAVIORAL CONSULTATION IN APPLIED SETTINGS
An Individual Guide
Thomas R. Kratochwill and John R. Bergan

THE CHALLENGE OF COGNITIVE THERAPY
Applications to Nontraditional Populations
Edited by T. Michael Vallis, Janice L. Howes, and Philip C. Miller

CLINICAL PSYCHOLOGY
Historical and Research Foundations
Edited by C. Eugene Walker

ETHNIC VALIDITY, ECOLOGY, AND PSYCHOTHERAPY
A Psychosocial Competence Model
Forrest B. Tyler, Deborah Ridley Brome, and Janice E. Williams

HANDBOOK OF BEHAVIOR MODIFICATION WITH THE MENTALLY RETARDED
Second Edition
Edited by Johnny L. Matson

HANDBOOK OF CLINICAL BEHAVIOR THERAPY WITH THE ELDERLY CLIENT
Edited by Patricia A. Wisocki

PSYCHOLOGY
A Behavioral Overview
Alan Poling, Henry Schlinger, Stephen Starin, and Elbert Blakely

USING RATIONAL-EMOTIVE THERAPY EFFECTIVELY
A Practitioner's Guide
Edited by Michael E. Bernard

Ethnic Validity, Ecology, and Psychotherapy

A Psychosocial Competence Model

Forrest B. Tyler
University of Maryland
College Park, Maryland

Deborah Ridley Brome
University of Massachusetts
Boston, Massachusetts

Janice E. Williams
Morehouse School of Medicine
Atlanta, Georgia
and
Stanford University School of Medicine
Stanford, California

PLENUM PRESS • NEW YORK AND LONDON

Library of Congress Cataloging-in-Publication Data

Tyler, Forrest B.
Ethnic validity, ecology, and psychotherapy : a psychosocial competence model / Forrest B. Tyler, Deborah Ridley Brome, and Janice E. Williams.
p. cm. -- (Applied clinical psychology)
Includes bibliographical references and index.
ISBN 0-306-43870-4
1. Psychotherapist and patient--United States. 2. Race--Psychological aspects. 3. Afro-Americans--Psychology. 4. Whites--United States--Psychology. 5. United States--Race relations--Psychological aspects. I. Brome, Deborah Ridley. II. Williams, Janice E. III. Title. IV. Series.
[DNLM: 1. Models, Psychological. 2. Professional-Patient Relations. 3. Psychotherapy. 4. Race Relations--psychology. WM 62 T981e]
RC480.8.T95 1991
616.89'14--dc20
DNLM/DLC
for Library of Congress 91-21237
CIP

ISBN 0-306-43870-4

A Division of Plenum Publishing Corporation
233 Spring Street, New York, N.Y. 10013

Printed in the United States of America

Preface

This book has grown out of our individual experiences as well as our shared ones; out of our differences as well as our commonalities; and out of our conflicts as well as our convergences. Among us there are differences in gender; in individual, family, community, and racial histories; in life experiences, identities, and career paths; and even in reasons for writing this book. Of course there are also commonalities. We enjoy one another's company; we enjoy working together; and we feel enriched from our collaboration. We have written this book out of our complete selves, not just our professional selves.

The original objective of our book was to present to practitioners of psychotherapy, trainers of psychotherapists, and psychotherapy students a model of conducting psychotherapy that actively acknowledges and builds upon the ethnic and racial heritage of both therapist and client. We have found that to fulfill that objective we need also to acknowledge and build upon the psychological ecology of the therapist and client; and we also need to outline the kind of research necessary if we are to develop and evaluate the perspectives presented here. Those perspectives are embodied in what we have come to call the ethnic validity model (EVM) of psychotherapy. This model serves as the organizing framework in this book for providing a comprehensive view of (1) cross-ethnic/racial psychotherapy; (2) Tyler's psychosocial competence model, the framework underlying the ethnic validity model; (3) the ethnic validity model itself, and its applications to psychotherapy; and (4) a discussion of training, supervision, and research issues. As we wrote this book, we realized that the issues and concepts we presented have usefulness that extends beyond their role in helping to understand the influence of race, ethnicity, and culture in psychotherapy. Who we are and the salient aspects of who we are—such as those based on religious preference, gender, physical condition, and social class—affect our self–world relationships not only in psychotherapy but in many other settings as well.

This book is designed to orient the therapist toward examining human competencies and coping mechanisms, as well as human frailties and dysfunctions, within a cultural context. It informs the therapist about the various ways in which culture plays a significant role in determining both client and therapist perspectives and levels of understanding. This book is directed to all psychotherapists, not just those who are from a minority group or who plan to work with minority group clients.

This book is also directed to all students learning to do psychotherapy, not just those who are from a minority group or who plan to work with minority group clients. Our cultural identity as well as our personal and professional identities are present, with their limitations as well as their strengths, even when we are interacting with someone from a similar background. The three of us are psychologists and build from that disciplinary perspective. Even so, it seems to us that these ideas are relevant to therapists and counselors across the range of helping professions. Two of us are black and one of us is white; we were all born and reared in the United States. Even so, it seems to us that these ideas are relevant to therapists, counselors, and clients from other racial, ethnic, and cultural backgrounds.

We have chosen to focus primarily on black and white ethnic/racial interactions in the United States. There are a number of reasons for that choice. One is that black–white relations in our society have served as a model, an exemplar, for other cross-ethnic/racial interactions. Sometimes they have served as a framework for defining a newly encountered group by inclusion, sometimes by contrast. In either case, black–white relations have provided the framework for the interaction. Another reason is that the unresolved nature of black–white relations constitutes the central ethnic/racial issue in this society today, and seems likely to continue as such into the distant future. Certainly there are distinctive elements to Latino–white, Asian–white, Native American–white, Asian–Asian, Latino–Native American, and similar relations, and we do not wish to diminish their importance. There are also distinctive elements to interactions among and between individuals of different social classes, different regions of any country, and disparate living contexts (i.e., urban, suburban, or rural). Unfortunately our time, space, and experience are limited. We will refer to some of these dyads throughout the book, but we will not try to do so in a comprehensive fashion. We encourage you to use these examples as a guide to build on this framework and extend it on the basis of your own experience, needs, and context.

Issues of gender are as important as and even more pervasive than the ethnic/racial issues we are emphasizing here. We refer to them also. They need to be explored in the depth and detail we have sought to achieve in this book with regard to ethnic/racial issues, because they raise an additional set of important questions. Each of us is either male or female. To write a book that presumes to present a comprehensive portrayal of gender issues requires a two-gender collaboration. Perhaps our approach in this book to converging across racial and gender differences can serve as a guide to others wishing to undertake that task, but it is beyond the scope of this book. Writing on gender will challenge and extend existing perspectives in ways that will inform us all about gender issues as well as the utility of the EVM perspective.

We have sought to use nonsexist language. In fact, that task has seemed easy compared to the task of choosing nonracist words to refer to ethnic/racial groupings. In particular, the decision about whether to speak of African Americans or blacks has important political implications to many people. We have chosen to use the terms *black* and *white* uncapitalized as descriptive terms. We have not capitalized them as they are not proper names as are Asian, Latin, and so forth. We have chosen them rather than Caucasian or African American because they are the comprehensive terms in use. We hope that as a reader you will accept our choice as a good faith one to highlight the importance and complexity of racial/ethnic issues, not as an effort to assert a particular position on how they should be viewed. Also, the people we describe in this book, as is true of everyone, have a multifaceted heritage. We have described them first in each instance in terms of the aspect of that heritage that has seemed the most salient, whether that be race, ethnicity, place of origin, or some other characteristic. It has not been our intent to imply that any of these characteristics is inherently more significant than the others.

We are aware that the examples we cite are taken primarily from work with people in outpatient settings. It has not been our intention to ignore those more severely dysfunctional individuals who require inpatient care. Rather, we have included examples in which it is easier to illustrate the issues of ethnic validity. The underlying life issues that have contributed to the current state of severely dysfunctional persons are no different from those in the lives of less dysfunctional individuals. They may well have been harsher and more traumatic. Responding to the effects of those traumas requires sensitivity to the issues we are seeking to emphasize. Helping those individuals to attain more meaningful lives may be a more difficult task; it is not a task that can be accomplished by being insensitive to ethnic validity issues.

We want to call attention to one more aspect of our collaborative approach. To us it has been of seminal importance in developing a shared sense of the meaning of the concepts and perspectives we have sought to present. Specifically, we have written the chapters of this book separately and together. We have critiqued one another's work and probed one another's biases as well as insights. We have demanded that each of us write from the others' perspectives, present that material for review, and revise it until it was not only acceptable, but meaningful to each of us. We have not assumed that only people who are black can write about the black experience, that only people who are white can write about the white experience. On the contrary, we have said that our white author must write about black experiences in ways that have validity for our black authors. We have also said that our black authors must write about white experiences in ways that have validity for our white author. As you read, check your perspectives of us and our ideas against our perspectives of you and yours. As you try out these ideas, check your perspectives of them and of yourself against the perspectives of the people with whom you are trying out those ideas. We take full responsibility for points that are less than clear and for any errors we have made in translating the realities of others.

Acknowledgments

There are far more people who have contributed to this book than it is possible to acknowledge. We can note only a few of those who seem particularly important to mention. First and foremost are the clients who have trusted us enough to share their struggles and to suffer with us, even tell us, when we are blind to them. Much the same is true of students. They also must struggle against our limits as well as their own. Both clients and students take far more risks with far fewer protections than we do as therapists or teachers.

Each of us has had particular sources of support. Those are acknowledged in the following paragraphs.

I, Forrest Tyler, have been provided the basic institutional support needed for writing this book by the University of Maryland, especially the Department of Psychology. Further, without the assistance of the University Counseling Center staff I would never have been able to try out and develop many of the ideas that are central to the themes presented here. My graduate student research teams and students in my classes have helped incalculably by taking careful pains to help me understand my ideas and express them more clearly. Corinne Meijer and Dominicus So have also provided particularly invaluable editorial assistance. My colleagues Kenneth Pargament and Marianne Celano have read the manuscript carefully and encouraged us to struggle to express our ideas as clearly as possible. I also want to thank my parents, who gave me opportunities they never had. My work can most honor their memory by contributing to greater understanding of and more benign concern for people like them, those less favored. My wife, Sandy, has been both supportive and understanding in ways that have made this task easier, more enjoyable, and certainly better than it would otherwise have been.

I, Deborah Brome, would like to express my love and appreciation to my husband, Henderson, and my daughter, Leah, for their support and patience. This book and the work that it has demanded have always been a part of our history together, resulting in sacrifices for all. Your support, belief, and faith in me and in the vision of this book have been experienced through your willingness to accept these demands, yet assist me in balancing work with the treasures of life, our marriage and daughter. I also thank my parents for their lifelong encouragement, support, and insights, which have significantly contributed to my world view. In addition, I thank my colleagues at the University of Massachusetts, Boston, in particular Joan Liem and Cass Turner, for their encouragement; my research assistants Elizabeth Pike and Jacqueline McKinney; and Phyllis Doucette and Majid Zandipour for their technical support.

I, Janice Williams, gratefully acknowledge the support of Morehouse School of Medicine, particularly the Departments of Family Medicine and Psychiatry and the Academic Computer Network. I would also like to thank my family and friends, whose love and support have made my life and this task more manageable.

Contents

1

Ethnicity and Psychotherapy
Who Should Treat Whom?

Visualize, if you will, a community mental health center located in an urban area that serves a predominantly ethnic minority population. Seated in the waiting room are a middle-aged, black American couple; a young white Cuban mother and her two young children; a black Barbadian mother, her two latency-aged children, and one adolescent child. The health center receptionist is a young adult black American and a resident of the community. The therapist enters the waiting room to greet her client for the first time. The therapist is a middle-aged white Irish American, and her client is the middle-aged black American female. The client looks at her husband and slowly gets up to follow the therapist to her office.

For most mental health professionals, this multi-ethnic scenario is a familiar one. And given our stored impressions and experiences with various ethnic/racial and minority groups, this situation generates a host of associations about the persons described. We can readily create and form images of their attitudes, their characteristic ways of interacting, and their socioeconomic status. Accompanying these images are predictions about whether a white Irish American female therapist and a black American female client can develop an effective therapeutic relationship, a relationship based on trust and mutual respect.

For some professionals, to make such a prediction with any confidence would require more information. For instance, it would be important to know the therapist's qualifications and experience in working with black Americans, her racial attitudes and prejudices, her socioeconomic background, her comfort with herself and with those who are different from her, and her knowledge of black American culture and black personality theory. These same professionals would want to know the client's presenting problem and the duration of the problem; her therapist preferences in terms of ethnicity, race, and sex; her experience with white Americans; her racial attitudes and prejudices; her attitudes about the community mental health center; and her socioeconomic status. These variables have only recently been recognized in the psychotherapy literature as contributing significantly to therapeutic process and outcome.

Beyond our predictions about the probability of a successful therapeutic relationship lies a more general and fundamental question: Who should treat whom? This question directs our attention not only to the probability of success of a cross-racial/ethnic dyad, but also to the appropriateness of cross-racial/ethnic pairings given differences emanating from each person's world view and experiences. Embedded within this question lies concern about the ability of the psychotherapist and the client to relate to someone who is different from themselves. Also inherent in this question are underlying questions about the role of ethnicity and culture in shaping any individual's perspectives and assumptions about human functioning and in restricting any individual's ability to form and sustain relationships.

In spite of the diverse and numerous ethnic legacies in the United States, the study of the influence of ethnicity, race, and culture on therapeutic processes has been slow to emerge as a valid and legitimate issue within the disciplines that practice psychotherapy. Several reasons can be advanced to account for this situation. First, there is America's allegiance to the melting pot notion. Like all countries developed through the contributions of multiple nationalities and races, there is a struggle to define ourselves as a united group. The melting pot concept has been used to describe the process through which a multitude of nationalities have meshed to form one national identity, which is called "American." Essentially, this concept asserts that individuals from different nations, traditions, and legacies evolved to form the one culture and one ethos that defines the American personality and provides a sense of commonality among diverse individuals. That American identity and feeling of oneness in turn has been shaped by how the nation has viewed its psychological and sociological character. Psychological theory and research conducted in the United States have not escaped the melting pot phenomenon. As psychology has struggled to define itself within its cultural ethos, a universal and monolithic quest has ensued. The result for many years has been the proliferation of a single human norm by which all others have been measured. The standard has been thought by some to be white Anglo-American male and by others to be the white middle class. This standard has functioned as the basis of psychology's melting pot perspective. The major difficulty with this standard, as with the melting pot notion, is that all nationalities and ethnic groups and races have participated in shaping the standard, or the resulting "American" identity.

As pluralism has evolved as a realistic commentary on America's sociological and psychological character, issues of ethnicity, race, and culture have slowly arisen as avant-garde topics within mental health circles. The forces that have brought about the heightened necessity for a discussion of ethnicity and race have emanated from social reform movements, in particular the civil rights movement that crystallized in the 1960s. The civil rights movement addressed, among other things, the imbalance of power in this country; racism and its consequences; and self-pride, integrity, cultural identity, and accessibility to resources among ethnic and minority groups. From the civil rights movement other interests such as the women's and gay–lesbian groups were organized.

Civil rights movement advocates also addressed several key concepts that were replicated in mental health social reform. Psychology and mental health practices did not escape involvement in the context of change. One very early instance was the introduction of the Clark and Clark doll study in the 1954 Supreme Court Case *Brown v. The Board of Education.* Other topics documented in the literature have pertained to questions of racial pride, racial identity, and cultural integrity (J. Jones, 1972; Sussewell, 1981). In the 1960s and 1970s, black psychologists began to question and to conduct empirical research on black self-concept and identity development in an attempt to refute claims that the black self-concept was inferior to that of the standard (the white self-concept). These studies led to a new wave of thinking in the mid-1970s, again predominantly among black psychologists. That new wave focused on developing separate psychosocial reference frameworks for blacks and advocated the adoption of a more pluralistic than monolithic approach in psychology. Subsequently, there has been the emergence of literature among other ethnic minority groups calling for a similar pluralistic approach (President's Commission on Mental Health, 1978).

The social and civil rights question of the imbalance of power surfaced in psychology in the acknowledgment of the disproportionate number of ethnic minority to white psychologists in the country. For example, in the early 1970s, blacks comprised 11% of the population but less than 1% of the practicing Ph.D.'s (Gary, 1978). A strategy used to challenge the imbalance of power was an effort to obtain a representative proportion of psychology degrees awarded to blacks. Equally important to the goal of increasing the number of black Ph.D.'s was the hope that the black perspective would become an integral part of the discipline. Advocates within psychology for these positions felt that the academic research and professional interests of ethnic minorities would enrich psychological theory and play a significant role in social reform.

The emergence of the community psychology movement also involved an attempt to address the imbalance of power by introducing the notion of community input and control of mental health establishments. By including community input in the shaping of mental health practice, community psychologists attempted to balance the standards and world views used in identifying effective functioning and in treating dysfunctional behavior in community residents. Implicit in this thrust were the forces of social reform and psychological pluralism.

As the nation has addressed its monolithic approach to viewing its culture, so have psychology and other disciplines. The melting pot notion has been slow to take a backseat to ideas of pluralism in the country at large as well as in behavioral science. Yet, within the disciplines of psychology, social work, and psychiatry, one finds an ever-growing demand in the 1990s for research, seminars, and lectures that address the impact of ethnicity on mental health practice. Prior to the 1960s, ethnicity and race were rarely included as part of conference proceedings or represented in refereed research journals. When ethnicity was discussed, it was considered a variable that contributed to differences between individuals. These differences from the standard, normative group to which other groups were compared were seen as negative and counternormative. Ethnicity was not accepted as a variable that contributed significantly to the shaping of a different and legitimate way of understanding the world and how individuals functioned in it. Ethnic differences were to be accounted for statistically and thus were treated much like background noise on a tape recording. The richness of ethnicity factors in understanding the competencies and strengths of people was not recognized as a viable part of that discovery process. Instead there was a constrained use of ethnic variables that produced a blurred vision regarding their importance.

The recent introduction of ethnic factors as important in their own right has fostered the acceptance of ideas that support a pluralistic culture and that respect the legacies and traditions of a variety of peoples. The challenge we now face is advancing the study of ethnicity in mental health practice beyond its current avant-garde status. To capture the richness of ethnicity means that within mental health and psychotherapy circles we must develop methods of research and practice that respect the traditions and legacies of others. More importantly, these methods must recognize the conceptual and theoretical constraints embodied within many of our traditional paradigms and practices. This challenge requires more than a general understanding and acknowledgment of the perspective that views cultural differences as not equated with pathology. Many psychotherapists have reached that general level of sophistication. What is now required is that we move beyond our discipline's intellectualized response to the question of ethnicity, race, and culture. We need to incorporate our individual experiences, ethnic self-awareness, and organized collective knowledge about culturally diverse groups into psychological literature, research, and professional practice.

ETHNICITY, RACE, AND CULTURE: SHAPING THE INTERACTION

To discuss the role of ethnicity and race in addressing the question of who should treat whom, it is important to establish a framework for how these terms are conceptualized in the current context. *Ethnicity* characterizes a sense of connectedness that has been transmitted over generations by virtue of common ancestry. Ethnicity records a legacy of ancestral experiences, including those relationships that one's ancestors had with others. This historical legacy is incorporated at the unconscious (enculturated) and conscious (socialized) level of one's personal identity (McGoldrick, 1982).

Ethnicity is essential to the development of an ethnic identity. Ethnic identity is a sense of group membership based upon shared ancestral history, customs, and values. It is the conscious identification of an individual with his or her ancestral group. Some individuals are more in touch with their ethnic identity than others. Ethnic identity does not necessarily reflect the closest genealogical tie of an individual. To the observer, the ethnic group with which a person identifies may be only remotely related to what that observer expected. In such cases we sometimes find that the chosen ethnic group is the one which is seen as having the most status or prestige within a society. For example, a person may choose to identify with Swedish ancestors because there is a great, great grandmother from Sweden, when there is a grandmother from Germany who is two generations closer. Or, a person may choose to identify with a Native American ancestor versus an African slave ancestor. McGoldrick (1982) has argued that an ethnic identity is a basic psychological need. Certainly it is important for understanding ourselves and self–world relationships.

Ethnicity is a concept distinct from *race*. However, in most discussions of ethnicity, race enters the discussion as a viable and necessary conceptual counterpart. There is no consensus among scholars as to the definition of race. Some scholars, such as Ashley Montagu, consider the race concept to be "utterly erroneous and meaningless" (Thomas & Sillen, 1972, p. 26). They assert that race is a term that describes the characteristics of a group of people and at best is an "artificial averaging" that ignores intragroup differences (Thomas & Sillen, 1972). In American and European society, the race concept has been used to characterize groups of people based on physical (phenotypic) characteristics, yet for many these artificial groupings have taken on a genotypic meaning. That is, race has been linked with and thought to give some clues to a person's genetic endowment and baseline potential for intellectual ability and advancement in society.

Race does not provide the most detailed information about ethnicity. However, it may provide information about one's historical legacy as the oppressor or as the oppressed. In America, race has been used to align some ethnic groups and to disenfranchise a myriad of others. The Caucasian race represents a host of ethnic groups whose phenotypic characteristics include relatively white skin and whose ancestral roots are predominantly European. The Negroid, or black, race represents a host of ethnic groups whose phenotypic characteristics include black, brown, or bronze skin and whose ancestral roots are African. History reveals that the legacy of the black skinned–white skinned relationship has most often been one of slavery, colonialism, oppression, violence, and distrust. This legacy continues to color current black–white relations in America and to set a prototype for the relationships among the dominant majority groups and the dominated minority groups. Thus, in America the majority group is the *culture-defining group* in that it has taken on the role of dictating to other groups what standards and values shall be rewarded by the community at large. Minority groups do not define standards for the heterogeneous society, so they are non-culture-defining groups.

Non-culture-defining group (NCDG) membership and culture-defining group (CDG) membership are ascribed statuses that describe our ecologies and shape our personal ecosystems. These statuses also hold within them power relationships we inherit in our personal interactions. We are each born a member of one group or another, and in heterogeneous societies there is typically one group that sets the standards for that society. These standards typically do not reflect the diversity of that society or culture, but reflect the values, attitudes, beliefs, and meanings of the more powerful group. Thus, there is a culture-defining group and a non-culture-defining group legacy that the individual inherits by birth.

This status as a NCDG member or CDG member becomes part of

our self-system and is relatively stable and consistent. What this status means is that our self-perception as a NCDG or CDG member does not change significantly with the situation or environment. It is part of our identity. However, changes in our ecology or situation may have an influence on how this part of our self-system is experienced by us or by others. For example, when considering the American culture and what is considered normative behavior, the black American is aware that he or she is a member of the NCDG. He or she is conscious of the fact that his or her group does not dictate the standards for society at large. That understanding of one's power to set standards for the larger group is also translated to situations that involve one's own group. It is possible for this person to use his or her status to understand power relationships and to exercise this knowledge to bring about constructive change in his or her community.

In American society, race has defined one's status as a NCDG or CDG member. Furthermore, through race, people from various ethnic groups sharing the same skin color have been brought together voluntarily and involuntarily to create a broader-based, inclusive cultural framework. Race unified whites into Americans and blacks who had various ethnic legacies in Africa into black Americans. Whereas whites, due to their position of domination, have maintained aspects of their ethnic heritage within this framework, blacks have not. It is well documented that slavery and racist practices systematically ensured that significant aspects of culture would not remain intact for those African tribes brought to America (Billingsley, 1968; Hines & Boyd-Franklin, 1982; Nobles, 1980). Moreover, other peoples of color (e.g., Asians, Native Americans) also have fallen prey to the CDG–NCDG classification system.

Thus, race serves as a broader-based concept that joins individuals from various ethnic groups on the basis of external physical characteristics. It provides another way of understanding the legacy of group relationships and interpersonal interactions. Race cannot be interchanged for ethnicity, nor ethnicity for race. Consequently, these two variables are essential in understanding relationship patterns and interpersonal dynamics between individuals who are the same and between individuals who are different.

When we introduce the concepts of ethnicity and race into a discussion of psychotherapy we are also introducing a range of interactional patterns and ways of relating that are consciously and unconsciously embedded into an ethnic and racial past. This ongoing historical relationship exists for those who share the same racial/ethnic origin as well as for those who do not. Whites share a particular legacy with whites and another with blacks; blacks share a particular legacy with blacks and another with whites and so on.

To highlight this point further, let us use as an example an interracial social gathering. There may be some comfort felt by black guests and white guests in knowing that there are individuals who are like them at the party. They may make initial assumptions about individuals' social experiences, heroes, taste in music, intellect, style of dance, and other characteristics on the basis of race alone. These assumptions capture common experiences that resonate to what it means to be black and what it means to be white. In addition, they provide a basis around which to relate to those who are racially the same and different from oneself. With further conversation, one may learn that one person who is white is also French and Jewish, and another is of German and Roman Catholic background. As whites they will share a particular legacy that will influence their interpersonal dynamics and assumptions about one another, plus additional ethnic legacies that will enter into their interactions. Similarly, the black American and the black West Indian will have their racial and ethnic backgrounds enter into their interaction. What we find is that in addition to intergroup histories shaping assumptions and interpersonal exchanges, there is an in-group ethnic/racial history that significantly influences interpersonal exchanges and group dynamics. We often make assumptions about others based on differences. Similarities play an equally influential role in shaping our assumptions and interactions. Consequently, we find that each ethnic/racial dyad carries with it a host of possible ways of relating. Some promote further understanding about oneself, one's culture, and the other person; some promote misunderstanding or further entrenching of oneself into destructive ethnocentricity.

Culture is the final term of this triad to be discussed. For us, culture is what a group of people identify as being common to them, and it is represented by the shared creativities of that group. Culture refers to the person-made part of the human and physical ecology and includes such things as language, values, experiences, symbols, and art. This definition combines the perspectives of Herskovits (1956), Triandis and Lambert (1980), and Hilliard (1984). Herskovits contributes the notion that culture is person-made and is an artifact of our humanity. Triandis contributes the notion of the breadth of person-made influences. For Triandis, culture includes both the tangible products of a group of people and their subjective states and reality. And Hilliard contributes the idea of the collective, or the "shared creativities," of a people.

There are cultures within cultures, such that cultures may share such things as belief systems, rules of relating, and foods. Cultures are fluid and dynamic rather than fixed and insulated. They can merge, become further defined, or be nested within one another. Consequently, within a culture there can be multiple ethnicities and races who have identified a common set of shared creativities. Yet, these races and ethnic groups also distinguish and identify among themselves a shared set of creativities that have meaning for them apart from those of the larger, heterogeneous group. The term *subculture* has often been used to refer to the cultures of these groups. It denotes the status of a particular "shared creativity or belief system" as defined by the dominant group. Thus, CDG members often refer to themselves as having a culture and to NCDGs as having subcultures. Moreover, it is assumed that the CDG defines the ethos of all groups as well as the subjective and physical ecology.

As an alternative to referring to some groups as having cultures and others as having subcultures, we prefer to think of culture as representing multiple levels of shared creativity (both subjective and physical) that reflect the variety of ways in which human beings experience and define themselves in the world. For any heterogeneous group of people who share a particular territory or space, there are, for example, values, perspectives, tools, and symbols they share, and these things represent their culture. However, within this heterogeneous group there are racial groups that have their particular sets of shared values, perspectives, tools, and symbols that are significantly different from those shared by the larger heterogeneous group. And within these racial groups there are ethnic groups that have their particular sets of shared values, perspectives, tools, and symbols that are significantly different from those shared by the heterogeneous groups or by their racial group.

Cultures also interact with one another, and through their interaction they create symbols and subjective experiences that have common meaning to them or that further delineate how they differ from one another. Thus, when cultures interact they engage in a process of merging and differentiating, or to say it another way, of converging and diverging. This process, which helps to create a common ground as well as to clarify differences, can be rewarding and group enhancing, or it can lead to conflict.

In conclusion, culture is a complex, psychosocial descriptor that incorporates the symbols, life experiences, and realities of multiple ethnicities and races. Culture is the representation of individuals' shared experiences with one another and of groups' shared experiences with other groups. To some extent cultures are dependent on one another for defining themselves and for enhancing their development and growth.

UNIVERSALISM, PARTICULARISM, AND TRANSCENDISM: A REVIEW OF RACIALLY/ETHNICALLY RELEVANT RESEARCH

As psychotherapists are increasingly confronted with the possibility of conducting therapy with persons different from themselves and of justifying why they are or are not qualified to do so, the question of who should treat whom has stimulated much debate and controversy. Underlying this question and the responses to it are some fundamental assumptions. They pertain to whether people's ways of living and being human are a reflection of their common humanity, their unique individuality, or the social milieu and historical context in which they are socialized and live. Therapists conceptualize themselves, their clients, and their therapeutic efficacy and range within frameworks that seem to represent three relatively distinct schools of thought.

The first school emphasizes universal elements of human growth, development, and effective functioning. We refer to its adherents as *universalists*. Universalists believe there are fundamental constructs that represent a core of human experience that supersedes the importance of other variables such as race, culture, and life circumstances in determining how individuals develop and view the world. Consequently, to understand the therapeutic process universalists focus on convergent processes that they assume underlie all human conduct.

The second school emphasizes those unique elements of various groups of individuals that impact their growth, development, and patterns of effective functioning. We refer to advocates of this position as *particularists*. For them, differences in human experience and expression are thought to be the critical factors that determine the efficacy of therapeutic relationships and the success of therapeutic enterprises.

The third school recognizes, accepts, and respects similarities as well as differences between groups in regard to human development and experience. Advocates of this position are referred to as *transcendists*. For this group, emphasis is placed on both the commonalities and differences among people. To them, interactions may converge across such boundaries, they may diverge, or they may conflict. Therapeutic efficacy grows out of understanding these possibilities and of learning to utilize them to the benefit of the client involved.

Each of these schools of thought is represented by a body of psychological research that advances its position. Before discussing some of the empirical data that support each perspective, a general comment about the state of the art of cross-ethnic/racial psychotherapy research is needed. Atkinson (1985) has provided an excellent critique in what he calls a "meta-review" of four major literature reviews. These reviews were by Harrison (1975), Sattler (1977), Abramowitz and Murray (1983), and Atkinson (1983).

The impact of racial factors on psychotherapy has also been the topic of a number of other literature reviews (Bryson & Bardo, 1975; Butler, 1975; Garfield, 1978; Handy, 1978, Note 1; G. Jackson, 1979; E. E. Jones, 1978; Parloff, Waskow, & Wolfe, 1978). In general, these reviewers agree that there are relatively few studies that have focused on racial characteristics as they affect the therapy situation, relationship, process, or outcomes, or on therapy as it in turn affects those characteristics. Further, of that handful of studies only a few have not found racial differences.

Atkinson's meta-review and most of the above reviews have focused upon empirical research. However, of equal importance in understanding the origins of empirical research and the thinking behind it are theoretical articles written on cross-ethnic/racial/cultural psychotherapy. Much of the following section draws upon these bodies of literature.

Atkinson's analysis revealed three important features about cross-ethnic/racial psychotherapy research. First, most of the research that has been conducted has been done on black–white psychotherapy dyads. Research examining psychotherapy relationships with Asian Americans, Latino Americans, and Native Americans is limited, forcing individuals interested in cross-cultural counseling and psychotherapy relationships involving members of those groups to generalize their impressions from black–white dyads to other ethnic minority groups.

Further, most cross-ethnic/racial counseling and psychotherapy studies have utilized survey or archival research designs. In survey research clients and therapists are asked their opinions, feelings, or attitudes on a criterion measure such as counselor preference. In archival research, researchers examine client records to obtain data regarding aspects of the therapy or counseling relationship of interest. Analog research designs, which typically follow laboratory procedures with the random assignment of clients to treatment levels, are seldom used and therefore underrepresented in this research.

Third, Atkinson observes that there are two types of settings and, consequently, populations from which subjects have been selected. The majority of the early research studies used outpatient mental health clinics or inpatient psychiatric hospital settings. Recently, much of the research has utilized college counseling center settings.

According to Atkinson, a major obstacle in comparing the research reported in the four reviews has been organizational consistency. That is, there has been no consistent way to categorize the studies cited across all four reviews. Each reviewer used different descriptions in labeling the dependent variables about which research was reported. Atkinson settled upon seven categories of dependent variables as being the most efficient in summarizing the literature. They are client use, client preference, counselor prejudice, differential diagnosis, differential process, differential treatment, and differential outcome. In the discussion to follow, these categories are used to present research supporting or at least consistent with the universalist, particularist, and transcendist perspectives.

Universalism

In the research and psychological literature the universalist perspective is represented by those studies and conceptual articles which purport that ethnic and racial variables do not significantly alter the process and outcome of psychotherapy. The universalist's perspective is predicated on the assumption that all human beings possess the same personality configuration and fundamental characteristics. Given this basic assumption of commonality, it is concluded that world views and dilemmas faced in functioning in the world are not significantly altered by cultural or racial factors. Universalists acknowledge that the environment does influence human development. However, they argue that the core elements of self-definition and personality are the same for all individuals and supersede the racial, cultural, and ethnic influences. Typically, we think of our traditional models of personality development and of psychotherapy as exemplary of the universalist perspective. For example, Freudian theory of personality development and its psychotherapy counterpart, psychoanalysis, are examples of a universalist perspective. Both assume a universal foundation to human behavior and psychotherapy and propose specific ways to bring about change on that basis.

In psychotherapy, universalism is a perspective that uses as its foundation an assumption about what is the same among individuals. The therapist enters the therapeutic relationship with a fixed framework about the components of the client's personality and how they operate. Furthermore, the therapist guides the intervention process and decides whether the intervention has been successful on the basis of these assumptions.

At another level, we can think of the universalist process in psychotherapy as a process of convergence. That is, the therapist seeks to capture the commonality of experience between himself or herself and the client. Once this common focal point has been found and the therapeutic connection has been made, the process of change is ready to begin. Universalist perspectives provide a means to search for commonality in human experience and to manage the diversity among people in the world. They provide a framework and guideline for understanding human behavior. The major difficulty with these perspectives is that they are monolithic, often represent one cultural framework, and may be quite foreign to the way the client articulates and understands his or her world and functioning.

Enrico Jones's (Griffith & Jones, 1979; Jones, 1978) appraisal of black–white psychotherapy relationships is an example of a predominantly convergent or universalist position. Jones notes that race alone and the influence of race and culture cannot dictate therapy outcome. Rather, he believes that the therapist's sensitivity to the client and to the client's circumstance is the universal dimension that determines therapy outcome. That is, it is the therapist's ability to be open and in tune to the client's needs, lifestyle, and values that is the crucial variable.

Another rationale advanced in support of a universalist view is that personality functioning and therapeutic interactions are universal since they focus on the basically universal nature of individual psychodynamics. Korchin (1980) supports this point when he argues that there are (1) universal laws that govern human behavior, (2) a universal nonbiased set of scientific concepts and methods, and (3) unique ethnic characteristics that are the products of social conditions of learning, but that are secondary derivative human characteristics. The arguments outlined by Korchin reflect psychology's more general belief that there are universal laws. That belief has probably also served to justify a lack of commitment to investigating the presence of ethnic/racial factors that may bear on our concepts and the realities of human pathology, therapy, and well-being. In short, the large body of existing psychotherapy research conducted almost exclusively by white therapists with white clients stands as a testament to the universalist position as well as to implicit and explicit racial/ethnic biases.

There have been client preference studies as well as psychotherapy outcome and process studies that support the universalist school. For example, with respect to client preference research, Alston (1974) found no differences between blacks and whites in their willingness to explore problems in therapy with him. Cimbolic (1972) studied black clients paired with white counselors and with black counselors and did not find any significant differences in racial preferences. Similarly, in regard to process literature, Weiss and Dlugokinski (1974) did not find race related to length of treatment for children. Stevens (1945) reported that black professionals established rapport more quickly with black clients, but that the therapeutic resistance encountered was essentially similar to that of blacks with white professionals.

Jones (1982) has reported an outcome study concerning whether dynamic, insight-oriented therapy is appropriate for black clients. His outcome measures were therapists' ratings. Half of the clients were white; half were black; half of the therapist–client matches were racially similar; half were racially diverse. Clients were young adults who ranged from welfare recipients to professionals. The gender distribution was approximately equal for whites, but low for black males (36%). All of the clients improved with therapy and without any significant differences as a function of therapist–client racial match.

Similarly, Kaduchin (1972) feels that there is a "happy medium" between empathy and understanding that influences therapy outcome. In his study, this medium was achieved in all racially paired therapist–client relationships. A short-term therapy study by E. E. Jones (1978) also found both commonalities and differences. Specifically, in a study involving black and white therapists and carefully selected and matched (for age and education) black and white female clients he found some overall similarities in the evolution of the therapy process and found no differences in outcome as a result of racial matching. He did find race-related process differences. He emphasizes that bringing up race issues in an appropriate nonthreatening way is crucial to effective therapy and assigns to the therapist's clinical sensitivity the responsibility and power for transcending race-related issues. He also noted that in all cases there were substantial differences between the first session and subsequent ones. Thus he warns against generalizing from analog studies based solely on an initial session.

In spite of the fact that the E. E. Jones (1982) study supported the conclusion that the dynamically oriented therapists felt there were no race-related outcome differences, there were race-related therapist and client differences found in other aspects of their ratings. White therapists (in contrast to black therapists) rated their clients, especially the black ones, as more impaired psychologically. Yet, they were more favorable in their descriptions of black clients than of white ones. In contrast, black therapists viewed white clients more favorably. Black clients were seen by both white and black therapists as somewhat wary and detached in the therapy relationship, as if warding off intimacy or the therapist's power. However, white clients were seen as cautious and worrying, but more flexible. These findings, although limited, suggest that the degree of therapist–client cross-race commonality has some significant limits. E. E. Jones's findings suggest that what degree of commonality there is may be a function of therapist sensitivity, therapist–client matching, and a focus on convergent versus ethnically distinctive characteristics of therapeutic process and goals.

The limited findings supporting the absence of therapist–client cross-race differences may be even more striking in view of G. Jackson's (1976) argument that racial bias may have led to the conduct of such studies in a search for findings to support the absence of racial differences. Specifically, he argues that "color-blind" theory in the early post-World War II period led to a few studies designed to demonstrate that Euro-Americans could work successfully with blacks and also led to the justification for not including blacks in psychotherapy studies. He argues also that more recently, in response to a heightened outcry about the relevance of racial factors, there has been a backlash movement that has led to efforts to argue that racial differences found are in fact nominal or more a function of social class factors than racial factors. That is, in his view, there has been an effort to discount significant cultural/racial factors to obscure the facts of racial oppression. Whatever may prove to be the merits of Jackson's arguments, it is true that there are few relevant studies, and most of these are seriously confounded in design and relatively few find no racial differences. Clearly, more research is needed. These studies and analyses should at least in part be oriented toward assessing whether similarities found rest on experiential commonality (ethnic convergence) or on the presence of underlying universal psychological processes (basic universal dynamics).

Particularism

The particularist school of thought is represented in the literature by those empirical and conceptual papers which assert that ethnic, racial, and cultural variables significantly shape the world view of the therapist and of the client so that they become the most salient variables in determining cross-racial/ethnic therapeutic effectiveness. Particularists assert that in America, sociocultural factors such as race and ethnicity significantly alter the way human beings experience the world and view themselves.

Particularists are so named because they purport that there is a "particular" variable that supersedes other universal or common experiences in developing concepts of self, self–world relationships, and conceptions of human competence and effective functioning. In the literature, a number of variables have been identified as significantly shaping an individual's world view. They include race, ethnicity, culture, gender, and social class.

The commonality of human experience sought by the universalist is not thought by the particularist to extend from one ethnic/racial framework to another. That is, commonality of human experience cannot always be achieved. Divergence, which refers to the notion that all human experiences are not directly translatable into one another, captures the essence of a particularist perspective. Furthermore, to disrespect the divergence among people breeds conflict and violates the reality of a pluralistic society. Many of the studies which suggest that minority group members leave therapy prematurely and prefer same-race/ethnic therapists represent studies that support the particularist position.

There are several examples of the particularist position on interracial/cultural psychotherapy. For example, G. Jackson (1976) asserts that one's racial history provides the perceptual basis for how one experiences reality. He argues that blacks and whites have different perceptual experiences. These differences are seen as reflecting the cognitive style of blacks versus that of whites. For example, he discusses how the European (white) world view emphasizes a cognitive approach to life that is man-to-object oriented and individually focused. In contrast, the African (Afro/black) approach is affective, man-to-man and group focused. Jackson goes on to posit that these differences need not be all or none (i.e., pro Afro, con Euro, and vice versa). Instead he asserts that to the extent to which blacks have adopted aspects of European bipolar thinking in their way of viewing the world, they have come to share similar realities to whites.

Handy (1978) argues for "divergent validity" in his discussion of black mental health in this country. He notes that concepts of mental health have been used by society as social control mechanisms and that the mental health professions using them have served the status quo. Like his colleague Joseph White (1970), Handy argues that white mental health does not address the reality needs of black Americans and has not incorporated aspects of Third World mental health in its conceptualization.

Underlying Jackson's (1976), White's (1970), and Handy's (1978) arguments regarding the necessity of black concepts in mental health is the assertion that American psychology lacks pluralism. Various arguments have been advanced by psychologists as to why a pluralistic view is needed: (1) America is a heterogeneous society and American psychology should reflect this diversity; (2) ethnicity and culture significantly shape how individuals view the world and construct characteristic ways of functioning, and these unique characteristics will only be most accurately reflected in a pluralistic psychology; and (3) pluralism is the medium through which psychologists can design assessment and intervention techniques that promote optimal perceptual flexibility. That is, pluralism promotes a multicultural rather than a monocultural perspective, thus enhancing the psychologist's ability to make perceptual shifts in understanding the meanings, import, and relevance of various human behaviors.

Basic to the argument that black clients need to be seen by black therapists in order to engage in effective, supportive, and worthwhile psychotherapy is the belief that establishing rapport with clients is the key to successful psychotherapy outcomes. The nature of the rapport considered essential by these psychologists goes beyond the ability to empathize with the client. It includes the therapist's ability to know about the client's culture, to feel and experience what it is like to be black in a white society, and to know how this status in America compounds the client's presenting problems. It also assumes that the client is part of a valid culture, one that does not just deviate from a white norm, but that is separate from the white norm. A number of psychologists believe that the only persons who possess such a "cultural fine tuning" of the black experience are other blacks. More importantly, they also assume that the client is likewise attuned to the cultural sensitivity of the therapist.

There are several process studies that support these particularist views. The first studies of this kind were done 30 years ago, in the 1960s. These studies are representative of current literature in that they find that race and ethnicity influence the process of psychotherapy. What has changed is the interpretation of the finding. In the 1960s such a finding was used to endorse same-race/ethnic psychotherapy pairs, whereas in the late 1980s these results have been used to assist in sensitizing therapists to cross-cultural issues. For examples, Phillips (1960) found significant attitudinal and behavioral changes in black students assigned to black therapists and little change in those assigned to white therapists. Carkhuff and Pierce (1967) examined self-exploration in a southern female client population. They found the clients most similar in race and socioeconomic status to the counselor tended to explore themselves most, and those most dissimilar explored themselves the least. In regard to therapist–client rapport, Banks (1972) found that black therapist–client pairs achieved the highest rapport among middle-income and low-income blacks. Like Carkhuff and Pierce, he found that blacks are more willing to involve themselves in self-exploration at a much deeper and more meaningful level when seen by a black therapist than by a white therapist.

Other process studies that support race as a salient therapeutic influence address client variables. For examples, some investigators note that blacks in America are preoccupied with "the Negro problem"

(Heine, 1950; Shane, 1960). Also, it has been suggested that black clients are more submissive and suspicious with white therapists (Frank, 1947; St. Claire, 1951). Sue, McKinney, Allen, and Hall (1974) found that black clients with white therapists attended fewer of their sessions and were terminated after a smaller number of sessions.

In sum, studies of racial pairs in psychotherapy have reported differences in self-exploration, therapy attendance, therapeutic rapport, therapy outcome, and therapist preference. The reasons given for these results are varied. Generally speaking, they range from the idea that whites have been so ingrained in thinking that their culture is the correct way of knowing the world that they are unable to respect the culture to which their client belongs (Jackson, 1976, 1979), to the idea that whites are biologically different from blacks and they therefore see the world from a reference point that is inherently different and cannot be transcended (Nobles, 1976).

As previously stated, most of the research to date on culturally different and racially different pairs has been done with black–white therapy pairs. However, it has been hypothesized that heterogeneity of therapist–client pairs is ineffective for other groups as well. For instance, Acosta and Sheehan (1976) found that Mexican American students (as well as Anglo college students) stated a preference for therapists of their own group. More recently, Acosta and his colleagues (Acosta, 1979, 1980; Acosta & Sheehan, 1978) have found ethnically related differences between Anglo-American and Mexican American college students in self-disclosure and attitude toward therapists but not in reasons for therapy termination (the latter finding held also for black Americans). Roll, Millen, and Martinez (1980) reviewed the reasons for underutilization of mental health services by Chicanos. They report that their underutilization of psychotherapy is directly related to the stereotypes and myths of the Chicano culture. This view has been supported by Cortese (1979), Comas-Diaz (1981), and Bernal and Flores (1982) in their discussions of intervention techniques with Hispanics. Similar views have been presented by Tinloy (1978), Toupin (1980), Li (1980), and Lin, Inui, Kleinman, and Womack (1982) in relation to forming and maintaining therapeutic relationships with Asian Americans.

With respect to client preferences for counselors, Harrison (1975) found that black clients tended to prefer a same-race therapist. Also, Atkinson's (1983) review of client preference research tended to support Harrison's conclusions. Similarly, Sattler (1970) found that black clients preferred black counselors and that more positive relationships resulted when clients and therapists were of the same race.

This group of studies provides considerable support for the views of particularists. The client–subjects in these studies prefer therapists with similar racial/ethnic backgrounds, establish better rapport with them, become more involved, and change more. Reasons offered for these findings range across a spectrum of divergent validity and conflict validity considerations. Included are divergences of world view, experiences, lack of trust, and inadequate training based on an assumption of universality or convergence. As with the studies that found no cross-ethnic differences, these studies are few in number, limited in scope, and point strongly to the need for much more research on these issues.

Nevertheless, in addition to the sentiments expressed about differences in world views and realities for various ethnic and racial groups, there is the sentiment that white counselors, as they are presently trained, are for the most part unable to counsel ethnic minorities effectively (Bryson & Bardo, 1975). This sentiment relates directly to the training models currently employed, and the assumptions upon which they depend, including the assumption that techniques and strategies that are successful with one group will work effectively with another group. This argument is essentially a criticism of current training practices. Its relevance has been supported to some extent in a study by Turner and Armstrong (1981) of the racial and psychotherapeutic views of white and black therapists. They found that the black and white therapists in their study did not see themselves as "better" able or "more" able to establish good rapport with opposite-race clients, but that white therapists take less cognizance of a black client's race and experience more subjective discomfort with other-race clients. Black therapists, in comparison to white therapists, see white therapists as more prejudiced and as moving slowly on a wide range of issues. These findings, while raising important questions, do not tell us whether these differences affect the actual conduct or outcome of therapy, or whether clients should be racially matched with their therapists. Rather, they leave open the possibility that more appropriate therapeutic training can permit therapists to overcome ethnic/racial differences or that they can overcome those differences in spite of inadequate training and their own prejudices.

Transcendism

Transcendists view ethnicity, race, and culture as variables that significantly impact therapeutic processes. However, they do not view these variables as obstacles that cannot be hurdled. Instead, with the right combination of skills and therapist attributes (e.g., racial sensitivity, warmth, democratic style, etc.), the therapist is thought to be able to transcend the barriers presented in therapy by racial or ethnic differences. To transcend these barriers means to overcome them in such a way that the ethnic/racial integrity of the client and the therapist are maintained. Moreover, the differences in world view between the therapist and the client are appreciated and integrated into the therapeutic exchange. Possible outcomes from such a process are (1) the achievement of a common vision that reflects both the client's and the therapist's world views (convergence), and (2) the resolution that there are strengths and limitations inherent within both the client and the therapist's world views, yet no common perspective need be achieved (divergence). Therapist–client conflict, from the transcendist perspective, need not be a unique by-product of cross ethnic/racial dyads.

In recent years, several models representing transcendist perspectives have been developed. They include, but are not limited to, E. Smith's (1985) stress, resistant, and delivery model, D. W. Sue's (1978) cross-cultural model based on locus of control theory, Ibrahim's (1985) theory of cross-cultural counseling based on humanistic theory, and Comas-Diaz and Jacobsen's (1987) discussion of ethnocultural identification and assessment. A common theme in all of these models is the import of the cultural and psychosocial environment in shaping how information is shared, understood, and processed in therapeutic exchanges. But, many of these models and papers focus on explaining the ethnic minority client to the therapist in an effort to communicate how the cultural ecology shapes relationships and human interactions. Less is written about the therapist and what the therapist needs to do to assess his or her world view as a product of his or her environment. More models that address the therapist are needed.

The literature reflecting the transcendist perspective consists of a number of research articles that identify those therapist traits associated with either satisfaction in cross-ethnic/racial therapy or with nonconflictual cross-ethnic/racial therapy. These therapist variables were not specifically outlined by Atkinson (1985) but subsumed under other categories such as process studies and outcome studies. More recently, a number of studies (Gordon & Grantham, 1979; Jackson & Kirschner, 1973; Parham & Helms, 1981; Sanchez & Atkinson, 1983) have examined within-group differences. For the most part these studies have attempted to examine counselor preference, therapeutic process, and outcome by examining the complexity of the ethnic/minority client. Researchers assume an interaction between various aspects of a client's ethnicity (such as racial identity development and degree of acculturation) and other variables such as gender, social class, and education. In making this assumption, researchers are acknowledging the heterogeneity of a particular ethnic/minority group and respecting the range of differences within that group. The result is a more complex perspective of therapeutic process and of reasons as to why a particular cross-ethnic/racial dyad is effective or destructively conflicted.

As previously stated, there are several studies that examine therapist variables. For example, Lerner (1972) argues for a more democratic approach to therapy that permits the sharing of power between therapist and client. She found this therapist variable particularly important in treating lower-class clients, some of whom were black and some of whom were white. In a study of therapist characteristics hypothesized to contribute to dropout rates among lower-class clients, Baum, Felzer, D'zmura, and Shumaker (1966) found that therapists who tended to have the most success with lower-class clients were those who were more clinically experienced, more comfortable with the psychotherapy task, more able to use appropriate strategies, and more flexible in therapy. Similarly, Terestman, Miller, and Weber (1974) found that the more skilled therapists were more successful in treating lower-class clients. They were better able to deal with differences in class, race, and religion than less skilled therapists.

Yamamoto, James, Bloombaum, and Hattem (1967) studied the issues of race and ethnicity and how these can be transcended in therapy. They found that therapists who were more accepting of ethnic diversity (but not those who were less so) saw as many black as white clients for six or more times. Ewing (1974) compared client evaluations of pre-college counseling interviews in which black and white students were randomly assigned to black and white counselors. He found that the counselor's degree of helpfulness was more related to the training and experience of the counselor than to the racial similarity of student and counselor.

These studies suggest characteristics of the therapist that relate to differential outcomes in therapy with patients of ethnically diverse backgrounds. The therapist variables supported in these studies as yielding more positive outcomes included experience and skill level. Taken as a group, these studies are limited in number and scope and need substantial augmenting. Nevertheless, they point to the possibility that social/ethnic differences can be constructively transcended in the therapeutic context. This possibility is argued for by Bryson and Bardo (1975), who maintain that students preparing for the counseling profession must be provided opportunities for direct experiences with individuals from diverse ethnic and socioeconomic backgrounds. They suggest that counselors must be willing to accept that some individuals have needs, values, and attitudes different from their own. Acosta, Yamamoto, and Evans (1982) also have studied the factors that impinge upon and improve on the capability of low-income and minority clients to profit from therapy.

The transcendist literature attempts to instruct the therapist on how to achieve a greater sense of convergence between the therapist and the client (Beale, 1986; Benesch & Ponterotto, 1989; Borus, Anastasia, Casoni, Russo, DiMascio, Fusco, Rubenstein, & Snyder, 1979; Ford, 1987; Hector & Fray, 1987; Moffic, 1983; Ponterotto & Casas, 1987). This literature also highlights the therapist attributes that assist with achieving this level of convergence. What it does not discuss directly, and what we want to emphasize, is the role of ethnic/racial and cultural similarities and differences of the client and therapist in shaping the therapy relationship. The transcendist literature provides us with some understanding about what personal characteristics of the therapist and of the client can lead to positive (and negative) evaluations of each other and of their therapeutic relationship, but not of how to move beyond them to promote mutual personal growth.

CRITIQUE OF FINDINGS

The research studies bearing on the relevance of ethnic factors in psychotherapy are few, some of them are limited in scope, and some are not well designed or well conducted. Nevertheless, they provide a basis from which to critique the issues of ethnic validity, universalism, and particularism. One of the issues raised by the limited number of studies is the role of one's heritage in forming and sustaining a psychotherapy relationship.

The universalist orientation bypasses two major questions. First, are there in fact diverse conceptions of individual's relationships to their own lives that have internal and external validity? Second, are there diverse conceptions of individual's conceptions of their relationships to those around them that have internal and external validity? That is, the approach overlooks the possibility of divergent validities. Since the possibility is not admitted, it is not likely to be studied.

Another salient issue that arises is whether the research approaches used can identify cross-racial issues apart from therapist–client issues. That is, treatment and research approaches have focused primarily on client difficulties in therapy as an outgrowth of the client's individual psychopathology. Proponents of process-oriented and humanistic approaches as well as those advocating traditional pathology-oriented approaches to therapy have shared in rejecting the possibility that their identities and world views as well as those of their clients are psychosocially formed. Consequently, there has been no compelling rationale to develop methods for identifying the presence of ethnic validity factors. Nor has there been a rationale for interpreting results in ways that would support a conception of ethnically valid, but different, ways of being human.

It is important to acknowledge the possibility that these conceptual, methodological, and ethnic biases may have inhibited relevant research and obscured the presence of ethnic factors in psychotherapy. Even so, the available findings are instructive. They can be summarized by saying that some studies report that race differences between therapist and client do not make any substantial difference, some report that they constitute a crucial difference that cannot be transcended, and some report that they make a difference, but under certain circumstances it can be transcended. It is this apparently contradictory set of outcomes that suggests the advantage of adopting an ethnic validity perspective.

The studies that found no differences in cross-race matching of therapists and clients are limited in number. Even assuming their findings to be valid and generalizable, they may reflect ethnic convergence rather than universal psychodynamics. The studies themselves do not provide grounds for making that differential decision. That issue can be studied only as it is allowed as a possibility. Unfortunately, without substantial exploration and study, the concept of universal dynamics may be maintained simply by default.

Findings of racial/ethnic differences and the reasons proposed to account for them challenge our conventional patterns of thinking about pathology, well-being, therapy, and the training of therapists that focus on universal individual dynamics. In short, such findings force us to acknowledge the possibility that people have validly different world views that grow out of their unique natures and/or their psychosocial experiences. Consequently, we are confronted more directly with the necessity of incorporating those factors in theories about individual functioning, about therapist effectiveness, and about the possibility of valid but different patterns of therapeutic interaction. Both ethnic validity and particularist perspectives incorporate these perspectives.

In some of the studies it has been found that racial differences can be transcended in the interests of effective therapy. Findings from these studies suggest that the therapists who can transcend these differences are more democratic, more experienced, more skilled, more comfortable, more flexible, more able to use appropriate strategies, and more accepting of ethnic diversity. Evidently, an important component of effective transcendence of ethnic differences is the capacity to understand and accept ethnic diversity. In short, the more effective therapists are the ones who are more capable of grasping the client's internal and eternal perspectives on life and the world, and of understanding and accepting the validity of the client's world view and of helping the client to work with that world view in problem solving. It is the findings from these studies that provide the strongest support for adopting an ethnic validity perspective.

Fortunately, a few studies have begun to appear that are sufficiently comprehensive and detailed that they provide more specific information about the similarities and the differences of black and white therapists and clients interacting with one another. They also provide an illustration of the kind of detailed work and attention required to enable us to understand the issues involved in therapeutic interactions.

WHY WE NEED A NEW MODEL

Given our current knowledge of cross-ethnic/racial psychotherapy, what type of model is needed to further advance our thinking, training models, and skill base? First, we need a psychotherapy model that permits acceptance in the therapeutic process of different ways of living as valid. This model should also view people as capable of integrating individual and social experiences and contexts in defining themselves, their worlds, and their ways of living. Consequently, it imposes the same requirements on the formation of psychological theories and research designs, on the interpretation of findings, and on their applications. Such an approach seems particularly crucial to any effort, including therapy, that is aimed toward helping people solve problems in living.

Second, we need in America a perspective that addresses America's heterogeneity and the historical relationships that have evolved. We need a model that demonstrates how these relationships can be conceptualized and worked through in psychotherapy. Moreover, in this model we need to address the power relationships between individuals that result from ethnic relations, as well as from our traditional conceptions of psychotherapy. Third, we need a model that addresses how to understand and work with these similarities and differences in the therapeutic relationship.

Fourth, we need a model that helps therapists to examine their unique sociocultural attributes and how these attributes relate to their role of therapist and helper. In particular, we need to redefine traditional definitions of countertransference and transference. At present, traditional definitions of these terms refer to aspects of an individual's personal history that become a part of the therapeutic relationship and shape client–therapist interactions. However, our current discussion suggests there is another level of history and experience that enters into and shapes the therapeutic relationship. This level is the sociocultural historical level. The sociocultural historical level is ingrained in our ecological existence and binds us to our social and political realities. This level of experience is not accessible to our conscious level of understanding of ourselves and feels far removed, abstract, and symbolic. However, it is real and provides a basis for at least some of the therapist's subjective and perhaps irrational experiences in therapy relationships, especially in cross-racial relationships.

In order for a model to meet these requirements it must incorporate a reassessment of what is meant by human functioning and competence in such a way that it allows for divergences of experience and of conceptions about the nature and goals of life. It must also integrate the role of ecology and socialization in shaping an individual's self-view, world view, and relationships. The ethnic validity model of psychotherapy meets these needs and requirements. It is predicated upon three assumptions: (1) that there are a variety of ways of being human and that these ways are not directly translatable one into another, (2) that there are characteristic patterns of relationships and exchange among people who differ with regard to such characteristics as ethnicity and race, and (3) that the integrity of an individual's heritage and identity must be respected at the individual and group level. This model also incorporates Tyler's model of psychosocial competence as a framework for conceptualizing human functioning and growth from a nondeficit and pluralistic perspective. The psychosocial competence model and the ethnic validity model are presented in Chapters 2 and 3, respectively.

2

The Ecology and Psychosocial Competence

As do all living creatures, human beings develop, survive, prosper, are destroyed, or destroy themselves within the context of their ecology. In a fundamental way the very nature of our existence, both psychological and physical, is inextricably linked to the environment in which we live. Our goals, aspirations, values, as well as our adaptational outcomes are keenly responsive to our interaction and experience with elements of the ecology. Studies are now showing that ecology is relevant even *in utero* and that neither the idea of genetic determination nor the idea that each of us is born as a tabula rasa is entirely justified.

Who we are and what we become are very much a result of the dynamic interplay between the ways in which we manipulate the environment and are manipulated by it. Let's take, for example, the relationship of our physical health to the things we eat. We manipulate the world of food by choosing those things that become a part of our diet. If we choose nutritious and healthy foods we will probably enhance our physical well-being. In contrast, if we choose the foods that are not nutritious and are unhealthy for us, we stand a good change of destroying our health. The same can be said of psychosocial stress. We make choices about how we organize and respond to life's events. To the extent that our efforts to handle stress are adaptive, we can maintain some degree of psychological health. In both physical and psychological matters we can also make random choices. The upshot is that we can respond to the environment in ways that minimize or maximize our well-being, haphazardly or in a more focused manner. Random responding allows the environment to wield its power and influence over us unabashedly. So potent is the influence of ecology that a passive orientation to it can lead to products that precisely reflect the forces of that environment, be they intentional or unintentional. In the end, the way in which we construct patterns of survival is functionally related to our general knowledge of the world as well as to our specific knowledge and perceptions of the supports and threats within the environment.

When we speak of *ecology* we refer to the composite of living and nonliving objects within an environmental system that are interrelated and dependent upon one another for sustenance and balance. Included in the total ecology is the human ecology, consisting of people, the relationships among them, and their unique social characteristics. An *ecosystem* is a smaller self-sustaining unit within the ecology. Among people, ecosystems are defined in terms of the specific characteristics that group people and determine their distinctiveness. Throughout this book we refer to such ecosystems as human ecosystems, ethnic ecosystems, therapeutic ecosystems, culture-defining versus non-culture-defining ecosystems, and majority versus nonmajority ecosystems.

To some extent ecology is destiny because there are some aspects of who we are and where we are that are fixed and immutable. There are other aspects of our ecology that are less fixed but that, nonetheless, are enormously influential in our lives. For example, we cannot change our gender, our racial and ethnic heritage, our national origin, or the generation of our birth; but, we can shape their psychological meaning for us, we can educate others to influence their perceptions of us, and we can define the limits of acceptable discourse and the parameters of acceptable behavior relative to these enduring characteristics as we and others relate to them. We are unequivocally who we are relative to these attributes. Not only that, but there is typically a well-formed general opinion and reaction to what they represent. When individuals who embody that opinion are in highly visible and powerful positions, they usually take the lead in setting forth the cultural ethos relative to us as well as in providing a model for how most others will respond to us. In effect, politically powerful individuals help to shape another aspect of our ecology, the attitudes and reactions of others to us.

People sometimes choose to exercise self-control over their lives and to some extent modify their destined ecologies. Within limits each of us has some freedom for self-definition and self-determination, but clearly the responsibility for initiating those freedoms is ours. Consider individuals who live with substantial adversities such as disabilities, traumas, and deprivation. They exercise some control over their lives and do so in a way that attempts to minimize the deleterious effects of those circumstances. In many instances no one puts forth an effort to deal with those situations until the affected persons marshal and use their own resources to redefine themselves, seek help, and demand changes in their conditions and the way others respond to them. More generally, history teaches us that the catalyst for social change usually is not voluntary benevolence on the part of societal members but the demands made by those who are most directly affected by inhumane and unjust practices.

How do people manage an ecology that is dealing them hardships? Some people join with others of a different ecosystem in order to form a new one. In so doing, they experience a different world view and way of negotiating life that is potentially useful to them in managing their own lives. For example, a person experiencing difficulties around a particular set of issues may consult a friend or a trained helper and thus form a supportive, therapeutic ecosystem. When a person joins another ecosystem he or she may also benefit by gaining the opportunity to define further or even redefine his or her own ecosystem and its relative merits. Moreover, some people extract important life skills from their experiences with difficulties—skills that may help them handle similar situations in the future. For example, a person who successfully handles a plant closing and the attendant loss of gainful employment may be better prepared to handle a job relocation at a later date. That kind of "baptism by fire" provides what has been termed in the literature a *steeling* effect on one's personality (Garmezy, 1983). The mere experience of dealing with difficult situations often makes a person hardier, and that hardiness provides the individual with a stronger capacity for coping in the future.

Ultimately, what becomes of people and other living creatures is to a significant degree determined by their ability to negotiate their ecology as well as by the ecology's favorableness toward them at a given time and within a particular ecosystem. This latter point conveys the message that sometimes no matter how strong people are or how assiduous and tenacious their efforts, if the environment is overwhelmingly unfavorable toward them, the psychological and tangible returns on their efforts will be diminished. We would indeed be in error if we were to assume that people can exert unmitigated influence over their environment. That, of course, is not the case at all. For example, in the ecosystems of wildlife there are dynamic states in which the roles of predator and prey, hunter and hunted, change because of the nature and actions of the inhabitants of the ecosystem and their physical location. Everyone's opportunities for prosperity and even survival are jeopardized when a species is preyed, hunted, or otherwise oppressed.

Social groups are shaped by ecologies with their own versions of predator and prey, hunter and hunted, usually ordered along economic, political, racial, ethnic, religious, and gender lines. If we follow the analogy from wildlife mentioned above, a group of persons may prosper at a given point in time if they are members of the more powerful ecosystem. Conversely, they may suffer at that time if they belong to a subordinating ecosystem. As regards the human ecosystems, shifts in the cultural ethos can create changes in the existing social order and thus changes in social relationships. For example, in the United States, women have achieved higher status in the late 1970s and 1980s than they had done previously and by some barometers are better off than they were before. Human ecosystems, owing much to the initiatives taken by women themselves, have changed. Women have greater opportunities for developing an autonomous sense of self, a related pattern of self–world relationships, and more effective coping strategies. Even though women still are not the culture-defining group within the ecosystem, public opinion and expressions have changed, many policies that affect women have been revised, and women have been afforded the opportunity to participate more fully in society in a self-actualizing fashion.

American society is somewhat stratified so that one layer of the ecology takes the form of dominant versus nondominant, majority versus nonmajority, culture-defining versus non-culture-defining ecosystems. Individuals who are the nondominant and non-culture-defining inhabitants of the American social ecology experience the effects of their negative power position in many ways. One way is through the constraints placed on their opportunities for self-actualization. This set of circumstances does not mean that members of nondominant culture groups do not realize a sense of psychosocial competence but that they must do so within, and in spite of, a context that systematically impedes this undertaking. The construction of those patterns of competence and their eventual outcomes are keenly responsive to a constraining ecology.

ORIGINS OF A COMPETENCE ORIENTATION

Human beings not only try to survive the natural and social order but they also try to do well and even try to change that order. Within people an intrinsically rewarding and unique motivational force has been identified. The early psychoanalytic and behaviorally oriented writings suggested that this motivating force is the reduction of tension, whereas more recent thought suggests that it is the need for competence, or effectance. Whether the motivation is innate or learned is the subject of debate as well. The origin notwithstanding, it does seem as though individuals strive for personal effectiveness and mastery over the environment, not just the reduction of tension or the satisfaction of drives.

Our discipline has not always concerned itself with the study of competence. It is unfortunate that for so long we focused almost solely on detecting and refining our knowledge of abnormal behavior, to the exclusion of other adaptational outcomes. Traditionally, the search for personal deficiencies has pervaded the domains of clinical psychology and clinical psychiatry. We now know that there are other equally legitimate areas of inquiry and that the earlier emphasis on deficits was myopic in scope. Clinical psychology and clinical psychiatry took their philosophical direction from the medical model upon which they were founded. That model rests in a major way on the premise that disorder resides within the individual. It then follows that the responsibility of the helping professional is to treat the person with a view toward uncovering pathology. This focus is highly individualistic and disorder oriented, and it naturally leads to a search for pathology within individuals.

The focus on personal efficacy and its role in psychological well-being is a relatively recent endeavor—that is, it has arisen within the last three decades. To this extent, the emphasis on psychosocial competence represents a major paradigm shift. It coincides with newer conceptions of mental health in which well-being is no longer equated with the absence of pathology but rather is seen as the presence of a positive sense of self and a capacity to negotiate the complexities of life. In his book *The Structure of Scientific Revolutions,* Kuhn (1970) discusses catalysts for scientific change. He states that we have fertile ground for the emergence of new scientific models when an existing paradigm proves to be no longer a viable problem-solving tool and is incapable of subsuming new problems. So it is with the emergence of the study of competence.

The focus on psychosocial competence has arisen from several events. Specifically, most individuals cope reasonably well with hardships. There are more who overcome these conditions than who yield to them. Therefore, we have had to revise our considerations about the nature and strength of human personality. Competence as a psychosocial construct represents a shift in our perspective on human effectiveness from the more pathological aspects of personality to a focus on more positive, forward-going aspects. The idea of psychosocial competence also stands in contrast to earlier conceptions in which well-being was synonymous with an absence of pathology and was defined with reference to a standard of "normal" behavior. Mental health professionals have observed personal characteristics that do not fit these models but that are effective nonetheless. Therefore, we no longer embrace those earlier criteria exclusively.

There is a domain of human functioning that lies outside the quest for freedom from pathology. In the tradition of Hartmann (1958), an ego psychologist, there is a "sphere" of the personality that is "conflict free." That domain is involved with personal effectiveness and environmental mastery—thus, it embodies a more positive and a more proactive focus. The newer criteria for health also include the presence of a positive sense of self and the capacity to negotiate the complexities of life.

There were several harbingers of this new orientation to mental health. Jahoda's (1958) seminal work, as reported in a monograph to the Joint Commission on Mental Illness and Health, is one. Her work laid the foundation for future investigations of the nature of competence. In that document she reviewed existing criteria for mental health and on that basis outlined six dimensions of positive mental health. Briefly, they are (1) self-attitudes, (2) level and quality of personal growth and development, (3) degree of personality integration, (4) level of autonomy, (5) adequacy of perception of reality, (6) degree of environmental mastery.

Silber, Hamburg, Coelho, Murphey, Rosenburg, & Pearlin (1961), described the coping styles of competent high school seniors preparing to go to college. As a follow-up to that report, Coelho, Hamburg, and Murphey (1963) described the competence characteristics of this same group of students during their first year of college. The sample was a group of high school students from middle-class families of a Washington, D.C., suburb. Participants were high achievers who demonstrated competence in several areas of their lives, including peer relationships, school work, and their involvement in broader social activities. These adolescents were interviewed periodically from their senior year in high school through their first year of college.

After intensive study, Silber *et al.* (1961) and Coelho *et al.* (1963) reported a number of common characteristics in this group of competent adolescents. They held a favorable view of themselves and of novel situations. They found problem solving to be intrinsically rewarding, so they actively sought out challenging events. They mastered their immediate situations by taking a great deal of initiative and responsibility for their lives. They mastered future situations by becoming actively planful and by setting goals and outlining strategies for achieving them. Finally, these adolescents coped with their fears and apprehensions about their college experience in a way that did not compromise their functioning.

Grinker, Grinker, and Timberlake (1962) described the attributes of a group of "healthy" males attending a midwestern Christian college.

Grinker referred to this group of men as "homoclites," meaning that they were ordinary people with little ambition. They did not hold the typical American middle-class value of upward mobility and success. Rather, Grinker's homoclites strove for "happiness, a family, and service to others" (p. 422). Further, they aspired "to do well, to do good, and to be liked" (p. 445). They grew up in a tradition in which it was important to be happy with what you had and in which you were expected to use your skills and talents in the service of the common good. Grinker's study is instructive on a number of different counts. It underscores the point that at a time in the not so distant past, the notion of health and well-being was somewhat foreign to the way in which we thought about people. Grinker, who seldom interfaced with a group of individuals who were not struggling with the ravages of pathology, expressed surprise at the existence of these apparently well-adjusted men. He went on to say that when he discussed his findings with colleagues and others, they would say, "those boys are sick, they have no ambition" (p. 446). This illustrates a reluctance to accept health in whatever form it happens to come. Grinker's study also says to us that here is a pattern of competence quite different from our usual conceptions, but it is a pattern that is adaptive and functional in its context, nonetheless. Further, his study drives home the importance of taking into consideration the ecology and how it shapes adaptational patterns.

The work of M. Brewster Smith (1965) provided an early framework for the study of competence as well. He examined dimensions of competence among Peace Corps workers in Ghana who were the first to perform a tour of duty abroad. The Peace Corps workers submitted to several measures of psychological functioning including questionnaires, field and psychiatric interviews, and personal narratives. Some of the more salient analyses, and those that form the basis for many of Smith's conclusions, are the results of the field interviews. In these analyses, Smith was concerned with characteristics of the workers' personality and performance that contributed to an understanding of their overall competence. Using a combination of the Q-sort technique and factor analysis, Smith found a main personality attribute, which he called "Self Confident Maturity," and a main performance attribute, which he called "Competent Teaching," that characterized the Peace Corps workers. Also, within the category of "Competent Teaching" there were two different, yet equally functional, patterns of competence. They were "Involvement with Africa" and "Exclusive Commitment to Teaching." The dimensions of personality that were related to competent performance among the workers were "Interpersonally Sensitive Maturity," "Intellectualizing Future Orientation," and "Controlling Responsibility."

Ezekiel (1968) provided a detailed analysis of the relationship of the Peace Corps workers' personal narratives to their performance. These narratives were judged on the basis of Differentiation ("description of a complex and detailed mapping of the future"), Agency ("description of the future self as prime agent in determining the course of the future life"), and Demand ("description of a life perceived by the respondent to demand long-term continuing effort"). In general, Ezekiel found that the greater the workers' ratings in these three areas, the more competently his or her performance was rated on several objective indices. Further, the competent Peace Corps workers, as judged by job performance ratings, were active persons with a strong belief in their own skills and abilities; they maintained an optimistic view of the future; and they saw themselves as playing a major role in executing their present and future plans.

The attributes that provided the basis of competent functioning among the young men in the Grinker study, the young adults in the Smith study, and the adolescents in the Silber *et al.* study are quite similar to one another. They are also consistent with those delineated by Jahoda. Taken together, they suggest that competence consists of characteristic ways of viewing oneself and the world, and of negotiating the demands of one's ecology. These studies, particularly the Grinker and the Silber *et al.* studies, illustrate the impact of ecology in shaping patterns of competence. Ecology's role seems especially vivid when we compare the different contexts of the Grinker study and the Silber *et al.* study. The lack of ambition and lack of a need for increasing stimulation characteristic of the homoclites would not have been adaptive for the adolescents from middle-class families in which emphasis was placed on achievement and upward mobility; and neither would the search for challenge and novelty have been adaptive for the homoclites. Each pattern of functioning was legitimate and realistic for its context.

Stress-Illness Models

By now, few people doubt that the experience of stressful life events can place an individual at risk for developing psychological and physical problems. When the demands of life exceed an individual's abilities to cope with them, he or she becomes particularly vulnerable to depression (Byrne, 1984), heart disease (Connolly, 1976; Theorell, Lind, & Floderus, 1975), cancer (Bahnson, 1980, 1981), streptococcal infection (Meyer & Haggerty, 1962), sudden cardiac death (Rahe and Lind, 1971), and a host of other disorders. However, not everyone exposed to stressful life events experiences prolonged assaults on or even threats to his or her psychological and physical well-being. There is not a direct relationship between the experience of life events and the onset of illness. In light of these facts, the stress-illness model has been elaborated to include characteristics of the individual and of the environment that may enter into the equation and mitigate impairment.

Embedded in the reformulated stress-illness model is the notion that there may be individual differences in personality and characteristics of the environment that mediate psychosocial stress and illness, making a person more resistant and resilient in the throes of life's events. These attributes account for a much larger percentage of the variance in individual outcomes than had been previously considered. The inquiry into these stress resistance factors has provided another catalyst for exploring competence. For example, in the personal domain, we have begun to look into the attributes that make some people more resistant than others and to determine whether those attributes may be akin to something known as individual competence. It is true that people differ in their psychosocial makeups. It is also true that they differ in their attitudes toward themselves and the world, as well as in how they bring these characteristics to bear on their coping efforts.

There are several *protective* factors that have been identified, some of which are personal and others of which are environmental. In the personal domain are such attributes as self-efficacy (Bandura, 1982), self-esteem (Fleishman, 1984), internality (Anderson, 1977; Parkes, 1984; Werner & Smith, 1982), personal hardiness (Kobasa, 1979), and an easy-going personal style (Holahan & Moos, 1985, 1986). Collectively, they refer to a concept of self concerned with the degree of personal integrity, efficacy, and fortitude.

There are several environmental conditions that can protect people from the impact of stress. They include, for example, the timing of an event (Charlesworth & Nathan, 1982; Lazarus, 1966). Singular events are easier to deal with than are multitudinous ones. Prior experiences with the same or a similar event provide some protection (Charlesworth & Nathan, 1982; Lazarus, 1966), as does social support (Cobb, 1976; DeLongis, Folkman, & Lazarus, 1988; Holahan & Moos, 1981). Studies of social support indicate that the absence of supportive relationships is strongly associated with psychological and physical impairment and even increased mortality rates (Berkman & Syme, 1979). The presence of support can be protective as well as therapeutic. It modifies the stress-illness link by inoculating people against the damaging effects of stress and by facilitating coping before and after the onset of an illness. Social support therefore helps people to negotiate life's events and to forestall some of the potentially negative consequences of them.

The research literature consistently demonstrates that individuals who are more self-efficacious are less likely to become disorganized by stress than those who are relatively lacking in efficacy. Likewise, certain environmental conditions can help to deflect life-change events and to ease their severity. In brief, the intrapersonal and social ecologies of an individual contribute greatly to the way in which he or she fares in life.

In his review chapter "Stressors of Childhood," Norman Garmezy (1983) illustrates how many studies, due to methodology or investigator bias, magnify the horrors of children subjected to unrelenting ecologies. He cites studies of children subjected to the vagaries of war, racial discrimination, poverty, and family disorganization, which provide a contrast to these earlier conclusions. These studies indicate that not all children subjected to adversity succumb to it. There are, in fact, diverse adaptations to stressful circumstances. Garmezy found three common attributes that consistently accounted for better coping among children who experienced unusual life stressors. They included personal characteristics of the children themselves as well as familial and extrafamilial support. Among the personal traits that inoculated children against stress were a positive regard for oneself, a sense of active agentry in one's life, and a sense of control and responsibility for the outcome of events in one's life.

Longitudinal studies conducted on the island of Kauai provided an opportunity to investigate the physical, psychological, and emotional outcomes of children under stress over an extended period of time (Werner, Bierman, & French, 1971). All children on the island were followed from immediately after conception until they reached the age of 10. Of those who were described as having been born and reared in abject poverty and as beset with unusual life stressors, Werner and Smith (1982) found that only one-fifth of them developed serious emotional and behavioral problems. In fact, most of these children, though significantly disadvantaged by their ecology, fared well through their early years. In the words of Werner and Smith, they "worked well, played well, loved well, and expected well."

What made these children invincible? Werner and Smith reported that certain personal attributes were crucial. They indicated that the resilient children showed problem-solving ability and a healthy sense of mastery over their environment, evident as early as infancy. They were active, independent, trusting, and they related well with other people in their environment. With increasing years the resilient ones had a more planful and active approach to their lives as well as a more robust sense of self-esteem, and they made more appropriate use of their social supports. Once more, the basis for competent functioning consisted of a characteristic view of oneself and of the world, and a characteristic way of interacting with events and other people.

Beyond Stress Resistance

In the literature the concept of competence is variously termed effectance motivation (White, 1959), maturity (Heath, 1977), personal soundness (Barron, 1963), personality integration (Seeman, 1959, 1966), psychological effectiveness (Poe, 1973), and ego development (Loevinger, 1976). The different names notwithstanding, the basis of each concept is that within people there is a need and a desire, as well as a capacity, to master their environment and to function optimally within it. White's term *effectance motivation* embodies the notion that people are motivated to acquire a sense of personal competence by interacting with their environment. He states that we derive intrinsic pleasure by acting upon the environment, by discovering its potential for change, and by making actual changes in it. Seeman's (1959, 1966) research among college women indicates that a high degree of personality integration is characterized by a coalescence of cognitive and affective processes whereby the individual has a positive evaluation of himself or herself, a high degree of actualization in self–world relationships, and a strong intellectual capacity. Heath (1977) developed a model of maturity that consists of characteristic self–world relationships, values, self-evaluation, and intellectual style. In addition, the work of Goldfried and D'Zurilla (1969) and of Spivak and Shure (1974) emphasizes the importance of problem-solving ability and means-end thinking, respectively, as important ingredients for psychosocial competence. They have developed corresponding techniques designed to foster these attributes in psychotherapy.

The role of competence in health and well-being is solidly documented. The casualties of an ill-defined sense of self, self–world relations, and way of negotiating life's events abound. Everywhere there is evidence of psychosocial competence preempted by personal stress and distress. Behavioral scientists for some time now have asserted the value of personal and environmental mastery in man's quest for well-being. More and more these notions are being upheld in other arenas—medicine for instance. Most vocal are those practitioners who no longer believe that the locus of responsibility for physical health rests solely with the physician. For example, the very crux of behavioral medicine, a relatively new interdisciplinary specialty, is that individuals must become ambassadors for and managers of their own bodies and health in order to survive over the long haul. In this regard they must achieve a health-related competence. Recent statistics show that the major cause of death among most Americans today is not the infectious diseases of 70 and 80 years ago, but the illnesses inspired by faulty lifestyles. In a major way we fail to minimize our exposure to some of the most robust predictors of disease and mortality. For example, we overeat and are too sedentary, and we abuse substances (e.g., tobacco, alcohol, drugs) and are indifferent to the nutritional value of the foods we consume. Moreover, in a fast-paced and often confusing postmodern era, we are failing to handle the anxiety and psychological distress that can accompany life in these times. An underlying theme in all of this is that we actively participate in our own destruction and we must actively participate in our survival. We have to begin to see ourselves as somewhat autonomous units capable of exercising a certain amount of control over our bodies with a view toward health and well-being, and toward a strategy for relating to the environment in a manner that enhances our well-being.

The concept of competence has significance for both psychological and physical well-being. Of particular importance for achieving competence in either domain is the active involvement of the individual and a reasonable stance with respect to the environment. Tyler (1978) has developed a model of psychosocial competence that builds on earlier definitions of this construct but that goes beyond them. A basic assumption of Tyler's model is that mastery is neither absolute nor universally agreed upon. There is considerable debate over what this phenomenon is, who possesses it, and to what degree. Competence mirrors to a large extent the variety of ecosystems of which a person is or has been a part. Therefore, no matter what the outcome of those debates may be, the criteria for determining mastery must reflect, at least in part, those criteria that are derived from a person's relevant ecosystem(s).

Tyler's model, as described below, outlines the components and patterns of competence with respect to the limiting and delimiting potential of the environment. The supporting research indicates that there are different, yet equally legitimate, ways of being an effective coper. Tyler's psychosocial competence model provides the conceptual basis for the ethnic validity model (EVM) described in Chapter 3. The EVM incorporates the principles of psychosocial competence and argues for the existence and validity of diverse ways of being human on the grounds that each of us has evolved in relation to his or her ecology. Thus, the patterns of psychosocial competence may change depending upon varying ecological characteristics (e.g., a person's gender, race, culture, or ethnicity) without creating qualitative changes in competent functioning. The patterns of competence that each person embodies have by their very nature advantages and disadvantages, as well as strengths and limitations. Further, because people are different, any two individuals can put together for themselves a set of rules for living that have the potential for diverging, converging, or conflicting with one another. It is therefore incumbent upon us as therapists to give special recognition to these interpersonal dynamics and the way in which they affect the process and outcome of psychotherapy.

Also, with respect to psychosocial competence, we assert that each person is a psychologically autonomous unit within his or her ecology. Knowing an individual's ecology is instructive, but it is only partially adequate with respect to understanding him or her. We must also know how that particular person has attached meaning and priority to various ecological parameters and how he or she expresses that meaning. Not only that, but we must know something about his or her unique life experiences. For example, individuals typically make one aspect of their identity more salient than others. Let us take for example a woman dentist who considers herself first a dentist and secondarily a woman, as compared to another woman dentist who considers herself first a woman and secondarily a dentist. These two women assign different ranks to their professional and gender identities, and although they share similar ecosystems they are likely to have put their lives together quite differently. Even if the two women dentists were to rank their professional and gender identities similarly, in order for us to get a better understanding of them, it still would be important to know how their unique life experiences have shaped who they are.

We do not suggest that there are universal norms for competence. Rather, there are norms based on geographical, political, racial, cultural, and ethnic ecosystems, and even individual norms for any given person. Each person has considerable freedom to put together for himself or herself a way of being that is adaptive and functional within his or her world. Some of the ways of being converge, some are distinctly different yet compatible, and others are different and incompatible. Unfortunately, in the past many authors who have written about psychosocial competence have done so from a highly enculturated point of view. That is, they have assumed the prevailing attitudes, lifestyles, and behaviors of the more dominant group to be the only truly valid way of being, the ultimate paradigm of competence, and the one against which all others should be judged. Their corollary is that any divergence from this way of life is deviant and necessarily less valid. Many mental health practitioners have unwittingly adopted this view and by doing so have fallen short of therapeutic helpfulness. In the context of psychotherapy and other approaches to human well-being, the ethnic validity model deals specifically with diversity and supports the acceptance of different ways of being as valid in and of themselves.

TYLER'S PSYCHOSOCIAL COMPETENCE MODEL

Tyler's psychosocial competence model for conceptualizing human functioning consists of three components: self efficacy, self–world relations, and behavioral attributes. These are personal characteristics that, in a coordinated fashion, underlie more and less competent functioning. It is assumed that all patterns of competence are shaped by a person's ecological environment and the rules for effective functioning dictated in part by his or her particular ecosystem. Even though the patterns of competence among individuals may differ, each is assumed to be legitimate for that person in that context. Those patterns may not always be the most adaptive. Each individual interacts with the world on the basis of his or her own personal history and acquired knowledge, as well as on the basis of his or her most accurate perception of a particular situation. People vary on all of these dimensions as well as in their abilities to bring them to bear in everyday functioning.

Thus, a full description of a person requires an account of that person's past and present ecosystems as well as an account of that person's psychosocial characteristics. The ethnic validity model outlines in greater detail some of the characteristic patterns of competence and relevant issues that may arise among people who are ecologically different and the same, specifically in a psychotherapeutic context. The ethnic validity model is based on Tyler's model of psychosocial competence. To provide a basis for understanding the ethnic validity model, Tyler's model is outlined and the relevant supporting research literature is presented in the following sections.

Self-Efficacy Attributes

In Tyler's model, the self-efficacy dimension is the degree to which individuals view themselves as being valuable, as causally important people, and as effective in shaping the events and outcomes in their lives. The self-efficacy dimension here is based in part on Rotter's (1966, 1975) concept of locus of control and DeCharms's (1968) related notion of origin versus pawn. To that extent, these two constructs combined provide the conceptual underpinning for the self-efficacy component (Tyler, 1978).

Locus of control can be conceptualized as the extent to which people believe they are causally important in their lives. It is based on and measured in terms of the degree of expectancy that one's efforts to shape life's outcomes will be reinforced. According to expectancy theory, people engage in those behaviors they believe are most likely to produce the desired outcome and whose outcomes are highly valued. The locus of control construct is assumed to be a continuous variable ranging from an internal stance to an external one. An internal locus of control refers to a belief in personal control and responsibility for one's own life, and in a generalized expectancy that one's actions will be reinforced. An external locus of control refers to the belief that the responsibility for and control over one's life resides largely with fate, luck, chance or powerful others, and that therefore it is relatively fruitless to put forth personal effort in the service of goals or in actualizing them (Rotter, 1966).

DeCharms's concept of origin versus pawn is akin to Rotter's notion of internality and externality. Origins see themselves as free to make choices in life and perceive the causes of their behavior as originating from themselves. Pawns see their behavior as being controlled by outside agents and the causes of that behavior as originating from other sources. Thus DeCharms emphasizes choice aspects of control, while Rotter emphasizes the role of reinforcement.

Locus of control is an important psychosocial construct that has generated large amounts of research over the years. Studies indicate that individuals who are more internal tend to engage in more proactive, more constructive, and healthier behaviors with related positive outcomes. For example, internality is positively correlated with help-seeking in times of distress (Grace & Schill, 1986), active coping (Tyler, 1978), interpersonal trust (Tyler, 1978), smoking cessation (James, Woodruff, & Werner, 1965), contraceptive use among females and males (Hendricks & Fullilove, 1983; Lundy, 1972), marital satisfaction among women (Bugaighis, Schumm, Bollman, & Jurich, 1983), academic achievement (Stipek, 1980), and healthy adaptation to chronic pain (Crisson & Keefe, 1988). A detailed discussion of the literature is beyond the scope of the present volume, but for the interested reader, two excellent reviews of this research are by Phares (1976) and Lefcourt (1984).

James Dyal (1984) reviewed the cross-cultural research with this construct. The most consistent finding was the presence of an external orientation among American blacks, Asians, individuals with lower socioeconomic statuses, and women. These data support the notion that locus of control is constructed with reference to a person's life circumstances. The sense of control is tuned to reflect a person's cultural milieu, as well as the supports, threats, opportunities, advantages, and disadvantages a particular society doles out to its culture- and non-culture-defining members.

More recently, Tyler and his colleagues have conducted cross-cultural studies that compare the patterns of attribution in locus of control in Indian and Puerto Rican college students with those of American students. Tyler, Dhawan, and Sinha (1989) found some important areas of divergence and convergence when Indian males and females were compared with American males and females. For example, there were differences across the two cultures in their beliefs about externality. The Americans, to a greater extent, held the view that people do not get adequate recognition for their deeds and that time equalizes the misadventures and triumphs that people experience in life. The Indians, on the other hand, had a greater sense of external control over becoming leaders and over a person's exposure to desirable life events. There were also important distinctions across cultures in the way they organized their locus of control attributions. The leading factor for both samples pertained to a sense of personal control over the outcome of life events. A sense of personal control was also the secondary factor for the Indian group. The secondary factor for the American group pertained to "confronting or yielding to the system." The two cultures differed on the third, and final, factor as well. The Indian group stressed "being a victim," whereas the American group stressed "luck versus hard work in individuals' lives." There were cross-cultural similarities and differences between males and females in both cultures.

The work of Tyler, Labarta, and Otero (1986) further supports the notion that locus of control is constructed with reference to the cultural context in which the attributions are made. In a cross-cultural study, they found that a more internal locus of control was related to better grades, lower levels of symptomatology, and higher active planfulness scores in Puerto Rican and American adolescents. At the same time, the factor structure of locus of control attributions between those two groups of adolescents differed. These differences were based on the very nature of the factors themselves as well as on the relative influence of demographic variables. For example, there were sex differences in the factor structures for American adolescents, but not for those from Puerto Rico. The factor structures consistently contained conceptually similar items with loadings in opposite directions for Puerto Rican adolescents, but not for Americans.

The self-efficacy mechanism operates among people in such a way that more competent individuals think of themselves as being valuable, as effective agents in their lives, as causally important people, and as responsible for shaping the outcome of events. In contrast, less competent individuals do not see themselves as being particularly valuable, important, or responsible for affecting the outcome of events. A person's functioning can reflect back on his or her sense of self-efficacy as well. For example, an individual who performs tasks poorly, who has difficulty negotiating life's events and demands, who performs in a capacity incommensurate with his or her skills, or who is relatively inactive in everyday life can develop a sense of worthlessness.

A person's sense of self-efficacy affects competent functioning in many ways. In a review of related research, Bandura (1982) reports that self-efficacy will influence a person's level of motivation for setting goals and initiating tasks, his or her level of personal commitment and investment in the service of those goals and activities, and the extent to which he or she will persevere when confronted with roadblocks. In this same paper, Bandura describes studies that suggest a sense of personal efficacy is related to many behavioral outcomes. For example, self-efficacy is related to a person's aspirations for achievement, as well as to the kinds of career choices he or she makes. Personal efficacy is also related to differences in how people respond to stress such that more efficacious individuals are less physiologically responsive than less efficacious ones. People with a strong sense of self-efficacy are less likely than others to become depressed; and they are more likely to develop interest in activities for their intrinsic value.

Self–World Attributes

While the self-efficacy component of Tyler's model pertains to self-evaluation, the self–world component of the model is the extent to which a person is optimistically trusting of other people and of the world in general. In a somewhat predictable and benign environment, more competent persons possess a moderate degree of optimistic trust that serves as a springboard for developing constructive interchanges with other people. Less competent persons are pessimistically distrusting and, in contrast, tend to develop relational patterns that are unproductive at best and self-destructive at worst. The self–world component of the model is based on Rotter's (1967) concept of interpersonal trust. He gives primacy to this dimension in building and preserving the social order, for without trust we could expect little in the way of long-term effective functioning among individuals and institutions. Rotter's definition of trust is derived from social learning theory and is thought of as being established in the context of our relationships with other people. It is defined as the generalized expectancy that other people are reliable and dependable. Rotter's research with this construct indicates that people who trust are more capable of being trusted themselves. They are liked by their peers, make friends easily, and are more autonomous in making and executing life plans. Rotter's (1980) review of research on interpersonal trust further indicates that people who trust are happier, more honest, and better adjusted than those who are less trusting; moreover, trusters are more likely to forgive other people and to regard others with dignity.

Interpersonal trust is one of the essential elements of human relationships. It helps to bring us into orbit with one another. It is also the cement that keeps us there. The literature is replete with examples of behaviors rooted in the absence of trust. The recent controversy over whether psychotherapeutic pairs who are ecologically dissimilar can effectively work together is an example. One of the major thrusts of that debate is the question of whether these two individuals can trust one another enough to establish a meaningful and viable relationship. Sometimes people are so untrusting that their orientation to the world is one of hostility and hypervigilance. They trust almost no one. Typically, past experiences have helped to shape this stance.

Without a healthy degree of interpersonal trust one's overall degree of competence is substantially diminished. The kind of trust of others that is most adaptive, at least in a general sense, is that which is moderate in nature and reality based. Too much trust suggests that a person is failing to use his or her own judgment and capabilities and is creating an unhealthy dependency on others. Blind, unexamined trust suggests an unhealthy degree of vulnerability. It might also suggest an unrealistic view of human nature. Unfortunately, not all human beings behave with each other's best interest in mind. On the other hand, too little trust stands as a roadblock to building relationships and developing a sense of competence and well-being.

Behavioral Attributes

Self-efficacy and interpersonal trust, when put together with characteristic behavioral attributes, round out the psychosocial characteristics in the competence model. The behavioral attributes dimension refers to an individual's coping orientation, that is, whether he or she assumes active or passive agency in his or her life. More competent persons take charge of their lives, make plans, set goals, and initiate activities designed to actualize those plans and goals. They are able to delay gratification of short-term rewards for long-term achievements or enjoy short-term rewards when delay is not meaningful. More competent persons can actively enjoy their positive outcomes, grieve their negative ones, learn from both, and then redefine themselves and their worlds and move on to new events and experiences. Less competent persons assume more passive agency in their lives and have a much less crystallized life plan. Life is lived in a more unorganized and random fashion and outcomes are similarly achieved.

The configural pattern of self-efficacy, optimistic trust, and active coping underlies a mastery-oriented problem-solving approach to life. Competent individuals are more self and goal directed than less competent individuals and believe more that the world can offer relatively benign possibilities within which to actualize themselves. This pattern of competence is more likely to take place in a relatively benign and predictable environment. In a malign and unpredictable environment, competence will be modified accordingly; for example, people learn to live with lower expectations of self-efficacy and cope within a framework of realistic caution and protectiveness. Such adaptations limit people's well-being, but competent people are not unrealistic.

Research to date on Tyler's psychosocial competence model has demonstrated it to be a useful framework from which to conceptualize individual competence across the life span and across cultures. Studies have included populations from four major developmental periods—children, adolescents, young adults, and seniors—and from three different cultures—American, Indian, and Latin. These studies, collectively, suggest that a mastery-oriented problem-solving approach to life's events and tasks is evident as early as childhood and is related to higher levels of effective functioning throughout life. These studies also suggest that the competence model is a framework common to many people who negotiate their lives well. Further, as these studies show, there are varieties of competent functioning. The differences in functioning are shaped by the various aspects of a person's ecology (e.g., gender, culture, race, ethnicity) as well as by the generation of a person's birth. The next several sections summarize research on the competence model at different developmental periods.

Research on Developmental Periods

Children

Mondell and Tyler (1981) examined the model among groups of exemplary, average, and marginally functioning 7- to 12-year-olds to determine whether the configural variables could predict membership in the criterion groups. To assess the attributes of the model, they used the Psychosocial Competence Incomplete Stories Test (PCIST) and the Nowicki–Strickland Internal–External Locus of Control Scale. Their findings indicated that more competent children were more internal, more trusting, and had a greater penchant for active coping. The levels for the configural variables decreased for each descending level of competence. Children in the exemplary groups were higher than children in the average group, who in turn were higher than children identified as marginal in their level of functioning.

Additional evidence of the model as a valid construct for competence in children is obtained from an evaluation of a psychotherapeutic day camp. Mondell, Tyler, and Freeman (1981) evaluated the effects of a camp for clinically disturbed 7- to 12-year-olds on their competence attributes and their levels of goal attainment. As compared to controls, at posttest, camp participants gained significantly more than nonparticipants in internality, trust, active coping, and in attaining goals set at the beginning of camp. The controls showed no change on these measures.

Tyler and Varma (1988) examined the attributes of the psychosocial competence model and their relationship to help-seeking and helping behaviors among 8- to 10-year-old children in India. They were particularly interested in examining the constructiveness of these behaviors among high- and low-competence children. Constructiveness was defined by the extent to which help-seeking and helping behaviors were initiated by the child, by their relevance to the task, and by their appropriateness. Tyler and Varma's sample consisted of four groups of children in which each child was paired with another of the same gender; one child was given the role of help-seeker, while the other child was given the role of helper. Groups were counterbalanced for help-seeker and helper among high- and low-competence children. Each group was given a block design task that provided the setting for help-seeking and helping. Tyler and Varma found that more competent children put forth more effort than less competent children in solving the problems presented, and they displayed more constructive help-seeking. There was an additional interaction for girls. They also exhibited more constructive help-seeking in the presence of a highly competent helper. Further, with respect to helping, the more competent children, both boys and girls, displayed more constructive helping than less competent children.

A study of street children (*gamins*) in Bogotá, Colombia (Tyler, Tyler, and Echeverry, 1985), further demonstrates the usefulness of the competence model in understanding the constructiveness with which children put together their lives. It also illustrates the relationship of the competence characteristics to the ecological context in which they occur. These *gamins,* who ranged in age from 8 to 17 years, had typically left home because of unremitting family problems. They were uneducated or undereducated with respect to formal schooling. Most of them had lived in an institution at some point in their lives against their will. The investigators examined the ways in which they organized their lives with respect to their perceptions of the supports and threats of home, institutions, and the street.

In general, psychosocial well-being among the *gamins* was directly related to the degree to which the environment supported their psychological and physical well-being. The *gamins* saw home and institutions as more benign places that posed fewer threats to them than the street. Accordingly, they had more favorable evaluations of themselves and believed that they could be more trusting of people in the two former contexts. When in the street, they had the least favorable evaluations of themselves and were least trusting of others, but they rated themselves as more self-efficacious and most actively planful there. In institutions, they were least actively planful but more trusting than when on the streets.

The social ecology of the *gamins* is not monolithic. It comprises at least three dimensions—home, institutions, and the street. Each demands a different way of constructing a sense of psychological and social competence. As these findings suggest, the *gamins'* attempts at mastery are made with regard for the supports and threats they perceive in each context.

These studies of children suggest that the psychosocial competence model provides a useful way of discriminating among children who, on the basis of objective criteria, demonstrate varying degrees of mastery over their lives. In this regard, greater mastery is associated with greater self-efficacy, more active coping styles, and greater interpersonal trust in benign and predictable environments. It also embodies realistic wariness in hostile or unpredictable environments. In addition, the competence attributes are shown to be positively related to such prosocial behaviors as goal attainment, help-seeking, and helping. Further, among groups of latency-aged children, the psychosocial competence model has value in a cross-cultural context. Finally, for the street children in Bogotá, psychosocial competence attributes are related to the different realities of their various ecologies.

High-School Students

Research conducted with adolescents bears on the relationship of individual psychosocial competence to the ways in which they handle the developmental tasks of this period. These studies also suggest that there are important race and gender differences in the psychosocial competence configuration. One of the early studies by Tyler (1978) examined the competence model among eleventh and twelfth graders to determine whether the configural variables could distinguish a group of exemplary students ("getting their lives together well and handling school well") from marginal students ("having trouble getting their lives together and managing school"). Exemplary and marginal students were identified by their school counselors. Counselors were instructed to choose students on the basis of their overall functioning as opposed to simply on the basis of academic performance.

In general, the results showed that the psychosocial competence attributes distinguished more and less competently functioning adolescents. After partialling out the effects of social desirability, the most robust predictors were a strong sense of self-efficacy and an actively planful coping style. The relationship between the configural variables was stronger for exemplaries than for marginals. For exemplaries, these variables were positively related to their response to situational demands such as scholastic achievement. Further, among the exemplary students these psychosocial competence variables were positively related to their general aptitude scores. A relationship between the configural variables and external factors or aptitude scores was not found for the marginals. Social desirability emerged as a significant component of the competence configuration for the exemplary group, indicating that mastery, for them, included conformity to certain standards set by authority figures. Social desirability ordinarily reduces predictability, but in these studies it increased predictability. This orientation seems to be an adaptive survival skill in the school setting. It was related to each of the configural variables, and when placed as a component in the competence matrix, along with self-efficacy, coping style, and trust, social desirability significantly differentiated the exemplary students from the marginal students. These data suggest that exemplaries have a stronger sense of personal effectiveness consisting of self-efficacy, an actively planful behavioral orientation, and to a lesser degree, trust. Further, they suggest that these adolescents are putting their lives together with respect for the demands and realities of their academic environment—one in which conformity and achievement are central.

Having established an empirical basis for the validity of the psychosocial competence model among adolescents, Tyler and his colleagues used it to evaluate a 3-year group counseling program at the high school level. This project included males and females, exemplary and marginal, black and white. Studies originating from the project are varied and illustrate the point that race and gender significantly shape the ways in which these adolescents put their lives together.

Tyler and Gatz (1977) reported the precounseling and change characteristics of the first phase of this project. All students who participated in the intervention were counseled in each phase of the project. Before counseling, exemplary students were better copers and more internal than marginals. Black students, both exemplary and marginal, were less trusting than whites, higher in social desirability, and more sensitive to the adverse effects of racial discrimination on their coping efforts. At the end of the intervention, all counseled students made gains in their behavioral attributes and self-efficacy, but exemplary students gained more.

Tyler (1979), analyzing the cross validation phase of the project, again reported that at the beginning of counseling, exemplaries were more internal and more active copers than marginals and that these attributes were intercorrelated with social desirability. As a group, the females were more external than the males. Black students were more social desirability oriented, more active copers, and more systems blaming than whites. However, they were no more external and no less trusting than whites.

Tyler and Pargament (1981) reported significant changes as a function of counseling on all the competence variables, especially by race and by student group. All participants gained in internality, trust, and active coping orientation. White students became more systems blaming, more social desirability oriented, and more active copers than blacks. On the other hand, blacks became less social desirability oriented, less actively planful, and more trusting than whites. Additional group and race changes were noted as well. For example, exemplary whites and marginal blacks became more external as a function of counseling, and exemplary blacks and marginal whites became more internal. Exemplary whites made modest gains in active coping; marginal whites became substantially more active; exemplary blacks became somewhat less so; and marginal blacks became substantially less active.

In summary, the high school studies showed that exemplary students were consistently higher than marginals on internality and active planfulness before and after counseling and that social desirability was a part of their psychosocial configuration. Thus, it appears that in a teacher controlled, highly structured environment, social desirability functions as a significant psychosocial variable. Psychosocial competence is constructed in reference to the realities of the context. In the school setting, impression management is an adaptive survival skill.

Further, some of the other findings also suggest that males and females are constructing a sense of their responsibilities for their lives that is consistent with their divergent psychological and social realities. There were gender-specific differences on locus of control. Whereas males and females were alike in their composite levels of internality, they endorsed quite different items to make up that sense of internality (Tyler, Gatz, & Keenan, 1979). Females were more internal in a *passive agent* sense. They endorsed the view that they would get a fair number of chances, and once life situations had been set up by external factors, they saw themselves as responsible for accomplishing desired outcomes. Males saw themselves as more responsible for creating their opportunities as well as for accomplishing their goals in those situations. Also, the males' sense of control of their lives was focused more on tasks. In contrast, the females' sense of control was more generalized.

Counseling increased students' sense of internality, active planfulness, and level of interpersonal trust. Nevertheless, black and white students entered counseling differently and they changed differently. All of the black students were actively planful, whereas only the exemplary white students were. The white students who gained most on the goals they set for themselves in counseling were more internal and actively planful. The black students who gained more on their goals were moderately external and actively planful. These findings suggest that there are different patterns of competence that stem from divergent ecologies. In order to function effectively, black students had tailored their world views to incorporate the realities of an oppressive environment. Those realities led them to attenuate their perceptions of and expectations for control in certain areas of their lives. Therefore, optimal functioning for black and white students differed because their psychological and social realities differed. Yet, each pattern of competence was related to external criteria of effective functioning (e.g., grade point average as well as student and counselor evaluations of gains in counseling).

Among the black students, the more strongly they felt discriminated against the more external and distrusting they were. Among the white students, the more trustful they were the more strongly they felt that the black students were discriminated against. These findings are correlational and provide no basis for judging the causal directions. However, these suggestions are consistent with the historical context of the study (recently integrated schools by court order) and with informal observations made during the study.

In another arena, Young (1975) examined the relationship of black power ideology to self-concept and competence among black adolescents enrolled in a special college preparatory program. She divided the students into three subgroups on the basis of their level of commitment to black power ideology, yielding a high, a middle, and a low group. She hypothesized that students high in black power orientation would have a more positive self-concept and exhibit a more active coping orientation than those who were less convinced about black power ideology. Young did not find significant differences between these two groups. However, there was a nonsignificant trend in the predicted direction. The high group tended to have a higher self-concept and tended to be more active copers than the other groups. Contrary to prediction, students in the middle group were less active copers than the low group, and the low group nearly equalled the middle group in self-concept. These findings, inconclusive as they are, suggest that the more aware black students are of issues related to oppression in their lives, the more actively they cope, set goals, and actualize them. They also have positive perceptions of themselves. The competence attributes do not cohere in this manner for students who are less convinced about a black power ideology.

Williams-McCoy and Tyler (1985) compared unmarried adolescent fathers and nonfathers to determine whether the configural variables could distinguish these two groups of young men. They found that, in addition to being older and with a tendency to have been born out of wedlock themselves, the fathers were less trusting of others than the nonfathers. In a general way, these findings support other research which shows that low levels of interpersonal trust are related to negatively sanctioned social behavior (e.g., shoplifting in high school students; Wright & Kirmani, 1977). Precocious fatherhood can be compared to shoplifting on the basis that they are both disapproved of on a larger societal level and they both can carry significant negative social, personal, and legal consequences. The findings regarding interpersonal trust may also suggest that after becoming teenage fathers, these young men reevaluate their environment as being more threatening than before. Perhaps they perceive themselves as having transgressed against societal norms and fear the social and legal reprisals. They then construct a defensive world view to cope with a new ecology, one which they perceive as threatening to them.

The adolescent studies, like those reported about children, suggest that the psychosocial competence attributes discriminate among individuals who vary in their levels of mastery. The adolescent studies provide further evidence that patterns of competence reflect the characteristics of an individual's ecology (e.g., gender, race, and school setting). Further, among those adolescents, a sense of psychosocial competence was positively related to achievement, aptitude, and social desirability.

These studies also indicate that psychosocially competent individuals benefit more from their experiences, at least in a counseling setting. Finally, higher levels of interpersonal trust were related to not becoming an unmarried teenage father.

College Students

Studies of psychosocial competence among college students are varied and also support the positive role of the competence attributes in effective functioning and well-being. Further, this group of studies supports the cross-cultural validity of Tyler's psychosocial competence model as well as the notion that there may be divergent ways of organizing a sense of competent functioning. These differences may mirror the ways in which individuals organize their lives in order to surmount the obstacles within their ecology, minimize the threats, and utilize the supports available to them.

In a sample of Puerto Rican college students, Otero, Tyler, and Labarta (1986) reported that the components of active planfulness and locus of control within the competence configuration were useful concepts for understanding effective coping and well-being within this Latino group. These attributes were found to be related to one another, as had been the case in the American samples (Otero, 1982; Tyler, 1978). Other findings showed that students who believed in a greater sense of internal control and who were more actively planful were less distressed than students who were more external and less active. Students with the former profile also obtained better grades in their academic subjects.

Maish (1977) examined the relationship of black power orientation to political activism and psychosocial competence (self-concept and active planfulness) among black college students, professionals, and nonprofessionals from a wide range of vocations and occupations. She hypothesized that more politically active persons would be more actively planful, have higher self-concepts, and have a greater conviction about black power ideology than less politically active persons. Further, she hypothesized that college students would have a stronger black power orientation than professionals and nonprofessionals. She found that the more politically active persons were indeed more actively planful with superior evaluations of themselves. However, she found no significant differences between students, professionals, and nonprofessionals in black power orientation.

Otero (1982) investigated the ways in which more and less competent college students handle stressful life events. Four groups of students, exemplary and marginal, in experimental and control conditions, comprised the subject pool. The students were differentiated into exemplary and marginal on the basis of an overall profile, with exemplaries more internal, more trusting, and more actively planful. Otero tested the hypothesis that more competent persons possess greater adaptive abilities than less competent persons and bring those skills to bear in stressful situations. He also explored the ways in which exemplary and marginal students felt and thought about the negative and positive events in their lives. Each participant completed a life events questionnaire; after 3 weeks the experimental participants viewed a psychosocially stressful film; immediately afterwards all subjects completed the life events questionnaire again.

Otero's study showed that in the conditions before and after viewing the film, exemplary and marginal students were different from one another with respect to their experience of recent life events, their feelings about them, and the degree to which they were immersed in thoughts about those events. At both intervals, exemplary students, as compared to marginal students, reported fewer life events in total and also fewer negative ones. Exemplaries thought less about their past, particularly their negative past, than did marginals. In the condition before viewing the film, exemplaries were happier about the events in their lives and were less immersed in negative thoughts about them. In the post condition (after viewing the film), marginal students, as compared to exemplaries, reported a larger number of negative life events as well as an increased amount of worry and unhappiness about them. Exemplaries were less immersed in thoughts about their past in general, and less about negative events that had occurred in their lives. In fact, exemplaries had a greater number of thoughts about the positive events in their lives, whereas marginals had even fewer thoughts about the positive events in theirs. In addition, after viewing the film, exemplary students reported more happy feelings about the past events in their lives than did marginals.

These data support previous findings which indicate that a sense of personal effectiveness can moderate the subjective experience of stress. In this instance, personal effectiveness was defined in terms of a core set of characteristics that included internality, interpersonal trust, and active planfulness. It appears that more competent persons, as compared to less competent persons, organize their experience differently; they worry less about negative life events, and they become less emotionally distressed after the experience of stressful situations. Rather, they turn more to positive past events. Personal effectiveness, as demonstrated in this study, can shape one's perceptions of and feelings about past events in life, and it can buffer the negative effects of a new life event.

Tyler, Dhawan, and Sinha (1989) questioned whether a particular attribute of the psychosocial competence model—active coping—could distinguish between Indian college students of a higher and lower social standing. They also asked whether this attribute was related, more than other elements of the competence configuration, to the need for achievement and level of persistence among less privileged Indian students. They found disconfirming evidence for both of these particular questions, but found support for the validity of the competence model as a useful conceptual tool among Indian college students. They also found support for the presence of a different pattern of competence when Indian students of a lower caste were compared with another cultural/ethnic group disadvantaged by its ecology, black American students. Their findings indicated that, among the disadvantaged Indian students, interpersonal trust was a better predictor of the need for achievement and an active planful coping stance was a better predictor of persistence. In academic settings, active coping made the difference in achievement for American black students. As with American white students, the need for achievement among Indian students of a higher social standing was dependent upon an active planful approach to life and a belief in their self-efficacy. Their level of persistence, on the other hand, was related to moderate interpersonal trust and active planfulness.

Wood (1979) conducted a study in which he examined the role of the configural variables locus of control, coping, and interpersonal trust on the speed with which black and white male college students fall to same- and different-race catchers. Each participant was placed in an experimental condition where he or she was instructed to close his or her eyes and fall backward to a catcher. There were notable racial differences in the time to fall. Overall, black students fell more slowly than whites. Further, blacks fell more slowly to a black catcher than whites to a white catcher. In this experimental situation of interpersonal trust, it appears that whites are more trusting generally and that blacks are less trusting of persons from their own race than whites are of members of their own race. Relative to the psychosocial variables, the study indicated that white students who were more internal, who viewed themselves as being less controlled by powerful others, and who were less active copers, fell more quickly to a white catcher. Black students, on the other hand, fell more quickly if they were less internal and more actively planful. These findings underscore the point that ecological characteristics (e.g., race) interact with the competence attributes to determine behavioral outcomes. That is, for black students, falling quickly seemed to be an active coping response in a threatening situation in relation to an elevated sense of being controlled by powerful others. For white students, falling quickly seemed to be a passive response triggered by a sense of being in control and having a low sense of being controlled by powerful others.

In summary, these studies suggest that there is a positive relationship between active planfulness, high self-esteem, and political activism. Further, personal efficacy moderates the effects of stressful life events and attenuates the preoccupation with past events, especially the negative ones. The individual attributes of active planfulness, self-efficacy, and trust interact differently for black, white, and Indian college students. These differences seem to be the result of psychosocial functioning based on diverse ecological realities. There are also similarities among diverse cultural/ethnic groups (black, white, Indian, and Latin) on the competence configuration as a whole. For each of these groups, the attributes of active coping, internality, and interpersonal trust are correlated; and for each group, these traits are related to successful adaptation in the academic setting.

Adults

The next group of studies involves older and younger adults, and they too suggest that individual psychosocial competence makes a distinctive contribution to well-being. As is true in the previous studies, the nature of the ecology and one's relative position in that ecology significantly shape patterns of well-being. For example, Evans and Tyler (1976) found that the personal attributes of internality, trust, and active planfulness influenced the way in which middle-aged black women coped with the demands of life, apart from the positive effects derived from their ability to negotiate the labor market. Evans and Tyler studied exemplary and marginal workers and nonworkers to determine the presence of the configural variables and the extent to which they contributed to the well-being of these black women. Exemplary workers, as compared to marginal workers, were more effective in their families and in their communities; they received more favorable evaluations from their supervisors; they saw themselves as more responsible for their own lives; and they were more actively planful and more systems blaming for racial discrimination. Also, they were more social desirability oriented. On interpersonal trust, exemplary workers were somewhat less trusting than marginal workers. This different did not, however, reach statistical significance. A similar nonsignificant pattern existed for exemplary nonworkers as compared to marginal nonworkers. Therefore, among these black women, both working and nonworking, more competent functioning was related to a higher degree of internality and active planfulness, a moderate amount of trust, an external orientation to racial prejudice and discrimination, and a greater concern for social approval. The exemplary workers and exemplary nonworkers were more similar to one another in locus of control, trust, and in active planfulness than the exemplary workers and marginal workers were to one another. These findings suggest that it is the personal attributes that distinguish the women who were functioning more competently from those who were functioning less so, and not their work status alone. Evans and Tyler concluded that while work plays a vital role in promoting a sense of competence, it alone is not enough to account for psychosocial well-being in this group of middle-aged black women. They suggested that in addition to the intrinsic value of work, internal locus of control, interpersonal trust, and active coping constituted a common set of personality traits that undergirded effective functioning.

Pargament, Steele, and Tyler (1979) studied church and synagogue members of Protestant, Catholic, and Jewish congregations to examine the relationship of church attendance and religious motivation to psychosocial competence. Their subjects ranged in age from 24 to 63 years. The results of their study suggest that the role of religious motivation on psychosocial functioning is complex and varied, and they lend additional support to the notion that ecology plays a crucial role in understanding characteristics of personal competence.

Church attendance either alone or in combination with religious motivation can both enhance and detract from a person's psychosocial well-being. For example, persons who attended church frequently had belief systems, views of themselves, and levels of satisfaction that were different from those of individuals who did not attend church regularly. Frequent church attenders believed more that God controlled their lives and less that they themselves or chance occurrences did. Also, they were less critical of themselves, saw themselves as less effective managers of their lives, and were more satisfied with their fellow church members. Individuals who attended church service regularly with low intrinsic motivation for religious activities believed that their lives were primarily under the control of chance and powerful others. They had unfavorable perceptions of themselves, a low level of interpersonal trust, and an acquiescent coping stance. They, on the other hand, were not particularly self-critical and were satisfied with their congregation. Apparently, religiosity, a contextual variable, influences patterns of competence in different ways. With respect to achieving the theoretical ideal of internality, interpersonal trust, and active coping, religiosity has advantages and disadvantages for the individual.

These studies of adults indicate that psychosocial competence attributes are related to objective indices of effective functioning above and beyond differences that can be accounted for on the basis of employment, a factor typically thought of as promoting a sense of self-efficacy. Further, they also confirm the existence and importance of ecological variables (e.g., religion) in shaping patterns of competence and well-being. In sum, these studies seem consistent with and supportive of the general findings from studies with other age groups.

Seniors

Gatz, Barbarin, Tyler, Mitchell, Moran, Wirzbicki, Crawford, and Engleman (1982a) studied a group of elderly individuals to determine the validity of the psychosocial competence attributes at this developmental period. They also examined the role of ecological variables (e.g., race, age, and participation in the labor force) in shaping these patterns. Their sample included black and white subjects, mostly women, between the ages of 50 and 79. Their findings indicated that the competence attributes were related to an overall sense of contentment about life among the elderly. They found that, in general, persons who were more satisfied with their lives were more internal, more actively planful, and somewhat more trusting than those who were less satisfied with their lives. Components of the competence configuration also varied according to personal-social dimensions. For example, blacks felt less in control of their lives and were less satisfied with their lives than whites, but they were equally active in their approach to handling the demands of life. In other words, black elderly individuals were managing their lives well but were doing so with a different set of self-attitudes and with less enjoyment. Further, individuals who worked were more actively planful and more trusting, but they were less satisfied with their lives than individuals who did not work.

Starting from the premise that ecology significantly shapes these patterns, Gatz, Gease, Tyler, and Moran (1982b) examined the influence of age and race as ecological variables that have potential constraining effects. They compared black and white women—older (55–78 years) and younger (adolescents), marginal and exemplary—in their individual competence characteristics. Participants were identified as marginal or as exemplary using independent criteria. All groups were compared in self-efficacy, interpersonal trust, and coping style.

The findings from this analysis indicated that blacks as a group were more actively planful than whites, and exemplary black seniors were more active than any other group. There were some other important subgroup differences. For example, exemplary black seniors and exemplary white adolescents were more actively planful than marginal black seniors and marginal white adolescents, respectively. With regard to locus of control, seniors were more internal than adolescents, and exemplaries (seniors and adolescents) were more internal than marginals (seniors and adolescents). Blacks, as a group, were more systems blaming than whites, and black adolescents were the most systems blaming of all. In contrast, white seniors were the most individual blaming (least trustful) of all groups. Seniors were more concerned about social approval than were adolescents. Exemplary blacks were less social desirability oriented than marginal blacks; and exemplary whites were more social desirability oriented than marginal whites.

These patterns of competence among the different racial and age groups suggest that these variables do indeed influence psychosocial functioning. They also suggest that the interaction of race and age have important consequences as well. The pattern of competence among exemplary black seniors suggests that in a context of racial prejudice and discrimination, they have put together for themselves a life of activity and assertiveness with relatively little concern for broader social approval. As Gatz *et al.* (1982a) demonstrated in the study of seniors described earlier, black elderly women tend to be quite active in their orientation to the demands of life. These two studies also demonstrate that the psychosocial competence attributes of black seniors do not configure as they do among white individuals. Theirs is a quite different pattern, as theirs has been a quite different ecology.

The competence characteristics of internality, active coping, and interpersonal trust, clustered most strongly for the exemplary white adolescents. As predicted, they were least constrained by their ecology and therefore more closely approximated the optimal state of competence described in Tyler's (1978) model. These findings, as well as those for black seniors, suggest that the interactive effects of age and race are important ingredients in the psychosocial competence configuration. The effects of age and race can be understood, at least in part, in terms of how they bear on a person's chances in life and on his or her psychosocial realities. The white adolescents are part of a majority ecosystem and culture-defining group that is partial to them. Traditionally, their ecology operates in their lives in a relatively benign fashion and affords them more chances to discover and actualize themselves. They have the opportunity to construct a sense of competence that is relatively unimpeded by societal obstacles that confront many individuals who belong to a nonmajority ecosystem and a non-culture-defining group, and they seem to have done so.

SUMMARY

Competence is indeed an important and legitimate focus in the work of mental health professionals. Studies among the homoclites, the Peace Corps workers, and the children of Kauai; studies on health-related issues; and a range of studies on Tyler's model all support the presence of a shared constellation of personal attributes in individuals throughout the life span and across cultures who successfully negotiate life with all its vagaries and vicissitudes. They have an interrelated sense of personal efficacy, interpersonal trust, and an active planful approach to life that is functionally related to their broader ecology as well as to their personal experiences.

There is an internal struggle within each of us to survive and prosper, no matter what the circumstances may be. When one person's solution to that struggle does not coincide with another's or to a consensually validated notion, it does not necessarily denote pathology nor indicate the need to denounce that way of being human. The nature of an individual's survival is to a great extent ecologically determined. Prudent judgments and arbitrations about what competence is, who possesses it, and to what degree must be carried out with respect for the context of the individual. We must examine the norms, demands, limitations, and opportunities in a particular ecosystem, and the way in which a particular individual has been exposed to them and has related to them.

By its very nature, psychotherapy calls into question the validity of some aspect of how a person is relating to his or her ecology. The task of psychotherapy is a delicate undertaking, even when the parties are ecologically similar. When they have very disparate backgrounds and psychosocial realities, the process becomes even more precarious with the potential for destructive upheaval magnified exponentially. Our model, which we have called an ethnic validity model, provides a framework for conceptualizing psychotherapy between people who are culturally, ethnically, or racially different as well as those who are alike. Using as its conceptual base Tyler's psychosocial competence framework, the ethnic validity model makes explicit allowances for divergent and convergent competencies as people enter therapy, participate in it, and change from it. As illustrated by the high school studies, the individual change process in psychotherapy will be tied directly to a person's own psychological and social reality, and to his or her adaptation within the ecology. It is to the ethnic validity model that we now turn.

3

The Ethnic Validity Model

In many ways the ethnic validity model emerges in response to a crisis within the scientific community of psychotherapy. Thomas Kuhn (1970) states that accepted scientific models are questioned when they no longer are good vehicles for problem solving and are placed when competing models are proven superior. Kuhn further states that before an alternative is embraced there is typically a vacuous period during which several different models vie for acceptance. The traditional psychotherapy paradigms, ethnocentric in nature, are being examined with regard to their relevance for nonmajority and non-culture-defining groups. Their adequacy is being questioned as a basis for conceptualizing the adaptational status or the patterns and processes of therapy with individuals in non-culture-defining groups. They ignore or obscure the relevance of the cultural, ethnic, and racial background of the therapist and client and how these factors may substantially change the prescriptions and predictions of their paradigms.

Other questions, as we have discussed earlier (Tyler, Sussewell, & Williams-McCoy, 1985) and in Chapter 1, include such concerns as whether two ecologically dissimilar dyads can engage in a meaningful therapeutic interchange. For example, can each obtain an adequate grasp of and healthy respect for the other's world view? Can mutual trust be established between them? In response to these questions, there has been a proliferation of competing models of cross-racial/ethnic psychotherapy. One of these, the particularist view, may not be considered a model of cross-racial/ethnic psychotherapy since it does not recommend therapy between two people who are racially and ethnically different. The universalist model is intended to apply to all therapy pairings, no matter what the racial and ethnic makeup of the participants is. The transcendist model begins to confront these issues but falls short of offering practical solutions to them. The result is that these models are not altogether useful in guiding cross-racial/ethnic psychotherapy at this time.

We find the position underlying the particularist view indefensible on pragmatic, humanitarian, and ethical grounds. Cross-racial/ethnic pairings are inevitable given the ratio of the majority Anglo population to the nonmajority population, and given the dearth of trained therapists from non-culture-defining groups. If a nonmajority individual seeks help at a public facility or any setting in which therapists are assigned by the agency rather than chosen by the client, the likelihood of getting a majority therapist is high.

Cross-racial/ethnic pairings are also inevitable given the way in which clients are assigned to therapists. Clients are not necessarily paired with the same-race/ethnic therapist even when most of the therapists are Anglo and the client in question is also Anglo. Usually there are many other factors involved in the process of assigning clients to therapists. Some of these are the therapist's caseload, the nature of the client's presenting problem, the therapist's skills; sometimes the assignment is just plain random.

On the other hand, in settings in which clients are free to choose a therapist, not everyone chooses a therapist of the same race or ethnicity. Some individuals choose on the basis of a therapist's reputation and success in treating people like themselves, and the therapist may not be of the same race or ethnicity. Others choose a therapist of another race to preserve their privacy in the community, especially if it is a relatively small one. Still others choose a therapist different from themselves in order to get a new perspective on a particular problem and for the sake of diversity or curiosity.

Finally, aside from the question of clients' choices and agency assignments, we as human beings owe it to one another to use our skills in ways that have the potential for relieving suffering and for enhancing one another's well-being. We are all part of the human ecology and are therefore linked to one another by that which makes us human—the ability to understand, to reason, to feel, to care. Therefore, we see cross-racial/ethnic therapeutic pairings as an inevitable as well as a challenging reality. Admittedly, cross-racial/ethnic psychotherapy pairings can be destructive if not approached in a sensitive and thoughtful manner; but in legitimizing them we at least permit their viability. We do not believe that people of different races and ethnic groups are so different that they cannot work with one another and even gain in the process.

On the other hand, we believe that an approach to therapy like that of the universalists overlooks and understates the salience of race and ethnicity in the therapy process. A person's racial/ethnic characteristics, we believe, are an essential part of his or her psychological makeup.

They play a large role in how a person defines his or her humanity as well as in how he or she expresses it.

Paradigms can be very useful tools because they help us to organize our observations, and they serve as guides for our scientific pursuits. They can also have negative value since as guides they can constrain our thinking, stymie our curiosity, and even force us to interpret anomalous data in ways that fit our model. In many ways this is the case today with psychotherapy and the models we are currently using.

As is demonstrated in the literature, the scientific climate provides grounds for developing a new model of psychotherapy, and we have taken part of our direction from those grounds. However, it is also our view that the development of an ethnic validity model of psychotherapy is both a professional and an ethical imperative. No matter how much pain and agony it may create for us to acknowledge the salience of race and ethnicity, to deny it is to deny part of our own humanity as well as that of the clients we serve.

Unfortunately, it is typically assumed that issues of race and ethnicity are important only in reference to non-culture-defining groups and that culture-defining groups are deculturized in this regard. By culture-defining group we mean that group of individuals within a particular society whose values, rules, style of life, and criteria for competence set the standard for that society. This group is not always the majority, but it typically is. Culture-defining groups traditionally have assumed preeminence, and non-culture-defining groups have deferred out of powerlessness, hopelessness, or acceptance. Thus it is easy to see how ethnocentricity is spawned and nurtured. However, with regard to psychotherapy paradigms, some members of the professional community, including non-culture-defining groups themselves, are no longer willing to accept the sanctity of the traditional models.

Within the ethnic validity model we emphasize the point that sensitivity to one's race and ethnicity as well as that of others is important for everyone. Even culture-defining group members are shaped by an ecology with a distinct value system, way of life, and criteria for competence and dysfunction. Each of us is embedded in an ecology from which comes a perspective—not ultimate truth, but a point of view. Whereas one perspective because of historical, social, and political events has been culture defining, it is a perspective nonetheless. That perspective intrinsically is no more or no less valuable than a non-culture-defining one.

It is widely acknowledged that the accepted prototype of psychological development and health is the white Anglo-Saxon middle- or upper-middle-class male. In the literature there is increasing attention to and discontentment with the parochial nature of this view. But even with such expressions and acknowledgments in the public domain, some practitioners still use this framework to guide their work with nonmajority or non-culture-defining clients. One question that arises then is how do practitioners in their work with nonmajority clients deal with the anomalies that are inevitably created by an unqualified application of this model? Another question that may arise is why do practitioners continue to use it? As we explore the answer to the first question an answer to the second question emerges as well.

Many individuals downplay the significance of differences between people on the basis of their race, culture, or ethnicity. A person who does not see these issues as being valid in and of themselves could easily reframe those differences so they conform to a particular therapeutic model. That process of conformity, however, is an expedient solution on the part of the therapist—it provides an immediate way of dealing with anomalous data by leaving the basic conceptual framework of the model intact. The costs of this process can be enormously high. It runs counter to a style that emphasizes the well-being of the client, and it potentially destroys psychotherapy. For example, if a black person in therapy expresses a high degree of vigilance about his or her interpersonal relationships with white people or about his or her relationships with systems (e.g., judicial or governmental), that person could be perceived as being "paranoid." To a majority individual there is probably little need to doubt or fear societal institutions, but to many blacks that type of vigilance is adaptive and is a crucial component of competent functioning. Ridley (1984) refers to this phenomenon as "cultural adaptive paranoia" because it denotes the utilitarian value of articulating self–world relationships in this manner, given the realities of American society relative to black people. Yet, an interpretation of this nature and the use of the word "paranoia" by the therapist is foreign to the client's own perception of himself or herself. From the perspective of the client, vigilance has been incorporated and made a part of his or her way of dealing effectively with the world. From the perspective of the ethnocentric therapist, vigilance is construed as denoting individual pathology. Herein lie divergent conceptions of competence and the potential for conflict around what is considered to be normative. The problem is not with that appropriate vigilance. The problem lies in the broader ecosystem, which is not benign and predictable for members of a non-culture-defining group. To suggest that the goal of therapy is to make such people more trusting would be incongruent with their environment and would therefore make them more dysfunctional.

Ridley (1984) has raised another issue characteristic of the way in which therapists deal with client responses that are adaptive in the client's milieu but incompatible with the therapist's models. He discusses the tendency of black clients not to self-disclose, particularly in the presence of white therapists, since many blacks consider the sharing of personal information with whites to be potentially self-destructive. Since self-disclosure is considered to be the primary vehicle by which psychological health is achieved, an ethnocentric therapist may interpret this cultural dynamic as "resistance," as described by traditional models. In contrast, a therapist using the ethnic validity model will search for the unique meaning of guardedness for the client as well as examine the therapeutic ecology for further edification. In sum, the application of two different models of human functioning can yield quite different types of information about the meaning of the client's unwillingness to self-disclose.

If a black person in therapy holds societal institutions culpable for his or her inability to negotiate problems, an ethnocentric therapist may unwittingly interpret these attributions as unhealthy, since in some models a high premium is placed upon an internal locus of control. That therapist may be so enmeshed in his or her own view of the world or so guided by a particular model that he or she fails to grasp the meaning and value of this particular world view. For black people, some degree of externality is adaptive as well as indicative of health, for it represents a realistic assessment of the systematic and continual constraints that the white, culture-defining group places on the black, non-culture-defining group.

Further, if a client discusses issues of race and ethnicity in therapy and particularly with any degree of fervor, the therapist with a psychoanalytic bias may easily categorize that expression as "negative transference." The therapist may completely disregard the role of race and ethnicity in the client's life, and thus disregard a part of that client's humanity. That therapist also loses the opportunity to examine the therapeutic relationship as an ecosystem with racial and cultural elements and make that aspect of therapy a focus as well. Other individuals may not see such unexplained or difficult issues as legitimate and respectable anomalies, but rather as deficits or perversions endemic to the client's ecosystem. Labeled as such they do not permit the therapist to view them from a competence perspective. Instead they are seen from an individual disorder-oriented focus. To use a psychosocial competence framework requires an examination of the issues for their function and value in the client's particular ecosystem. This type of process can also serve as an opportunity for the therapist to begin to move away from his or her particular perspective, to see the world differently, and to learn from the client. This argument is not intended to imply that all anomalies are adaptive or functional. It is instead an indictment of a therapeutic process in which the therapist automatically assigns those client behaviors to the category of "deviant" when they do not conform to the consensually validated culture-defining-group model.

In each of the foregoing examples, the impediments to therapy have been couched initially in terms of client deficiencies in which the solution for each lies with the client. This approach does not foster an understanding of therapy as a collaborative process whereby the responsibility for constructing a sense of the problem, related issues, and outcome is shared by both therapist and client. Instead, it fosters a sense that the therapist is the ultimate knower of the problems and issues and the final arbiter of their solutions. Further, a view of this nature precludes the interpretation of the therapy context as a mutually formed ecosystem with its own set of parameters. It can be seen as a context that has gains and losses, and advantages and disadvantages; a context that has its own potentials for convergent, divergent, and conflicting ethnic validities.

A therapist with a universalist perspective can be expected to define racial and ethnic issues from the standpoint of a universal human experience. A therapist persuaded by this perspective may argue that any differences between therapist and client arising from race and ethnicity are no greater than those that exist between any two people, because no two people are exactly the same, their racial/ethnic heritage notwithstanding. Everyone has a separate ideology, world view, and way of life. Our response would be that the latter is undoubtedly very true; however, race and ethnicity carry with them historical legacies, survival value, stimulus value, and a particular way of life. Race and ethnicity are some of the basic windows through which people view the world and interpret reality. They operate in this fashion for clients, therapists, and everyone. It is therefore necessary to assign a more distinctive ecosystem validity to those windows.

Universalists may even argue that whatever the consequences of being a majority or minority group member, each of us experiences those consequences because each of us has experienced majority and minority status at one time or another. From their view, we all have a universal experiential reference base from which to understand others, albeit in a general way. To this view we say it is not the same as when status is based on fixed and immutable qualities such as race, ethnicity, or gender. In the latter instance, membership is automatically assigned at birth and the effects are potent, enduring, and far reaching. There are also unique experiences based on those fairly enduring characteristics of language, cultural, or national identification. In contrast, when status is based on less fixed qualities, especially those of a person's own choosing (e.g., ideology, professional identity, and other similar personal characteristics), the effects are more ephemeral, less strong, and less penetrating.

With regard to the historical legacy of domination and oppression of blacks by whites in this country and its manifestation in therapy, a universalist may argue that domination/oppression is a global experience—it is common and well known around the world. Therefore, the dynamics of working with a member of an oppressed group are the same no matter who the individual players are. The ethnic validity model argues for a consideration of the circumstances under which oppression takes place, wherever it occurs, as well as a consideration of each individual's unique experiences with it.

There are therapists who respect diversity and who continue to work from an ethnocentric framework. They may do so for lack of a well-articulated alternative. Until now there has not been a model to challenge tradition in the way the ethnic validity model does. The EVM is a shift in paradigm that challenges and responds to a historical limitation that has not respected ethnically diverse competencies in human functioning. It fully acknowledges the existence and importance of race, ethnicity, culture, and individual life experiences in human growth and development. Further, the model makes explicit allowances for the fact that individuals are active participants in their lives, constantly making rules and revising them in an effort to shape their own futures. The ethnic validity model requires the therapist to find out what those rules are and what that imagined future is. Without this kind of knowledge the therapist remains limited in his or her ability to assist the client. They may even be working at cross purposes.

The ethnic validity model is an alternative to existing beliefs about the nature of cross-racial/ethnic psychotherapy and its viability. Potential value of the model is suggested in the literature in relation to Asian Americans (Leong, 1986), Native Americans (Dana, 1986), gender (Brown, 1986), blacks and whites (Carter, 1990), and ethnic minorities in general (S. Sue, 1988). The model moves theorists and therapists beyond an existing impasse over the salient issues in cross-racial/ethnic psychotherapy and the question of whether it should take place at all. As discussed earlier, the current paradigms can be understood in terms of an emphasis on race and ethnicity as relevant in the therapy process and consideration of the degree to which these variables affect the therapy outcome. Three distinct models—particularism, universalism, and transcendism—have been identified in the literature and discuss in Chapter 1.

The ethnic validity model, a transcendist view, considers that the therapy pair forms a new ecosystem in which the therapist and the client mirror their referent ecosystems. To this extent there may be differences in world views and problem-solving strategies, as well as differences in their views on the bases for competent functioning. The ethnic validity model expresses the view that even though differences may exist in one or all of these areas, conflict and destructiveness do not necessarily follow. They may even provide fertile ground for a very rich and meaningful exchange.

Our ecosystems teach their members, implicitly or explicitly, the rules for living and apprise them of available life options. In addition to these facets of a person's existence shaped by the ecosystem, each individual embodies a uniqueness based upon his or her own circumstances. Each person has a sense of validity about himself or herself, his or her relationship to the world, and a way of negotiating life events. To the degree that the therapist and the client differ in their world views, the process of psychotherapy is potentially volatile, but as mentioned earlier, it doesn't have to be destructive. Particularists view the possibility of conflict as too risky to attempt psychotherapy. Universalists minimize these differences and the possibility for conflict and thus support psychotherapy between cross-racial/ethnic pairs. Transcendists fully acknowledge the differences and the possibility for conflict and support cross-racial therapy because they believe that the racial and ethnic differences among people are not necessarily stumbling blocks; they can be meaningful building blocks.

The ethnic validity model, in particular, acknowledges the potential for conflict. But within the model other patterns of interaction are examined as well. There are possibilities for finding common ground as well as for accepting discrepant world views. The model uses the concepts of convergence, divergence, and conflict to describe and to better understand the role of diversity and the myriad ways in which it can be manifested in therapy. Convergent ethnic validity in therapy refers to a pattern in which the criteria for well-being are similar between two people and are highly compatible. Divergent ethnic validity pertains to a pattern in which world views and styles are quite different from one another, yet compatible and tolerable. Conflicting ethnic validity refers to patterns of interaction in which the world views, the styles, and the bases for competence are not only different but incompatible, and the respective participants find the acceptance of each other's positions intolerable even as the basis for dialogue.

PROTOTYPICAL THERAPY DYADS

In a very detailed way, the model outlines some of the potential trade-offs inherent in cross-racial/ethnic psychotherapy. There can be certain gains and losses in cross-racial/ethnic pairings, especially given the differences in power, status, and influence ascribed to culture-defining groups as compared to non-culture-defining groups. There are certain gains, losses, and trade-offs in same-race/ethnic pairings as well. The ethnic validity model fleshes out some of the advantages and disadvantages of these pairings. At the same time it respects the uniqueness, integrity, and validity rendered by any or all of these commonalities and differences. The model permits the possibility that two ethnically different individuals can undertake psychotherapy without either compromising his or her sense of validity. The model also permits the possibility that the homogeneity rendered by same-race/ethnic pairings does not insure therapy success. In any ethnic pairing there is the potential for gains and losses. For purposes of illustration, the following sections provide brief discussions of some of the potential gains and losses associated with each of the combinations of culture-defining group (CDG) and non-culture-defining group (NCDG) therapist and client dyads. These dyads have been elaborated upon in greater detail by Tyler, Sussewell, and Williams-McCoy (1985).

CDG Therapist and CDG Client

As members of the culture-defining group, these two individuals are protypically middle- or upper-middle-class white males. They are ecologically similar with respect to race, ethnicity, and the context of their upbringing. They are likely to have similar values and world views, which make the potential for convergence between them relatively high. They have been socialized in, and customarily abide by, the same rules for competent functioning. Both have had similar access to society's major institutions and opportunities.

The gains for both therapist and client stem from the homogeneity of the pairing. Each party has an opportunity to have his values validated by another member of the culture, and there is comfort and pride derived from this kind of affirmation. The therapist and the client can learn more about how each other has interpreted and negotiated the culture. Each can learn from the other a variety of culturally congruent ways to cope with life.

The client, having as his therapist an effective coper and a role model who is similar to himself, can feel optimistic that his striving will not be in vain. He can also feel that his initiative and effort in the service of future goals will be rewarded. His chances for attaining goals and for happiness are within his grasp. His ecology, like that of the therapist, will be supportive.

The client and the therapist both lose the opportunity to articulate beyond the commonalities inherent in a homogeneous dyad. They may be constrained by a self-serving ethnocentric view of the world and approach to problem solving. Neither the client nor the therapist has the opportunity to learn from and share with a person whose values and way of life differ from theirs. In this they lose a chance for diversity.

Homogeneity between two individuals can facilitate communication, or it can hamper it. For example, since the therapist is familiar with the client's culture, he can assume an understanding of the client and his world other than what is actually true. The therapist can prematurely close off discussion of issues he assumes he understands. In doing so, the therapist treats the client as more *known* than he actually is.

If the client is not helped in therapy, he can become discouraged by not being helped by an effectively coping member of his ecosystem—someone to whom he looks for guidance. The therapist can feel incompetent and useless if he does not succeed in helping one of his own.

CDG Therapist and NCDG Client

The dyad is prototypically a white therapist and a black client. In a general way, the dynamics of this particular pairing are also applicable to other non-culture-defining groups so defined on the basis of social class, gender, race, or ethnicity. The common element is that in society at large, power is not shared and opportunities are not distributed equitably.

By working together the therapist and the client can each gain a cultural perspective different from their own. Each can learn about a different world view as well as about a different way to solve problems. They can learn from each other about cultural norms and about different ways of putting one's life together and functioning competently in society. If the client belongs to a group that is systematically discriminated against or otherwise oppressed, the therapist can benefit by obtaining a view of the injustices in society from someone who is directly affected by them. If the therapist is inclined toward social advocacy or activism, he or she gains a much better picture of where social change is needed. Yet, the client may not wish to be seen as representative of his or her group. Therefore, the therapist must distinguish his or her objectives from those of the client.

These two therapy partners immediately diverge on the basis of differences in race, ethnicity, gender, or ascribed status. The possibilities for divergence on issues are great, and the possibilities for conflict are even greater. Whether these partners can accept the divergent ethnic validities arising from their ecosystem differences will be at the heart of determining success or failure in therapy. If they are unable to understand and accept each other, the conflict mounts and communication breaks down. They both lose the opportunity to share with each other and to broaden their horizons by so doing. Also, the therapist can lose a sense of effectiveness as a therapist; the client can lose a sense of optimism. If the therapist uses this interchange as the basis for evaluating his or her ability to work with NCDG clients or their suitability for therapy, he or she can lose a sense of objectivity. Particularly, if the therapist interprets failure in this setting on the basis of whether his or her clinical skills are adequate for treating NCDG clients, he or she may erroneously regard those skills as being of no value in regard to other NCDG clients. Moreover, if the client uses this interchange as the basis for evaluating other CDG therapists or their effectiveness with other NCDG clients, he or she can also lose a sense of objectivity. The client may see the therapist's behavior as indicative of how that therapist interacts with all NCDG clients. The client may then view the therapist as an inappropriate therapist for any NCDG client. The therapist and the client can take it one step further and shun future therapeutic interactions with racially, ethnically, or socioeconomically dissimilar people.

NCDG Therapist and NCDG Client

As with other homogeneous pairings, the therapist and the client in this dyad can gain by having their values and world views supported by one another. Each knows what it is like to be a nonmajority member of the broader culture and has experienced its impact perhaps in poignant ways. They immediately converge around their relative positions in the ecosystem and the nuances of the related experiences. The therapist can readily empathize with the client. The client can feel relatively safe and at ease talking with another person whom he or she feels understands him or her. A disadvantage of this pairing is that these two individuals may not be able to look beyond their convergent perspectives and see the limitations of them. The client can lose the opportunity to grow beyond his or her own cultural framework. The therapist can be helpful only in a limited way.

As with other homogeneous pairings, the possibility for communication problems is increased if the therapist assumes that he or she knows the client better than he or she actually does. Here again is the possibility that the therapist considers the client as more *known* than is healthy for the relationship. If therapy is unsuccessful, they both lose the opportunity to share with and learn from a person different from themselves. The therapist can feel worthless and ineffective by not being able to help another member of a non-culture-defining group. The client can suffer greater pessimism by not being helped by someone like himself or herself who is an effective coper and role model.

NCDG Therapist and CDG Client

This dyad is commonly represented by a black therapist and a white client. Both therapist and client may gain from interacting with someone of a different cultural background. Each has the opportunity to learn new problem-solving strategies. Through these interchanges they can grow beyond their cultural commonalities, which otherwise may limit them in their coping options. The therapist can gain an understanding of what it is like to be an ineffective coper and member of the culture-defining group. The therapist can also gain a perspective on societal injustices as perceived by a member of the culture-defining group, which in part may be of a different quality and kind from those experienced by members of a non-culture-defining group. The client can benefit from the skills of an effectively coping non-culture-defining group member who, within all probability, has withstood a great deal of pressure and overcome the odds of achieving success.

Here again, whether each person can accept the divergent ethnic validities almost inherent in this pairing plays a key role in determining therapy outcome. If therapy is unsuccessful, they both lose a chance to increase their own understanding and acceptance of diversity. If the therapist uses this interchange as the basis for evaluating his or her ability to work with other CDG clients or their suitability for therapy, he/she runs the risk of dismissing his or her skills as being of no use with other CDG clients and of seeing CDG individuals as being unable to benefit from therapy. If the client uses this interchange as the basis for evaluating other NCDG therapists or their effectiveness with other CDG clients, he or she can also lose a sense of objectivity. Both therapist and client can generalize their experiences in this particular situation to all racially/ethnically mixed dyads.

ETHNIC VALIDITY AND ECOLOGY

As was stated earlier, diversity does not necessarily preclude constructive interchange in therapy. Equally important is the fact that homogeneity does not guarantee it either. Rather, from the perspective of the ethnic validity model, there are advantages and disadvantages, gains and trade-offs, in any therapeutic dyad. The EVM permits the possibility that there can be convergence, divergence, and conflict between any two people, be they ethnically and racially similar or different. The therapy context is an ecosystem with its own parameters of advantages, disadvantages, supports, threats, opportunities, and limitations.

One reason is that each person is a psychologically autonomous unit embedded within the ecosystem with considerable freedom to define himself or herself, his or her relationship to the world, and a related pattern of coping. That way of being may or may not correspond totally with that of his or her referent ecosystems. For example, two people of a shared ecosystem may attach varying degrees of significance to attributes of that ecosystem when they define themselves and their relationships to the world. One may experience his or her race as his or her most salient characteristic, whereas another may experience his or her humanity as the preeminent aspect of his or her identity. How they define their basis for competent functioning will be different. Their experiences in life will be unique because each will approach the world in a somewhat different manner. A person's primary identification with a particular race, culture, or ethnicity makes him or her a representative of that referent group. As such, the identification carries with it critical cognitive and affective components. For example, the person internalizes the explicit rules and tacit assumptions of the referent group. That identification also arouses certain emotional reactions. These may come from the value the person places on that identity as well as an internalization of its value in a broader social context. Further, a person's world view and interpretation of reality will be made on the basis of that identification. Similarly, how a person constructs a sense of self and self–world relationships is related to that identity. Therefore, on this basis, two people of a shared ecosystem who enter into a psychotherapy dyad potentially can have convergent, divergent, or conflicting ethnic validities. If they cannot understand and accept their divergent ethnic validities or contain their conflict, their potentially convergent therapeutic relationship is jeopardized.

Further, the way in which these two individuals manipulate supports and threats in their ecology may be different. For example, two majority group individuals may differ greatly on how they choose to use their power, influence, and status in society. One could use them in the service of personal gain and therefore perpetuate a threatening climate for non-majority-group individuals. The other individual could use these same attributes in the service of the common good and thereby diminish the threats to those who are not as powerful, influential, or high ranking. These two individuals, even though they are culturally similar, organize their lives in vastly different ways and are likely to be very different people despite their membership in a shared ecosystem. Their patterns of interaction in therapy can easily range from convergence, to divergence, to conflict.

Another reason why homogeneity does not ensure success is because of the increased ethnocentricity involved in same-race/ethnic pairings. Two ecologically similar individuals may have difficulty stepping outside of a familiar and shared problem-solving framework to consider a less familiar one. Their similar frameworks can provide an incredibly strong mechanism for self-validation. To this extent their interaction hinders an aspect of growth that takes place through interactions with individuals of a different culture, ethnicity, and race.

We reiterate that there are gains, losses, advantages, and disadvantages in any therapeutic pairing arising from the ecological attributes of the therapist and client. The therapist and the client bring with them a set of biases and limitations; they are to a large extent constrained by them. As they work within those constraints, they make trade-offs that lead to gains and costs. On the other hand, as they move beyond their individual perspectives to understand and accept divergent ethnic validities, they can be helpful to one another in ways not previously thought of.

A therapist gains and loses in therapy just as a client does. Although we are not accustomed to thinking of gains and losses with respect to therapists, they too are affected by therapy process and outcome. Their gains are typically thought of in terms of their efficacy as helpers when therapy is successful. Any potential losses are displaced and translated into client characteristics that the therapist perceives as inhibiting a good therapy outcome. Traditionally, the therapist is thought of as the expert whose job it is to "cure" the client. In this role, he or she is seen as removed from the hazards and from many of the benefits of therapy, especially those of a psychosocial nature. The client is seen as the most vulnerable member of the dyad as well as the one who stands to gain the most as a result of the interchange. However, the therapist is not immune to what happens in therapy, and he or she stands to gain and lose too.

The ultimate loss to the therapist and client is the failure of psychotherapy. The ethnic validity model requires us to examine responsibility for failure in a way not traditionally considered. Because therapists are presumed to be relatively neutral regarding therapy outcome, clients are singularly vulnerable to being blamed for unsuccessful therapy. For example, negative psychotherapeutic outcomes are usually attributed to the personal deficiencies of the client, without regard for the ecological characteristics of the therapist and client. These ecological characteristics significantly shape both therapy process and outcome. Therefore, an alternative framework for viewing the interchange is to examine who the client is, who the therapist is, the relative contribution of their separate ecologies, and the way in which they deal with their differences, commonalities, and conflicts.

The concepts of enculturation and socialization are important in more fully understanding ethnic validity in psychotherapy. Enculturation is the process by which members of an ecosystem acquire unexamined beliefs. These are the laws, rules, and axioms that we accept without question. Societal institutions (e.g., family, school, church) enculturate us. In contrast, socialization is the process by which we gain a distinctive perspective on ourselves, other people, our universe, and our place in it. We are socialized through life experiences, particularly through activities and interactions with people different from those to which we are accustomed. As a result of socialization, we gain a greater sense of autonomy and of our abilities to shape who we are and our way of being in the world. We learn that there is a range of options from which to choose. We also learn about other people and their ways of being. Some life experiences are consistent with our encultured views and some are not. When they are inconsistent, openness to accepting divergent experiences allows socialization to proceed more readily. Through socialization we can thus examine once unquestioned assertions and begin to see them as one view rather than as the sum total of reality.

Psychotherapy, as practiced from the perspective of the ethnic validity model, is a form of socialization. Both therapist and client are socialized within a newly formed therapeutic ecosystem. The client, having failed in some manner through the use of his or her familiar perspectives and coping skills, seeks the support of a therapist. In a collaborative fashion, they deal with those problems by exploring a new set of world views, meanings, and problem-solving options. In creating solutions to problems they arrive at mutually agreed upon options, some of which are new and some of which are old to both therapist and client. To the extent that the solutions are new, a kind of socialization takes place. The client learns a different understanding of his or her problems and a new way of coping with them. The therapist learns a new problem-solving approach—one that arises directly from the unique ecosystem created by him or her and the client. To the extent that traditional psychotherapy paradigms assume authority over the therapeutic domain, exclusive of input by the client, they are processes of enculturation. The client plays a somewhat compliant role by withholding his or her viewpoint with respect to the therapist's interpretations of behavior and suggestions for behavior change.

Training therapists to use the ethnic validity model is a process of socialization. It is a process that actively involves therapist in conceptualizing the therapeutic ecosystem, divergent patterns of adaptation, the patterns and processes of therapy, and therapy outcome. It rejects the approach of expecting therapists in training to dismiss their own viewpoints and life experiences without question.

The road to a shared understanding of the basis for the client's difficulties and a mutually agreed upon way of handling them is not always a smooth one. The degree of concordance between the therapist and the client at any given point can range from convergence to divergence to conflict. In the traditional sense, when the therapist and client diverge or conflict in their understanding of an issue, the responsibility for this lack of convergence is assigned to the client, and he or she is said to lack insight. The traditional concept of insight in psychotherapy as interpreted from an ethnic validity model is convergence between therapist and client—more specifically, a type of convergence whereby the client understands a particular issue from the viewpoint of the therapist. From the perspective of the EVM, convergence or "insight" is not the ultimate goal of therapy, nor is it desirable in all cases. A therapist or client who seeks convergence at the expense of other patterns of interaction does so at the risk of losing a sense of identity, respect, and ethnic validity. In the traditional sense, insight is a state only the client must obtain and is blamed for when it does not occur. We submit that clients need not be burdened unilaterally for the lack of insight. Insight and understanding flow in two directions—from therapist to client and from client to therapist. It is as important for the therapist to understand the client's perspective as it is for the client to understand the therapist's perspective. Moreover, it is important for them both to achieve a shared understanding of the issues.

SUMMARY

Traditional psychotherapy paradigms are limited in their ability to conceptualize divergent ethnic validities and their expressions in the context of therapy. These models either deny or give short shrift to the role of race, culture, or ethnicity in psychotherapy. They also fail to consider that these ecological parameters can fundamentally change the formulas, and therefore the predictive power, of their paradigmatic models. The usefulness of such ethnocentric models as a basis for individuals from nonmajority and non-culture-defining groups is being questioned, and new models are being developed. The ethnic validity model transcends the current crisis in at least two ways. One, it does not question whether differences of race, culture, or ethnicity among therapy dyads influence the therapeutic process. Rather, the model is predicated on the *a priori* assumption that ecology substantially shapes the process of psychotherapy and its outcome. The model emphasizes that ecology is important even when both members of a therapy dyad are relatively homogeneous with respect to their referent ecosystems. Two, the model, in a purposeful and concerted manner, addresses some of the salient issues that arise between prototypic therapy dyads. These issues pertain to the trade-offs in therapy with anyone—the gains, losses, advantages, and disadvantages. They also pertain to the possibilities for convergent, divergent, and conflicting ethnic validities. These issues will be explored in detail as we apply ethnic validity perspectives to understanding psychotherapy and learning to become ethnically/racially sensitive psychotherapists. The ethnic validity model provides us a way to implement and extend a transcendist perspective and to incorporate the valid components of universalist and particularist perspectives in doing so. In the chapters ahead we spell out the patterns, processes, and possibilities of psychotherapy as they have emerged for us as we have worked with an ethnic validity perspective and with each other. Before we start, we take a detailed look at the ecology of race and its implications for psychotherapy.

4

The Ecology of Race

In America today, the categories of *masters* and *slaves* are no longer directly applicable. Other labels are now used, such as majority and minority, upper class and lower class, male and female, able-bodied and disabled, and of course white and black. These labels in part connote a similar message, suggesting that the relationship dynamics emanating from a master–slave history remain and have influenced the ways Americans—blacks, whites, and others—experience their ecology and themselves. For these reasons we believe it is imperative to examine the influence of race on the human ecology. It provides a vehicle for moving beyond our ethnic ecosystems and reorganizing our perceptions of the world to acknowledge that there are a multitude of ways to be human and live competently. An examination of racial dynamics informs our understanding of human ecology by providing a prototype for examining the relationship characteristics among people who are similar to each other, among people who are different from each other, and in particular among people who hold different positions of power within a heterogeneous society. The examination of relationships among members of white and black America is particularly instructive because race relations, apart from ethnic relations, have played such a pivotal role in shaping the fundamental ways in which individual Americans perceive themselves and organize their lives.

Examination of the contribution of race to relationships also provides sociohistorical and ecological levels of analysis as aids to understanding how historical legacies influence intrapersonal and interpersonal processes. Consequently, this chapter continues to build upon and elaborate the ethnic validity framework. It does so by analyzing the influence of race as a salient variable in psychotherapy and as the prototypical example of the influence of other factors such as ethnicity and gender.

RACE AS A CONTEXT FOR PERSONAL LEGACIES

As a number of writers have documented (e.g., Bennett, 1964; Kovel, 1970), America's unique history of slavery has significantly influenced her human ecology by altering individuals' perceptions of themselves, their perceptions of others, and their psychosocial reality. In order for America to have accepted and legalized slavery for her first 200 years, the values supporting the master–slave relationship had to become an integral part of the belief structure of her society (Blassingame, 1979; Jordan, 1968; Meier & Rudwick, 1969; Oakes, 1982). Hence, those characteristics that defined the master–slave relationship had to be carefully and securely woven into the fabric of intrapersonal and interpersonal relationships. As a result, how Americans have formed relationships, what they expect from relationships, and how they view themselves and others in relationships have been significantly influenced by her participation in and legalization of slavery. More importantly, values developed to justify slavery have become a part of the human ecology and have been passed on to future generations through enculturation as well as socialization (Ezekiel, 1984).

In Chapter 2 we emphasized that enculturated values are beliefs and attitudes deeply rooted in a society. They are the often hidden beams with which a society builds its moral, legal, and ethical foundation. Enculturated values and beliefs are those for which members of the culture do not ordinarily know that there is an alternative. For instance, in the West we assume that the world did not create itself. Consequently, using religion or science, we search for an explanation for what external forces created our world. It is not part of our world view that the cosmos came into existence by natural means. Our belief in an external creative process is an enculturated view and one which is not necessarily held by people living in other parts of the world.

The processes through which we teach the more conscious rules of a society or group we call socialization. Enculturation provides the foundation of societal values; socialization assists us in consciously organizing our understanding of behavioral norms and enculturated values. For example, the notion that there must be a designated leader or group in charge of and responsible for the collective is an enculturated value. However, it is through socialization that we teach some children to be leaders and others to be followers. For example, historically the sex and race of children have been used as criteria to determine which children shall be socialized for subordinate or dominant statuses.

Enculturation and socialization processes work collectively to give each individual in a society a sense of cultural continuity and a way of understanding and making sense of his or her identity and environment. In that way the development of slavery necessitated that Amercians psychologically encode new standards for defining humanity. Both masters and slaves had to alter their understanding about themselves and about others to internalize their new status. For example, a master had to perceive himself as being powerful and as having the right to dictate the norms, values, and standards for slaves and by extension for other members of society. The master was taught to believe that others' realities had to meet with his understanding or perceptions to be authentic. Most importantly, in order to validate their inhumane treatment of human beings, masters found it of value to relegate slaves to a subhuman status. Those whites who chose not to be masters had to reconcile what it meant to belong to the master class and to be privileged. They also had to figure out a way to maintain, accept, or modify their relationships with others of their race who did participate in slavery (Elkins, 1968; Jordan, 1968).

Slaves confronted a different reality. They had to reorganize their psychosocial realities to maintain their sense of humanness, dignity, and legacy in the face of ecological pressures. Their challenge was to translate and to hold on to preslavery self-perceptions and feelings of humanness within the context of slavery.

There are a number of enculturated beliefs and values that have developed from, or at least been strengthened by, this pattern of master–slave relationships. These complex beliefs and values have been transmitted in various forms over generations. For example, one enculturated belief is the notion that in any society there must be dominant figures and weaker figures and, moreover, that "dominance is superiority." This perspective has provided continued justification for the domination of whites over blacks and allowed for the inhumane as well as paternalistic treatment of blacks (Breeden, 1980; Gossett, 1963; Oakes, 1982).

The enculturated values that Americans have demonstrated through their racial history have been demonstrated throughout history in other parts of the world (Kovel, 1970). Race has not always been the salient variable in defining one's ascribed status as a CDG or a NCDG. Socioeconomic status, gender, and ethnicity have all been used as either a source of empowerment or as the rationale for disenfranchising a particular group. For example, we can trace the idea of one group dictating to another group at least as far back as Plato's *The Republic* (fourth century B.C.). Plato divided society into three classes—gold, silver, and brass. Each class had an assigned role. The gold class comprised the aristocracy and the rulers. The silver class were the craftsmen. According to Plato, members of the gold and the silver classes merited training and education. The brass class were considered uneducable and were servants and slaves.

Gould (1981), in his classic *The Mismeasure of Man*, has elaborated on Plato's discourse. He has pointed out that Socrates, faced with the question of how to get the people to accept this hierarchical structure, fabricated a myth that they have different natures. He then asked his listener, Glaucon, whether the people would believe the myth. Glaucon said no, but that their children, grandchildren, and subsequent progeny would come to believe it. Gould then makes the point that

> The same tale, in different versions, has been promulgated and believed ever since. The justification for ranking groups by inborn worth has varied with the tides of Western history. Plato relied upon dialectic, the Church upon dogma. For the past two centuries, scientific claims have become the primary agent for validating Plato's myth. (p. 20)

It was this kind of view, espoused by Americans of European ancestry, that has taken on various forms in America. That is, the period of slavery in the United States contributed significantly to embellishing and solidifying existing values around superiority so that they became for the most part enculturated. Moreover, the master–slave relationship became a prototype both for black–white relationships in the United States and for how Americans respond to those who are different from them. Black–white relationships serve as exemplars of some of the ways in which individuals respond to differences. They serve as exemplars of the resulting psychological reorganization that takes place in order to maintain the oppressor–oppressed relationship. And most importantly for the purposes of our discussion, they also serve as exemplars of how individuals can transcend historical legacies and shape and create new relationships and experiences. Such experiences in turn influence individuals' ecologies and their perceived self–world relationships.

Many of the aspects of black–white relations described above have also been encountered by women in relation to men, between classes, and between ethnic groups. Each group has its unique experience, but the enculturated values that characterized the master–slave relationship seem to have characterized them as well. For example, in the Western world, women have endured oppression and subjugation from at least biblical times. As Burke (1986) has documented in *Women, Feminism, and Biology*, women have at times been considered biologically inferior, relegated to an inferior and even subhuman status, and often viewed as property. These enculturated values of male superiority and dominance have continued to characterize the self–world relationships between men and women. Furthermore, in America the subjugation of women has interacted with race to create a more complex dynamic in how black women and white women relate. In her paper on white privilege and male privilege, McIntosh (1988) discussed the multiple ways in which she experiences privilege in America because of her race. McIntosh, who is white, described how this sense of privilege is firmly implanted in her psyche. It impacts her world view, her expectations of life, and how she goes about the most routine aspects of daily activities. Moreover, she acknowledges that her sense of privilege as a white in relation to blacks is analogous to the sense of privilege that men experience over women. Historically, this sense of privilege was encoded perhaps most starkly in the patterns of black–white relationships in America. The generations that have followed have had to confront and reckon with the dynamics stemming from that legacy in forming and understanding relationships, not only white–black relationships but others as well. The consequence is that, in any relationship, race and/or racial dynamics enter as variables that contribute to the possible psychological gains, trade-offs, and conflicts that can result from an interpersonal interaction.

The attitudes and values that stem from such a master–slave legacy also influence the nature of the ecological evaluations made of one's surroundings. Ecological evaluations are the assessments that individuals make of their interpersonal and/or physical environment. When we examine ecological evaluations from the perspective of the master–slave dynamic, we find that they are made along a number of dimensions. These dimensions include psychosocial support, psychosocial conflict and threat, and physical support and harm.

We can examine these dimensions from two perspectives: interpersonal and intrapersonal. The interpersonal perspective pertains to the type of evaluations the master and the slave make about each other and about members of their respective groups. The intrapersonal perspective pertains to how the master and the slave organize their internal ecologies. Paolo Freire (1971) has explored these perspectives in far greater depth than we can pursue in this context. A number of writers from the social science and mental health fields have documented its development in the particularly American context (Blassingame, 1979; Breeden, 1980; Gossett, 1963; Jordan, 1968; Kovel, 1970; Meir & Rudwick, 1969; Oakes, 1982; Willie, Kramer, & Brown, 1973). We can only say that the reasoning we are presenting in this section parallels theirs as they have presented it in relation to dominant and subordinate class and race structures.

Both the master and the slave approach interpersonal interactions with caution. Even though the master is dominant, he remains concerned about and threatened by the possibility of losing his power and status. Thus, the master approaches the interaction by evaluating it for possible psychosocial supports (those factors that assist him in maintaining his status, position, and sense of self); for psychosocial threat or harm (those factors that can usurp his power base); and for physical support or harm (those factors that increase or endanger physical safety). Like the master, the slave also assesses the interaction or environment for psychosocial supports or threats, or for physical support or harm. However, in contrast to his or her master, the slave approaches the relationship concerned about his or her sense of self and physical safety rather than the loss of power *per se.* As the oppressed, the slave must become expert at understanding power, if he or she is to survive. In fact, the slave must learn to assess power relationships on multiple levels, including individual (personal power) and societal. For example, the slave may assume an equal sense of power when it comes to personal attributes such as his or her humanity; he or she may feel less powerful when it comes to his or her ability to challenge the master's humanity without bringing down group as well as individual physical and/or emotional reprisal. The slave may also feel less powerful in terms of having less societal support for his or her challenges to the master.

To some extent, relationships based all or in part on master–slave dynamics mirror those issues whether they are master–master, master–slave, or slave–slave, and whether they are same race or cross race. Major issues involved are those of sense of self and way of coping with such interactions. Perhaps even more central is the issue of trust, yet to have a positive interaction, both the master and the slave must take risks, however calculated they may be. The master must risk losing control, authority, and power. The slave must risk losing his or her perverse comfort with the status quo and risk emotional and physical safety (F. Jones, 1976). Further, the risks involved are ecosystem risks as well as individual risks. Both master and slave must assess them as well as decide whether they should trust each other.

These elements enter even in the master–master and slave–slave interaction in which there is a sense of sameness and of individuals making common assumptions about their ability to connect with one another. The two individuals are peers, yet their perceptions of themselves as masters or as slaves influence their ability to communicate effectively with each other. They may compete for power, try to oppress each other, or merge their views to the extent that they get lost in a narrow perception of the world from which they can no longer escape.

THE MEANING OF POWER

We have been emphasizing that the concept of power plays a pivotal role in formulating how both masters and slaves organize their experiences and relate to others in the ecology. Before we continue, we need to define what we mean by power and ask whether it is always negative. According to Wolman (1973) and E. Pinderhughes (1989), power is complex and multidimensional. They have identified several aspects of power. One is self-control, or the ability to determine and satisfy one's needs. Another is other-control, or the ability to determine, satisfy, or prevent the satisfaction of the needs of others. And lastly, they indicate that power is quantifiable and has a positive and a negative dimension. Power is positive when it promotes the needs of self and others and negative when it thwarts the needs of self and others.

Within the EVM framework, power is thought of as including not only the ability to achieve self-determination or other-control, it also includes psychosocial competence. The psychosocial competence aspect of power is positive in that it denotes one's struggle to increase mastery over one's life while respecting the diversity and rights of others. Within an EVM perspective, personal power also includes collective power in which help-seeking and prosocial behaviors, such as relatedness, are present. We consider these aspects of power to be positive. However, the self-determination component of power becomes negative when one's need for self-control infringes on the rights of others to satisfy their needs and disrupts community well-being.

As previously stated, the notion of control is a prominent aspect of power, particularly power over others. The control of others can be positive if it protects others or assists them in satisfying their needs. Within the EVM framework, power is positive if it assists self or others in achieving self-determination. Power becomes negative and violates EVM principles when it involves (1) having a person or group be unilaterally responsible for satisfying the needs of others; (2) thwarting others' ability to satisfy their needs and to determine their destiny in order to satisfy one's own needs; and (3) controlling one's own destiny, even if previously oppressed, by seeking unilateral control over others. Nobles (1990) has articulated one of the aspects of power in a way that parallels the EVM perspective on the self-determination and self-control components of power. He defines power as the ability to define reality and to have others accept that definition as legitimate and valid. In EVM terms, the degree to which people give up psychosocial power is the degree to which they forfeit their world view and understanding of the ecology and accept another's interpretation of reality. From this framework, the oppressed regain power as they reclaim their perspective of reality and define themselves.

Throughout history, in hierarchical societies one's position has implicitly and explicitly revealed one's worth or value to that society. In America it has also come to imply a person's degree of humanness. Thus, the label of master affirmed for whites their degree of humanness, as well as their worth and value to society. The label of slave communicated to blacks that they were not fully human members of society but were worthless and disposable.

In the following sections, we will focus on describing and analyzing the racially based master–slave ecosystem aspects of therapist and client pairings. To do so we need to look at therapist–client pairings as involving master–slave components. That they, at least to some extent, involve such ecosystem characteristics and that race is one of those characteristics has been asserted and documented by a growing number of writers (Bulhan, 1985; Fanon, 1967; Kovel, 1970; C. Pinderhughes, 1973; E. Pinderhughes, 1989). The extent to which such ecosystem characteristics are present in therapist–client pairings awaits far more research than is currently available. Nevertheless, there is evidence in support of the therapeutic efficacy of moving beyond such barriers (see Chapter 2 discussion of a transcendist perspective).

We want first to discuss therapist and client pairings from a racial ecosystem perspective. We will then consider some characteristic issues that may arise as a consequence of the racial aspects of different dyadic pairings. In doing so we are aware that therapist–client pairings can be viewed from other perspectives and that other aspects of such pairings are important. We are also aware that readers may disagree with our view of the general importance of racial ecosystem perspectives in therapeutic relationships. We are not seeking to ignore these other perspectives or emphases. We are trying to point out and illustrate why we believe there is a general presence of racially derived master–slave elements in therapeutic relationships. We are also trying to illustrate how those elements are manifested.

Race and Psychotherapy

In brief, each individual's historically ascribed status has master–slave elements built into it that become important in understanding the issues that individual confronts in forming, sustaining, and ending any relationship. This understanding has been incorporated in some way in how we understand ourselves and our values. It follows that as the client and the therapist form a new ecological unit, each person's understanding of his or her historical status is at least implicitly explored. That exploration results in mutual change, in growth or decline, in maintaining the status quo, or in some missed outcome.

Therapists as Racial Ecosystems

Therapists are not immune to enculturation and socialization. They too inherit the legacy of their ethnic and racial groups. Our experiences in conducting workshops with therapists and in teaching predoctoral clinical psychology students have shown us that therapists and therapists-in-training are often uncomfortable with the issue of race in psychotherapy. Their expression of their discomfort has varied, ranging from "I have my prejudices about people like everyone else, but these prejudices are not based on race" to "What are some techniques that I can use to provide my black clients with more culturally relevant treatment?" The latter question indicates that therapists often seem to be looking for a prescription of some kind, one that does not involve much personal exploration and emotional work on their part. The former remark indicates that therapists seem to be denying the role that race and their racial history have played in their own lives.

Therapists' reluctance to explore the master–slave dynamic or to consider the race issue is at least in part a reaction to the ugliness of oppression. America is unsettled and uncomfortable with the outward and visible ugliness of its slave history, both from the white and from the black perspectives. Some whites wish to banish from memory historical documentation of their potential for inhumane behavior toward blacks (even though they continue to support institutional forms of racism). Some blacks wish to suppress a history of oppression, since their lack of power and, more importantly, their loss of status as human beings are horrendous memories. These memories can fester and lead to a number of negative emotions, including anger, hatred, or depression. Yet, for blacks not to remember at all makes them vulnerable to further oppression and dehumanization. What seems to assist therapists in moving beyond their initial fears is to remind them of the role that enculturation and socialization have played in their lives. To understand these influences better, they must step back in time and examine what history can reveal about successful and unsuccessful relationships between races.

Recall that each person must formulate his or her ecological evaluation based on his or her racial history and personal circumstances. If we translate these expectations to a therapy relationship, they mean that in either a cross-race or same-race dyad, both the therapist and the client will make ecological evaluations of their environments, including the people in them, and will bring to therapy a set of expectations based on these evaluations. Furthermore, these ecological evaluations provide the initial framework for the therapeutic relationship and the foundations for convergence, divergence, and conflict in the therapy relationship.

Through self-examination, the therapist becomes equipped to handle the racial undertones and challenges in a therapeutic relationship. In traditional psychotherapy training programs, the therapist is taught that his or her background and personal life experiences can pose barriers and possibly interfere with the therapeutic process. Therapists usually interpret this intrusion of the therapist's individual characteristics as countertransference. Consequently, we find trainees spending much time in both their own therapy and in supervision, unravelling their psychological baggage and its origins. In these discussions, race is rarely introduced as an important variable for exploration. More importantly, if it is introduced it is more likely to be introduced with a nonwhite trainee than with a white trainee. The implicit assumption is that being nonwhite brings baggage and conflict and that being white is the norm and is baggage-free. Racial self-examination is crucial for both the white and the black therapist. Race is as much an integral part of who we are in America as is one's class, religion, or gender.

Establishing Your Racial Psychohistory

We would suggest, as have a number of people (Griffith, 1977; Helms, 1985; Sue & Zane, 1987), that the first task which confronts a therapist who wishes to increase awareness of how enculturated and socialized values have influenced his or her practice of psychotherapy is to formulate a racial psychohistory. That is, the therapist needs to examine his or her self-system as a racial being. Issues to explore include the role that race has played in shaping the therapist's philosophy of living, personality, outlook on life, patterns of interaction, and coping styles.

How does the therapist go about formulating a racial psychohistory? To do so, the therapist must ask himself or herself several different kinds of questions that pertain to three basic categories:

1. *The therapist's conscious understanding of his or her feelings about race.* Questions in this category pertain to the therapist's feelings about being black or white, conceptualizations of the ills and strengths of race relations, feelings about the importance of race in human and social development, and perspectives on prescriptions for rectifying racial disharmony and on who bears the responsibility for implementing these

prescriptions. Sample questions include: How do I define myself? Do I define who I am based largely on my experiences as a black (or white) person, as a male or as a female, and so on? Am I proud of my race? What are the strengths of my people? What are the weaknesses of my people? What is my philosophy on integration and segregation? What is my view on the ills of the black community and of the white community? Whose responsibility is it to rectify these ills?

2. *The therapist's earliest memories and associations concerning racial identification and stereotype.* Questions in this category are aimed at exploring the therapist's more implicit, covert, and/or subconscious feelings about race. They also explore the therapist's racial socialization. Sample questions include: What are my earliest memories as a black (white) child? What were the messages I received as a white (black) child, and where did these messages originate? How were race-related messages reinforced, and how were they challenged?

3. *The therapist's experiences with cross-race relationships.* Questions in this category pertain to the therapist's experiences in cross-race relationships and the therapist's appraisal of his or her success in these relationships. These questions also help the therapist gauge his or her history of engaging in and willingness to continue to engage in risk-taking behavior in cross-race relationships. Sample questions include: In general, how do I feel about members of the other race? What level of trust do I have in working with and befriending members of the other race? What have been my experiences in dealing with the white world and the black world? Collectively, these questions help the therapist to understand those aspects of himself or herself that will most likely be challenged in the therapy situation. As an example of the value of this process, one of us will share some aspects of her racial psychohistory with you.

An Excerpt from a Racial Psychohistory

I am a black female, born in 1953. In exploring my racial psychohistory, I realize that my definition of who I am is intricately tied to my race. My pride in myself, my values, my outlook on life, those things that I abhor or do not value in others are intertwined with my experiences as a black person. They are also intricately tied to the times in which I was reared. The historical context in which I have developed and continue to grow plays a crucial role in shaping my perceptions of my ecology and in defining those life circumstances I have confronted and that I will continue to confront. I was born during the latter years of segregation and was witness to the excitement and the violence that accompanied integration. This historical context has contributed significantly to my experiences and resulting world view.

My earliest memories pertaining to my race are more like unorganized snapshots. They include visits to the country that were well planned so that we knew where we could safely stop for gas and use restrooms, and where I first heard of the Ku Klux Klan. They also include an image of an elderly white woman looking at my mother with disgust as she allowed me to take a drink from a water fountain in a major department store. My most organized race-related memories are of my segregated, public elementary school. Two images are most prominent. The first is the amount of pride we had in our school. As Negroes we were taught to take pride in our environment, and we felt a sense of ownership about our school. The pride the community had in the school was seen at least twice a year, when we would have programs, plays, and musicals in which our teachers would dance and sing with us. The auditorium/cafeteria would be packed—standing room only. It was a great time.

My second image of my segregated school is of my teacher, Miss W., delivering a standard field trip message. The central theme of this message was that whites do not expect good things of you. "They do not expect you to know how to speak properly. They do not expect you to have brains, and they do not expect you to know how to behave. But we know that you have brains, and we know that you know how to do all of these things. Have pride in yourself. Negroes are proud people and behave nicely."

This message was really impressed upon me and my fellow classmates. It was especially emphasized the year before they closed our school because it was too old and physically rundown to participate in the forced busing plan. Each Friday afternoon during the last half of the school year, the sixth graders were divided into two groups, girls and boys. The girls would go with our only female sixth-grade teacher and the boys would go with the two male sixth-grade teachers. All the teachers in our school were black. For that 30 minutes, Miss W. would talk about having pride in ourselves and about how bright and wonderful and beautiful we were. She talked about setting our goals high and showing the world what we could accomplish. I didn't understand the purpose of these talks. However, once I was bused to the white school, the intent behind these talks was clear, and over the years these talks have become special memories.

The philosophies espoused at my segregated school mirrored and were compatible with those at home. I recall a natural transition from home to school. The color of the people was the same. They talked the same; they had the same expectations of me; the food was the same; and I felt protected and cared about. Two messages were also given at home. They were (1) you are beautiful (both inwardly and outwardly), and (2) you are brilliant. "The world may tell you otherwise but we know differently. Never give up or give in to others' negative assessments of you." Prior to my daily encounters with the white world through busing, I watched my father negotiate with the white world. I saw that he was "the only one" (Negro) on his job and that most of the time he felt respected at work.

But I also overheard his conversations with my mother and overheard his work-related telephone conversations, which revealed instances in which white individuals would attempt to sabotage his authority and efforts. It appeared to my parents that some of his colleagues had difficulty with his intelligence and competence. He would refer to these people as racists and continue to forge ahead, and do so effectively.

My mother, who would respond supportively to my father's race-related dilemmas, was the major warrior for me as I ventured off to the white academic environment and encountered overt racism for the first time. I was in the seventh grade. Early in the process, the struggles encountered by my father and the warnings of my teachers became real for me.

Prior to being bused to the white school, we (the black students) had to be placed academically. Tracking was the norm in those days. I was to be tracked in the slow group as a result of my poor performance on standardized tests. The major claim was that I was a poor reader and would be unable to comprehend course material. My parents, represented by my mother, fought relentlessly with the white system in trying to block this placement. The white system would not budge and placed me in a noncollege bound, slow track. Mother, however, did make it clear that I was to be moved to the college-bound track if I evidenced greater ability. Although I was not privy to this information or process for almost a year, I had noticed that in the white school I was separated from the few black friends being bused to that school.

As she knew I would, I received all A's and mother requested that I be moved to a more challenging group—the college-bound group. The school officials continued to resist, saying that I was too far behind and would not be able to catch up. I remember overhearing two white teachers discussing my mother's insistence that I had greater potential. They felt that she was pushy and out of line and that it would cause me considerable difficulty. Nevertheless, Mother persisted, and I was placed in the academically advanced, college-bound group and continued to receive all A's. However, I do not remember my teachers being at all pleased with my performance or celebrating my achievements with me the way my black teachers and my parents had done in the past. In fact, when one fellow white student commented on my straight A report card and how smart I was, the teacher quite angrily commented to her that they all (it was an otherwise all white class) could achieve all A's if they wanted to do so. Her comment was a negation of my abilities and very much in line with the warnings from my parents and segregated school of not being cared about or validated in the white world.

These incidents continued throughout my education in high school, college, and graduate school. The consistent messages from my parents were (1) do not accept others' evaluations of you; (2) check out messages from the white world with someone who truly cares about you; and (3) aim high in life. So, in high school, when a white teacher blocked my admittance to the National Honor Society when I had a 3.92 average, we fought the system and chalked it up to the never-ending battles with whites. When it was time to go to college and my guidance counselor told me that I should apply to a less rigorous community college instead of the Ivy League school where I received my undergraduate education, she was ignored. In college, when I did my honors project I was not dismayed over the lack of enthusiasm or support for my project by my advisor. I assumed it was par for the course. The message for me was clear. In this world, support and energy for my development would come from the black community. In addition, if I wanted to succeed, I had to be creative in my problem solving and in developing ways to assess my strengths and weaknesses because the white world would most likely provide a biased opinion of me or at least one which was not based on enthusiasm or caring for me as a person. Furthermore, I had to be a keen observer of all systems of which I was a participant and always approach these environments strategically. And finally, I had to stand up for myself and always maintain my pride and dignity.

All of my experiences with whites were not negative. Over the first 21 years of my life, I encountered three whites whom I felt were genuine in their caring about me. Two were math teachers, one in junior high school and one in college. They were excited about my abilities and consistently challenged me to reach for higher ground. They were not overly warm or verbally praising, but I knew that they genuinely cared about me and other students. The third person was a peer, a friend, Janice, whom I met while living with my family for a period in a New England town. Janice and I enjoyed writing prose and poetry. She was very talented and was very sensitive to the emotions of others. My family, one of three black families in this town, returned to our original home after a 2-year period. When I returned home, Janice and I continued to write. She later visited me for a day when I was in college, and for the first time she saw me with other blacks. Janice was very uncomfortable with my new ecological set; she was used to seeing me in all white contexts. After this visit, the friendship ended. I don't recall why. That is, I do not remember whether I reached out and she did not respond, she reached out and I did not respond, or whether we never made a point of contacting one another after the visit. Nonetheless, our racial differences were not discussed, and the things that once bonded us were not pursued.

These experiences have affected my relationships with black clients and with white clients and have influenced significantly the underlying race-related assumptions that I bring to any therapeutic relationship. For example, as a result of my past, I have assumed that genuine caring for a black person is most likely found only in relationships with other blacks. This assumption originates from my early childhood and adolescent experiences in which encouragement, caring, and confidence in my abilities came almost exclusively from blacks. However, this assumption may be contrary to my client's experience with black people or with blacks in the helping profession. Consequently, this assumption may interfere with forming a therapy relationship.

I also assume that whites, regardless of their wish to do so, find it difficult to unweave their psyches from the intricately woven fabric of racism. However, in order to work effectively with whites, I have to move beyond this assumption. I have to believe that it is possible for whites and blacks to develop a relationship characterized by genuine caring and respect.

A third assumption is that blacks are able to care genuinely about whites and can understand the experiences of whites. In my family, several of my aunts, in the role of servant, cared for (and nurtured) white children from preschool through adulthood. My aunts were genuine in their love for these children, despite the racism they encountered in the larger society. Their example showed me that the capacity to care genuinely about whites was attainable.

A fourth assumption is that to be an effective coper and psychologically healthy person, a black person must have a clear and strong black identity. This assumption is one I still believe. However, I have learned to be more understanding and accepting of those black clients who may not demonstrate all of these characteristics. Thus, when I question myself or a supervisee as to why a black person has no black friends or why an interracial couple only associates with whites, my awareness of this assumption provides me with an initial framework for understanding why this issue is important to me, when it may not be important to the client.

A fifth assumption is that race is more salient than ethnicity. That is, an African black and a West Indian black share with American-born blacks a history of oppression regardless of its form. Thus, I assume that, despite language and cultural differences, there is an underlying bonding around our common struggles with the white world. Although this assumption is true for some blacks, it is definitely not true for all blacks. In my experiences, the black–white distinction has been the most important human distinction. For blacks from other countries who are now living in America, it is my Americanness, as well as my blackness, that is important in shaping what impressions they form of me.

These assumptions do influence how I relate to my clients and my expectations of how they will relate to me. These are my intuitive, experientially based expectations based on my racial ecology. They may not be shared by my black clients or by my white clients. This assessment is strictly my own intrapersonal, racially based one. It is my responsibility to be aware of these assumptions and to evaluate my therapeutic relationships in part as a consequence of these intuitive and experientially based expectations.

Each therapist has a racial/ethnic psychohistory that brings with it a set of assumptions about how individuals relate to each other. If these assumptions are not explored by the therapist, they may shape the therapeutic experience in ways of which the therapist is unaware. The final result is always a loss of communication and of the opportunity to optimize levels of understanding. In our traditional modes of training, we systematically have trainees or supervisees explore how personal life events have shaped their relationships with others. We have been negligent in incorporating ethnic, racial, and cultural variables in our training of therapists. This process is equally important and merits special attention.

Before we leave this section, we want to note that we think a psychohistory is useful and important for anyone, particularly those who are going to become therapists. We realize that in giving only one example, that of a black person, we may be subject to the criticism that we, too, think that it is only blacks who need to look at their racial psychohistories. That is not the case. This psychohistory serves as a model for whites, Asians, Latins, other blacks, or anyone else, no matter what their CDG or NCDG status is.

The Client's Racial Psychohistory

The client also has a racial psychohistory, and information about it is needed in order for the client and the therapist to better understand convergent, divergent, and conflicting experiences in therapy. The therapist must become aware of this history and of those aspects of the therapist that are most important to the client in building a relationship. Is it the therapist's race, gender, sexual preference, ethnicity, and/or social class?

It is important to begin to obtain the client's racial contact history in the normal course of history taking and data gathering. This information should be ascertained whether the client is of the same or a different race than the therapist. Despite some underlying themes, each person holds a unique interpretation of the meaning of his or her race and of how it is integrated in his or her self-system. Therefore, to the extent that it is possible, the client and the therapist must comprehend the client's meaning of race as he or she proceeds to develop and sustain a therapeutic relationship.

Once each racial psychohistory has been at least somewhat established, the therapist needs to be aware of a number of characteristic issues that may emerge as a consequence of the racial legacies of the therapist and client. In the following section we will begin to examine the racial ecology of the therapeutic dyad. In particular, we will examine the characteristic issues that may arise and confront cross-race and same-race dyads as a consequence of the therapist's and the client's legacy as a master or a slave.

Characteristic Issues of Cross-Race and Same-Race Dyads

The types of expectations that can emerge from black and white racial pairings can be most broadly classified as (1) expectations that affirm one's psychosocial identity and context, or (2) expectations that challenge one's psychosocial identity and context. Expectations of affirmation refer to those beliefs that lead the client or the therapist to anticipate that he or she will experience validation of his or her humanness, self-worth, competence, and perception of reality. These expectations entail the affirmation of personal attributes as well as one's experience and one's understanding of the world. Expectations of challenge are those beliefs that lead the client or therapist to anticipate that he or she will experience obstacles to self-validation. These challenges range from fear of having one's perceptions unsupported to being viewed as less than human. Those expectations that lead the therapist or client to anticipate divergence or conflict stem from expectations of challenge. For example, the black client's expectation of being understood by a black therapist is an expectation of affirmation since it anticipates convergence; the black client's expectation of being misunderstood by a white therapist is an expectation of challenge since it anticipates divergence and possibly conflict.

There are at least five important ecological and individual areas in which expectations of challenge and/or affirmation are likely to be experienced in cross-racial dyads. They are as follows:

1. *Expectations pertaining to racial identity.* These expectations emanate from one's identification and affiliation with a particular racial group. Moreover, these expectations develop within a sociopolitical context of which the master–slave legacy plays an important part.
2. *Expectations pertaining to culture.* These expectations refer to those beliefs and assumptions that stem from the host of symbols, ways of communicating, styles of interaction, values, philosophies of life, interpretations of reality, self–world expectations, and belief systems that have been identified with racial groups, independent of their ethnicity.
3. *Expectations pertaining to coping skills.* These expectations pertain to the set of assumptions that clients and therapists have regarding each other's range of skills and degree of mastery over and harmony with the physical and human ecology. They include assumptions regarding knowledge of systems and of prescriptions for success.
4. *Expectations pertaining to self–world relationships.* These expectations pertain to those values, attitudes, and philosophies of life that contribute to how individuals perceive their relationships with others and their relationship to their ecology. They include assumptions regarding the nature of human relationships and conceptions of how they as individuals or as members of a particular group will be treated by others.
5. *Expectations pertaining to range of personal power and control.* These expectations focus on the perceptions of power and personal control. They include the prosocial and negative aspects of individuals' own perceptions of individual power and personal control and of their perceptions of power as ascribed to them by virtue of group membership or other special status.

RACIALLY RELATED EXPECTATIONS OF PROTOTYPICAL THERAPY DYADS

The form and nature of these categories of expectations are significantly influenced by the racial psychohistory and personal attributes of the therapist and the client. In the following sections, we will discuss the characteristic issues that arise from these expectations for four dyads, the black–black, white–white, white–black, and black–white therapeutic dyads.

Black Therapist–Black Client Dyad

Expectations Pertaining to Racial Identity

Both the therapist and the client begin the relationship expecting some validation of their experiences as black people. Indeed, in the EVM, we propose that same-race pairings can indeed provide that advantage. However, problems arise when these relationships contradict the client's or the therapist's understanding of their common racial reality. They pose areas of divergence that can result in conflict if they are not addressed effectively.

By virtue of the black therapist's position as "expert" and his or her shared racial history, the black client may assume that the black therapist may have a better grasp on race-related issues. Thus, the client may tend to look to the therapist for assistance and feedback in interpreting reality and in validating his or her experiences. For example, black clients may report a comment made by their boss or their child's teacher. What they ask of the therapist is assistance in framing the comment within its particular context and given who they are as individuals. The therapist is seen as the ratifier of their emotional experience and as an interpreter of racial reality. This expectation on the part of the client may be confirmed or it can be problematic and set the stage for conflict in therapy. The outcome will depend on whether the black therapist has sorted out his or her issues pertaining to race and formulated his or her racial psychohistory and its meaning in the same framework and fashion as the client.

The therapist can also have expectations regarding his or her clients as ratifiers of reality. Therapists learn from their clients, and in the course of doing therapy they create models of human behavior and development. Black therapists working with black clients may look to their clients to validate their models of black self-development and coping. Clients who do not subscribe to those models do not conform to the therapist's sense of the reality of human behavior. In such cases the client may be seen as being more dysfunctional than is the case.

A corollary to these expectations is the assumption that the therapist and client share a similar sociopolitical perspective about race relations and about same-race and cross-race interactions. For example, the therapist may possess a world view that values forms of segregation as a means to insulate blacks from the effects of racism. However, the client may possess a world view that values integration and that encourages black–white friendships.

A crucial variable in determining how "racial" and "sociopolitical" reality are perceived, interpreted, and communicated is the degree of racial consciousness of the therapist and client. Helms (1989) has used models of black and white identity development as frameworks for outlining a number of issues that may confront same-race and cross-race pairs and determine whether they will affirm or challenge each other's perspectives. She uses Cross's (1980) model of racial identity development to describe the formation of racial consciousness in blacks. The point Helms makes, and that we are making, is that the levels of racial identity development of the client and of the therapist are related to how they analyze, process, and experience psychotherapy.

According to Cross (1972), for black people, there are four stages of racial identity development, ranging from blacks' idealization of whites and the denial and denigration of blacks to their acknowledgment and tolerance of the values and perspectives of whites. What we emphasize through the EVM is a framework for moving beyond the obstacles presented within various racial identity pairs. We believe that therapists and clients can continue to develop a racial-psychosocial identity, one which is not defeated by diversity or initial conflict.

Expectations Pertaining to Culture

With a black therapist–black client pair, there may be an expectation on the part of each that the other person shares the same codes, symbols, and special ways of communicating that have been cultivated and used by blacks. Furthermore, there may be the expectation that the relationship will be mutually supportive and nurturing and that each will be accepted as a human being and a worthy individual. For example, black clients may communicate that race is important and indicate that they want a black therapist. Reasons for their preference may range from the hope of possible affirmation of their experiences as a black person to the belief that the therapist will serve as a black representative of the white world. Phrases that have been used include "A black person will know what I'm talking about"; "I don't want to have to translate"; and "I just feel more comfortable with someone black." In other words, the client perceives the therapist as culturally similar and as an ideological peer.

The difficulty posed by this expectation of similarity is that many black therapists and clients differ culturally, and they can make different choices within similar cultural contexts. To assume that the therapist or client will know each other's slang, foods, jokes, and sayings can seed the relationship for conflict. Moreover, to make cultural assumptions by virtue of skin color communicates to the client (or therapist) a judgment made about how that person has defined himself or herself as black. Also, within the American black community there are many ethnicities. Untested assumptions about the meanings of race and the importance of a "black culture" for any particular group are ill-advised and may become prejudices that are detrimental to therapy.

It is important to note, however, that many black therapists and clients do share a way of relating, have a common understanding about many aspects of life such as traditional foods eaten by blacks, and share a common vocabulary and set of proverbs. When these therapists and clients come together, their commonalities provide a source of affirmation of culture that can provide advantages for that same-race pairing.

Expectations Pertaining to Coping Skills

There is the expectation among some black people that those individuals who have had exposure to whites will have a better understanding of how to cope in the world. The client may assume that through educational attainment, the black therapist has successfully met the challenges and hurdles placed before him or her by the white community. Consequently, the black therapist may be seen as a model of a black individual who has made it in white America. The black therapist may also be assumed to have some understanding of the white world and of white values. The therapist is seen as a bridge between Afro and Euro cultures. However, these assumptions may not be valid. The therapist may be just as ineffective in dealing with his or her NCDG status as the client is. On the other hand, the black therapist may be a model or symbol of a black person who has achieved the white American dream. The outcome of these therapist–client interactions will be conflict and disillusionment unless they provide an effective basis for working together and do meet the client's needs.

Expectations Pertaining to Self–World Relationships

Their legacy from slavery and their African heritage provides the black therapist and client with a particular philosophy about life and a world view. For example, both may value the role of the group over that of the individual. However, they may have quite different views about sociopolitical perspectives that they feel support this notion and about how each should relate to his or her environment as a black person.

In order to build an effective relationship, both the therapist and the client must be open to the various ways in which each, as well as blacks and whites more generally, organizes his or her experiences and relates to his or her ecology. Therapists aware of their bias in perspectives are better able to help clients sort through how they wish to relate to others and to sort through the strengths and limitations of each of those options.

Expectations Regarding Range of Personal Power and Control

Some blacks enter therapy with the expectation of learning some specific skills and of being empowered. They also enter with some notions about how black people have used power, whether power has been used for prosocial reasons and for the collective, or whether it has been used for self-advancement and the oppression of others. Other black clients have formulated some specific thoughts about how black experts or blacks who have been empowered treat and feel about other blacks.

Some feel that empowered blacks will help other blacks. These black clients expect a prosocial use of power in their relationship with the therapist. For example, they see therapy as a point of information exchange, and a legitimate forum out of which can stem advocacy and community work.

On the other hand, some blacks feel that blacks who have attained personal power and socioeconomic gains are either unwilling to share their power and/or will oppress other blacks to maintain their position and control. In particular, some blacks feel that in the course of becoming credentialed, blacks tend to abandon their sense of brotherhood and sisterhood with other blacks, becoming individualistic in orientation. These blacks expect black therapists to either misuse or not use their power to assist them.

Conflict arises when the therapist and client possess different conceptions of what characterizes the prosocial use of power and these conceptions are not addressed or explored. A productive therapeutic relationship can be developed only if they can find a basis for convergence that is responsive to their expectations about power and control, and that provides a way for the client to resolve his or her difficulties in a constructive prosocial fashion.

White Therapist–White Client Dyad

Expectations Related to Racial Identity

The degree to which the white therapist and the white client achieve an understanding of their personal power, humanness, and competence is directly related to their implicit and explicit understanding of the meaning attributed to their race by themselves and by others in society. However, because of their position in American society, most whites do not examine their racial selves, nor do they see race as establishing parameters around their values and world views. Instead, we see their expectations related to racial identity and race consciousness manifested primarily when they express their philosophies, attitudes, and perspectives about various topics pertaining to race relations, such as interracial dating and marriage, affirmative action, black versus white intelligence, and concepts of beauty.

Nevertheless, the greater an individual's understanding of the meanings that he or she and broader society have about whiteness, the greater the experience of self-understanding and understanding of self in a pluralistic society. Implicitly, this understanding requires that individuals process (consciously or unconsciously) the meaning of their race. The era of slavery cemented the racial identity of whites by juxtaposing their humanness, superiority, and status against that of blacks and by creating the perception that reality and normalcy originate within the world view of the master. This view has led to some whites never processing their racial identity and disregarding differences because their identity is viewed as the norm for everyone. In addition, whites who are more knowledgeable about these aspects of their racial selves may lose power with other whites in regard to traditional concepts of the meaning of whiteness.

Until whites do confront their enculturated and socialized master–slave-based values about blacks and their relationships with them, their capacity to deal with their own identity and with diversity will be seriously impaired. The issue of racial identity playing a crucial role in psychotherapy among white therapy dyads has received limited attention in the literature. Helms (1990) has attended to the racially based dynamics of this dyad and has contributed a useful perspective for understanding how arrested racial identity development on the part of the therapist or the client results in particular dilemmas for the dyad. The psychosocial approach that we have been describing contributes a basis for understanding the contributions of our cultural and personal histories to our racial identities and views about individuals from other races. It also incorporates attention to our individual efforts at charting our destinies, the development of our racial identities, and consequently our approaches to the psychotherapy process.

Expectations Pertaining to Culture

Given their historical legacies as masters, the white client and the white therapist may expect to experience affirmation about their culture. These aspects of affirmation may come from their expectations that they each hold similar understandings of what it means to be a white American. Such relationships mirror the norms, standards, and enculturated values of American whites. However, either the client or therapist may feel alienated from their white reference group as a result of individual experiences, experiences with other races, or due to their ethnicity or religious beliefs. Such divergences experienced between the client and therapist can result in conflict. If these conflicting values are confronted, they can promote growth and understanding around different conceptions of what it means to be a white American, or an American of any hue or ethnicity, or perhaps just a human being. This therapeutic experience is going to be most productive to the extent that it does provide the opportunity to examine critically the values of the culture, particularly as they impact on the quality of the client's life.

Expectations Related to Coping Skills

The white dyadic relationship also serves as a forum for the development of coping skills from the point of view of American culture. This dyad can explore coping mechanisms and problems in living from a racially congruous base. The expectation on the part of the client that he or she will attain a prescription for successfully mastering the "American dream" or for making peace with self within the system may or may not be attainable. Nevertheless, both the client and the therapist are in a position to examine the functional and dysfunctional coping styles of their group and to develop more efficacious ways of living their lives.

Expectations Pertaining to Self–World Relationships

The legacy of master has influenced the white therapist's and client's perspectives of themselves as agents in their lives and in their environment which they have seen as supportive of their status but as threatening in many ways. They face in each other substantial constraints against forming the trust in relationships that is vital to effective psychotherapy and possibly to forming more meaningful human relationships. As with the black therapist and client dyad, the white therapist and client may have difficulty in acknowledging that there are diverse ways in which members of their group can define themselves and the nature of their relationship to the world. For example, both therapist and client may value individuality, yet have very different ways of relating to others. For the client, feelings of relatedness may grow out of association with others who are also anticonformist in their values and attitudes. For the therapist, relatedness may be associated with acceptance in the context of the status quo. Nevertheless, the legacies of individuality and of the master–slave tradition raise questions for both of them about the wisdom of trusting others, since any relatedness is something of a threat to their autonomy and mastery.

Expectations Pertaining to Personal Power and Control

Historically, when two masters met, there were a host of possibilities about the disposition of power. Power could be used positively or negatively. Power could be self-controlling or other controlling, or both. These possibilities were the products of their motives for relating and the position of the masters on the hierarchy. For example, when two masters of equal power and status would meet, one could have decided to become more powerful by thwarting the other (other-control and negative) or both could have decided to maintain or enhance their status through mutual support (self-determination and positive). Similarly, when two masters of unequal status and power would meet, the more powerful master could have chosen to either thwart or to assist the less powerful master in his efforts to satisfy his needs. The possibilities for the disposition of power for the white therapy dyad are analogous to those of the master–master relationship.

The issue of power for the white–white therapy dyad has been discussed in regard to social class and gender. For example, concern has been expressed about the ability of therapists to recognize and ignite the personal powers of their clients who are members of a less powerful group (e.g., women and the poor). There have also been discussions about some therapists' insensitivity to the realities of the client's socioeconomic status (Bergin & Lambert, 1978; Parloff *et al.*, 1978). Therapists reared in predominantly middle- and upper-middle-class homes are often evaluated as judgmental and unrealistic in their appraisals of the personal power of clients, particularly lower-status clients. In turn, this insensitivity is believed to be relayed to the client in therapy through the therapist's body language, verbal language, and interpretations.

One interpretation of this perceived insensitivity is that middle-class therapists are unable to reconcile why their white low-income clients are not functioning as masters. They consequently attribute their clients' lower status and psychological dysfunction to something intrinsic to the clients. White clients who are sensitive to messages about their failure as members of white society must then respond to this negative evaluation, of which they can accept in several ways. They can agree that they are not functioning up to their own expectations or to the norms of their group and may then choose to use the therapy relationship to become more powerful. Or, at another extreme, clients can agree with the negative evaluation and resign themselves to failure as intrinsic to themselves.

For the client to reject these negative evaluations, the client must have a sense of his or her personal power and be able to understand that there are various social realities that individuals face. Furthermore, these realities need not determine worth or degree of humanness, but they do require a different set of coping skills. To reject the messages of the therapist, the client must be able to reject the enculturated values and attitudes that are used to designate human worth, such as material possession and money.

Of course, not all white therapists are from middle- or upper-income backgrounds, nor do all white therapists from these backgrounds express class-related values (Mitchell & Atkinson, 1983; Parloff *et al.*, 1978). Nevertheless, the role of social class status is that it defines to a considerable extent whether an individual has a viable voice within society. The issue for us is whether it also dictates the extent to which the therapist's and the client's voices are heard in psychotherapy. The client may also have social class-based expectations about accepting the therapist's behaviors and assertions of caring, given the therapist's economic status and educational attachment. These expectations about the therapist can also limit or exaggerate the client's perspective of the therapist's humanness and variety of life experiences. Finally, the most basic issue is the importance of the therapist becoming aware of his or her heritage in a way such that he or she can hear the client's voice and work with the client to help him or her also overcome the problems that stem from that heritage.

White Therapist–Black Client Dyad

Expectations Related to Racial Identity

A key variable in our discussion of expectations pertaining to racial identity is superiority. The values and attitudes that emanate from the superiority belief in American society support a cultural norm in which there is a lower opinion of blacks and a level of hostility and unacceptance of them as peers. Moreover, these values and attitudes provide challenges for whites and blacks who seek to respect diversity and enhance self-awareness.

White therapists who exhibit enculturated values of superiority over blacks are often unaware of it. These therapists manifest their feelings of superiority in therapy, in case conferences, and in supervision. They tend to make statements about their surprise at the complexity of the personality of a black welfare mother or at the range of social interests and skills possessed by a black colleague. They may attempt to create a false convergence by expressing a value or behavior that is not truly part of their repertoire in an attempt to connect on a personal level. For example, a therapist may use slang words or phrases because the therapist has assumed that the black client has a limited range of emotions and verbal skills around which to relate to the therapist.

A white therapist may also exhibit superiority through paternalistic attitudes and behaviors by, for example, assuming that the black client is unable to learn to negotiate systems and the therapist must do it for him or her. A counselor who negotiated with the school around a black child's behavior and never included the mother, explaining that the mother felt overwhelmed and was unable to communicate effectively with the school or with her son, was being a "good master" and was unaware of it. He assumed that this mother could not learn to negotiate with systems or to advocate for her family, even though for 12 years she had negotiated with work settings and with social service agencies to obtain support and services.

A third way in which superiority is manifested is in some of the expectations that therapists have of their clients. For example, the white therapist may expect compliance and acceptance on the part of the black client and interpret the client's challenge as a problem of the client rather than as an indication of the client's ability to think about his or her therapy and the client's investment in the therapeutic process. On the other hand, the therapist may experience fear. The challenge of the black client may bring forth enculturated attitudes that blacks are dangerous.

In contrast, white therapists may also be sensitive to the dangers of replaying the master–slave relationship in the therapy setting. By acknowledging the history of white–black relations in this culture and by understanding that they are not immune to their culture's impact, they are able to learn from their black clients about themselves and about others. Moreover, they are able to use their socialized feelings as only one of the bases from which they assist the client in constructing an understanding of their self–world relations.

Like white therapists, black clients vary as to their belief in the superiority of one race over another, and their perspectives also significantly contribute to the nature of the therapeutic relationship. The black client who feels that whites are superior to blacks may enter therapy expecting to be helped or "cured" because the therapist is white and, therefore, take a passive stance. In contrast, clients who feel that blacks are superior to whites may not readily share their hostility, anger, or dissatisfaction with having a white therapist. They may choose to withdraw or to participate in a perfunctory way, which inadvertently results in their abdication of responsibility for their lives and a replay of the imbalance of power to which they may be reacting.

This nonevaluative trust or distrust on the part of clients puts therapists in a position of power and yet impedes them in their task of assisting clients to transcend such limited notions of themselves. In these situations, exploring the racial psychohistory of clients and therapists plus discussing the race differences of the dyad, with its strengths and limitations, seem particularly essential. For these clients, examining their enculturated limitations so that they can begin to transcend them in the therapeutic context is vital to improving the quality of their lives.

Expectations Pertaining to Culture

Most therapists recognize that individuals from different places have different customs, traditions, and ways of relating; they may, however, have difficulty discerning cultural differences among individuals born in their own country. Thus, white therapists may find it difficult to discern in what ways African traditions have been preserved in American language, food, and dress. They do not distinguish cultural differences from socioeconomic differences and what are considered to be genetic differences inherent in the make-up of black people. Culture is seen as being the same for both blacks and whites, and differences are seen as stemming from economic differences and different historical statuses.

For these therapists, convergence of standards and values with respect to self–world relationships and psychosocial realities is expected. There is some truth to this assumption. Nevertheless, it is limiting in that it ignores the various cultural and ethnic legacies of blacks and whites.

As we have noted earlier, there are therapists who do recognize cultural differences in American racial groups. Among them are some white therapists and black clients who view those cultural differences as severing any possibility of forming relationships or of understanding the other person's world view. To them the idea of differences obstructs growth rather than providing a context for exploring each other's humanness and approaching differences from an EVM perspective. To others, differences can be transcended. It is this latter expectation that provides a basis for working together in a therapeutic context to share their respective perspectives in a way that provides therapeutic gains for the client.

Expectations Pertaining to Coping Skills

Within a master–slave context, a white therapist who has little awareness of his or her racial self and of cultural differences can be expected to have great difficulty viewing an unfamiliar coping strategy of a black client as adaptive or creative. Instead, such an unfamiliar coping strategy is more likely be viewed as pathological. Likewise, a black client who has little insight pertaining to his or her racial self and little appreciation of cultural differences may have great difficulty understanding why coping strategies developed from only the white therapist's perspective make any sense, and whether these strategies are working or not.

A major barrier to overcoming these insensitivities is maintaining distance between themselves and thus remaining unaware of their different life experiences. This distance between therapist and client, which is most harmful therapeutically in its ignoring of the client's humanness, is manifested in several ways. It can be observed in the desire of therapists who work with black clients for prescriptions for understanding black culture. These therapists tend to appreciate workshops that delineate how blacks differ from whites and that offer in a cookbook fashion how to diagnose and treat black clients fairly and effectively. These individuals do not want to feel the "mess" of racial tension or deal with their bigotry and/or lack of knowledge. Furthermore, in understanding how to treat blacks, these therapists are not willing to struggle with the nuances of the ranges of social competencies that are needed to live effectively as a black person in America. To do so would require that they tackle their racial psychohistory, their white identity, and their prejudices. For them, those tasks feel unnecessary or irrelevant.

Second, the issue of humanness also arises in the philosophies and assumptions that some white therapists have about what it means to be black in America and about how blacks should cope with and approach their social status. A common one, the thick-skinned assumption, is based on the premise that in the process of living in America black people should, as a part of their development, form a tough emotional exterior, one that has been numbed to the more covert acts of racism. No one would question that all human beings struggle with unkindness, discriminatory behavior, and insensitivity from others. However, the thick-skinned assumption permits the therapist to avoid experiencing the client's reality and the emotional wounds (or joys) that are by-products of that reality. The therapist is denying the client's range of emotion, feeling, and humanness. Another assumption, that of assimilation, is based on the premise that for blacks to be "okay," they need to adopt white cultural norms and coping styles. These two assumptions often lead to therapeutic relationships riddled with conflict or marked by premature termination.

There are, of course, therapists who are genuine in their desire to get to know how the black person sees himself or herself culturally and psychosocially. They acknowledge the client's humanness by acknowledging the client's ability to know and to communicate who he or she is to the therapist. These therapists need not be knowledgeable of black culture, but willing to expose their lack of knowledge about the shared values, philosophy, legacies, rituals, and relationship patterns of many blacks, and to use the information provided by their clients to achieve the agreed upon therapeutic outcome. In a somewhat similar fashion, black clients who are willing to take the risk of exposing their biases and limited knowledge about white culture can work with white therapists and gain therapeutically in doing so.

Expectations Pertaining to Self–World Relationships

For this dyad, the manner in which the therapist and client perceive their own and each other's relationships to the world and the people around them is crucial to the formation and maintenance of the relationship. Given their historical legacies and ethnic roots, each has an organizing framework that involves a set of expectations about trusting or being wary of others, particularly others who are on the other side of the black–white racial barrier. They also have expectations about the extent to which the friendliness or hostility of the environment is individually or collectively oriented. For example, from the client's perspective and world view, it may be quite reasonable to feel a sense of responsibility toward black classmates when responding to questions posed in class, in spite of the stress this perspective brings, because of the feeling that the trustworthiness of the environment is going to be the same for all blacks. However, it may seem very unreasonable from the perspective of the white therapist for anyone to view himself or herself as a representative and agent of others. Each of these perspectives about self–world relations is legitimate, and each has its costs as well as its benefits. The degree to which the therapist and the client can work together depends in part on the degree to which they can together explore each one's sense of what perspectives are most congruent with the client's world view and realities.

Expectations Pertaining to Personal Power and Control

The expectations pertaining to personal power and control are difficult to distinguish from those pertaining to superiority and humanness. The white therapist's and black client's perspectives on superiority and acceptance of the other person's humanness shape their visions. They will see the range of personal power and control that they have over their lives and that they expect to influence each other's lives in the context of those visions. Moreover, their expectations shape their ability to see and recognize the multiple systems that influence how each other experiences autonomy and control. They will be able to work together more effectively if they can break through those limiting barriers.

Black Therapist–White Client Dyad

Expectations Pertaining to Racial Identity

The members of this dyad face many of the same issues faced by the white therapist–black client dyad, but their roles are reversed. The person who held the historical role as master and the most powerful is the person in need of help and is the least powerful one. For both members to work effectively with one another, they must address this historical role reversal.

The issue of inferiority–superiority remains a vehicle through which racial identity awareness is manifested. If black therapists have not successfully come to terms with their reality, then they will continue to struggle with inferiority issues. These therapists may look to their white clients for affirmation of their acceptance as part of the white norm and as an accepted participant of the majority culture. For these therapists, issues of convergence may have additional significance in that they represent affirmation of their understanding of the ecology of whiteness. On the other hand, these therapists run the risk of having their fears of inferiority affirmed when they confront divergence or conflict in therapy. As a result of their need for validation from the client, they abdicate their role and responsibilities as expert and give it to the white client, who is there seeking assistance from the therapist. These therapists may also expect to be perceived as less competent than a white therapist, never fully trust the client's acceptance of their expertise, and become impotent at fully examining the dynamics presented in the therapeutic ecosystem.

Another expectation is that of the perpetual test, in which the therapist expects to have to prove himself or herself repeatedly to be competent. If this expectation goes unnoticed by the therapist, then the therapist may become angry with the client and act out that anger in the therapy relationship. Also, if the therapist feels that this is a typical consequence of black–white interactions and that this expectation is the norm, then the therapist limits the degree to which trust will be established in the dyad.

Expectations Pertaining to Culture

Both the therapist and client may enter this dyad with expectations that both affirm and challenge. The expectations of affirmation are of two types. Both the therapist and client may expect to have their knowledge about the other person's group affirmed through processes of convergence and divergence. That is, they expect to confirm both cultural similarities and differences in relation to each other. They may also expect conflicts due to their cultural differences to interfere with their ability to form a relationship and work effectively with each other.

Each of these expectations is to some extent a function of the degree to which the therapist and the client have worked through their racial identity issues and have grappled with enculturated values stemming from the master–slave legacy. A key issue in these expectations is the degree to which both the client and the therapist perceive their respective cultures as compatible. It is also important for the therapist to be aware of how he or she and the client react to outward signs of cultural identity (e.g., the therapist wearing braids, type of music played in the waiting area, style of interaction, and office decor). Culture is experienced on many levels, and it may be that the client can accept cultural differences if they are not part of the therapeutic ecosystem but find them difficult to accept when they are visible.

Expectations Pertaining to Self–World Relationships

The issues related to self–world relationships for this dyad are similar to those of the white therapist–black client dyad. In this pairing though, it is the black therapist who needs to be particularly sensitive to the differences in expectations about the trustworthiness of the world and of blacks as experienced by his or her white clients. The therapist, given his or her world view and perspective, can help clients to modify their perspectives about themselves in the world. In turn, the therapist can learn from the client a different pattern of expectations about interpersonal relations.

Expectations Pertaining to Coping Skills and Range of Personal Power and Control

Many blacks and whites in this country have struggled to develop relationships among themselves that are not bound by the shackles of the master–slave relationship paradigm. That struggle arises in a particular form in a black therapist–white client relationship. To develop such a relationship, both parties must move beyond their social and historical legacies to an area of convergence that defines their humanness, their power, and their patterns of coping in other terms. The therapist must move beyond his or her enculturated expectation that the white client's relationship to him or her is to exploit or oppress him or her in some fashion. The client must move beyond his enculturated value of superiority. Otherwise, the possibility of their working together in a therapeutic relationship is quite limited.

Summary

In this chapter, we have highlighted the importance of race, separate from ethnicity, in discussing psychotherapy relationships. The point is that racial membership provides a separate and unique piece of information about who we are, how we are seen by others, and our position in society. This information interacts with our ethnicity and personal life history to create our psychosocial perspective and way of viewing the world.

We have used the black–white dyadic combinations to highlight the intricacies of racial membership and psychotherapeutic process. There are other racial groups and unique issues that arise, but we have chosen the black–white dyad as an exemplar for several reasons. First, it is a dyad that epitomizes, in the master–slave relationship, the role of history in shaping the ecology and world view of individuals ascribed one status versus another.

Second, the black–white relationship exemplifies the nature of the struggle to achieve balance or equality in relationships for a number of groups. It highlights and parallels the various struggles about diversity in a number of dyads, including those involving gender as well as cross-ethnic and other cross-racial pairings.

Finally, black–white relations provide the broadest available empirical base from which to analyze the issues involved. Conceptually, this racial dyad has provided a framework to entertain how we think about differences. For example, it was in the context of black–white differences that the concern about using whites as a normative sample arose. Consequently, at this juncture, other racial groups have a precedent upon which to advocate for a multiracial and cultural framework. It has now been fairly well established that white America is not the standard for assessing the behavior of other groups. Nevertheless, it continues to be the norm whose nature defines psychotherapy and the participants in it, unless we provide more compelling alternatives.

In sum, race in addition to, but separate from, ethnicity plays a significant role in the formulation of our ecology and psychosocial competence. It defines our sense of ourselves as well as our status on the power hierarchy, brings with it a set of coping skills, and fosters a particular world view. These factors are part of the therapeutic process, and we will endeavor to address their impact and provide guidelines for using them constructively throughout the remainder of this book.

5

The Processes and Patterns of Psychotherapy

We have been stressing that the nature of the processes and patterns of psychotherapy is determined by who the participants are as well as by what their purposes are in participating in that activity. We readily assume that both the therapist and the client bring their knowledge and experience about living to the therapeutic relationship. We also accept that both (and everyone else) live in multiple realities that they translate into more and less effective ways of negotiating the events in their lives. What we also need to know is the nature of the special characteristics of therapeutic patterns and processes and how they relate to our more general patterns of human interaction. Those topics are the focus of the present chapter.

Characteristics of the Participants

Who is the therapist? That question has most often been answered from the perspective of a theory or school of therapy. The therapist is a person who conducts himself or herself in a particular way consistent with a theoretical conception or with the agreed upon manner of the practitioners of a specific approach to therapy. That answer is at times deemed by its proponents to be the only "true" definition. Further, the validity of the answer is justified on the grounds of the theory or the shared consensus of the school members that "it works." That question can also be answered in a singular and personal way by any given therapist, although society and the therapeutic community impose constraints on individual deviations from generally agreed upon practices. An important aspect of these definitions is that they do not rest or depend on (except in the most indirect way) input from clients or the public at large. Yet from a broader perspective, a *therapist* is a person who fulfills a role defined by society as well as by the person in that society. When therapists assert that only they can define their role, they assume a special prerogative to define their own reality and that of the world, including that of their clients. They also assume that they are immune to the influences on human conduct that they believe affect other people, including their clients.

We find the belief that therapists are independent of their culture or immune to the forces that affect people indefensible. Rather, we have been arguing that therapists are as human as anyone and that the therapeutic process is continuous with ordinary human discourse, not totally different from it. We begin our consideration of the processes and patterns of psychotherapy with the statement that therapists need to ask themselves some very basic questions about their self-defined identities and roles to clarify the relationships of those roles to the rest of their lives. These questions include: Who am I as a therapist? Why do I want to be a therapist? How did I become a therapist? What am I trying to do as a therapist? What and whom do I represent as a therapist? How do my individual experiences and beliefs, heritage and identities influence me as a therapist?

Therapists do have unique perspectives and skills. They bring to the therapeutic context and relationship a repository of knowledge and experience that comes from their lives as individuals, their general education, and their training and experience as therapists. To the extent that therapists can come to acknowledge the interrelationships among those aspects of their lives, they can be integrated in the therapeutic approach so that they complement one another.

Clients also contribute to defining who therapists are. They may see their therapists as magical or uncontaminated figures, or they may see them as very human figures. We do not intend or desire to argue at length about the intellectual or empirical merits of any of these definitions. Rather, our goal is to place consideration of these questions about who therapists and clients are into an ecological and competence-oriented framework. We want to demythologize psychotherapy and conceive of it as a human enterprise from which all parties can benefit. We want to advance an approach that views psychotherapy as an interchange from which both client and therapist benefit, if it is indeed *therapeutic*. We can accomplish that objective only by placing both the therapist and the client in their respective ecological, ethnic, and personal positions in relation to themselves and each other.

Students who are undertaking their first psychotherapy cases often have tremendous difficulty seeing their life skills as relevant to the task they are undertaking. They seem to see therapy as discontinuous with any forms of human discourse of which they have been a part. Rather, their fantasy is that they are going to enter a strange new world, that therapy occurs in a different kind of ecosystem that has only tenuous and poorly understood ties to ordinary activities. Thus, their task of greeting a client in a waiting room assumes all of the mystery and unpredictability of descent from an airplane into a totally strange and unknown culture whose language and customs are unfamiliar but for whose welfare the individual is responsible. The neophyte therapist often acts as though the simple act of getting acquainted is inappropriate and an open invitation to the intrusion into the entire therapeutic enterprise of destructive transference and countertransference relationships. Yet the most important step for the therapist and client to take is that of getting acquainted with each other, and the therapist is in a more advantageous position to initiate and shape that process. The process of becoming acquainted is always limited and exploratory, but it does begin to establish the unique as well as the general aspects of their relationship.

When two people meet and begin to interact, each of them comes as a representative of a particular background and is also an individual with apparent characteristics such as age, gender, race, nationality, status (as expressed by appearance, dress, and manner), and specific role such as healer or friend (which may be more or less explicitly defined). In short, each of us is a manifestation of a psychosocial ecosystem as well as an individual, and that membership in a particular ecosystem becomes part of getting acquainted and interacting whenever its nature becomes evident to the persons involved. One aspect of that membership that is particularly important is each person's race/ethnicity. If the therapist is from a CDG and the client is not, then the therapist and the client bring that ethnic/racial relationship into the situation. The client may be less trusting of the benign potential of a therapeutic relationship. And, as some clients have noted, they may well wonder whether they will have to (and should have to) educate the therapist about their NCDG reality. The CDG therapist may wonder whether the client is capable of profiting from therapy or willing to work with a CDG therapist.

The implications of these characteristics and experiences for the effectiveness with which therapists can function can perhaps be highlighted by thinking of one's real or potential role as a supervisor/teacher of neophyte therapists. For example, as a supervisor/teacher one may not wish to know the issues in the sex lives of trainees, yet it is important to know whether and in what ways trainees have sorted out for themselves sexual competence and conflict issues that clients present in the course of therapy. Similarly, as a supervisor one may not wish to get involved with the religious and moral beliefs of a trainee. Nevertheless, it is important to work out with trainees whether they can deal with the possibility that clients may build their lives on different views of religion and morality and/or question and abandon views that are fundamental to the trainee. Similarly, it is important for therapists to work out for themselves how to deal with sexual, moral, ethnic/racial, and other such differences.

Another issue that must be considered is that of how much a therapist and client will or should know of each other's lives outside of therapy. For example, in urban settings in the United States, white middle-class-oriented therapists may live in relative anonymity and have little contact with or exposure to their clients outside of the therapy setting. In a minority ethnic/racial community, the preservation of anonymity is much less likely to be possible, and particularly so if the therapist's clients include other professionals, community leaders, or their families. For example, a therapist may be a partner in a mixed ethnic/race relationship or marriage. If the therapist is a member of the predominant white group, that aspect of the therapist's marriage is not likely to be known to clients unless the therapist shares that knowledge. On the other hand, if the therapist is a member of an ethnic/racial minority, that information is quite likely to be known in the minority community. The client's knowledge, or lack of it, about the therapist's relationships will influence how the client will interact with the therapist, and particularly so with regard to marriage or relationship issues. Further, whether the client knows it or not, the therapist's relationship will impact on how he or she interacts with clients, and particularly so as issues of relationships enter into consideration.

More generally then, within various cultural or ethnic/racial groups, the client–therapist sphere of interaction may be small, but in others it is extensive. This difference is partly due to the size of the community and the more limited social, religious, and cultural outlets available for members of minority ethnic groups. Further, in some instances it runs counter to the community's definition of the helper–helpee role relationship for the therapist not to be part of the community. Therapists and clients of ethnic or racial minority groups in many communities must utilize the same ethnic ecosystem and ecological sphere in order to meet their personal life needs. Their social networks, family activities, political interests, and neighborhoods often overlap with those of the client.

This overlapping of systems may create a particular source of tension for the neophyte therapist (or any traditionally trained therapist) because it does not conform to the traditional notion of the therapeutic relationship. After all, traditional notions of relationships are more often defined by the majority community and tend to be consistent with their role patterns. Moreover, it is often seen as complicating the presumed therapeutic transference and countertransference processes since the client and the therapist see each other performing "real life" activities. Yet, helpers or healers in ethnic minority communities may be seen as models within the community and more importantly must be seen as having personal knowledge about and an investment in the community and its members in order to acquire credible community status.

Perhaps we need to pause at this point to note that the concepts of "transference" and "countertransference" are based on the traditional detached impersonal therapist–client relationship. The therapist and client are presumed not to know each other outside of therapy, and it is presumed that any personal qualities that they assign to each other, or personal reactions they have to each other, are inappropriate and countertherapeutic. It is our view that such a perspective is culturally based and does not bear serious scrutiny. The point we are trying to illustrate is that therapists enter their therapeutic sessions with the following elements as part of who they are: (1) personal values, (2) cultural values, (3) ethnic/racial characteristics, and (4) ethnic/racial as well as other beliefs and prejudices. It is unwise to enter a therapeutic situation as a therapist without being aware of the potential inappropriate, as well as appropriate, intrusion of those personal characteristics. In therapy situations, therapists do embody power, status, and a certain aura of mystery. They are ordinarily not expected to, or suspected of, interjecting personal considerations into their behavior and judgments. However, it is misleading to assume that there is some magic by which individuals can become disembodied, disenculturated, "neutered" therapists.

Therapists can become sensitive to who they are, what skills and capabilities they have as individuals, and what realities, including their ethnic ecosystems, are part of them and/or may be called on in the therapy context. That awareness can be useful as a basis for interacting with, understanding, and helping clients who are admittedly different from therapists in some ways, but similar to them in others. Clients are in search of some contact, some understanding, and some assistance in reorganizing their inner and outer realities and in dealing with those realities more effectively. As therapists can come to see their individual and ethnic/racial characteristics as attributes in therapy (as in life in general), they are in a position to build on them and employ them more effectively in conjunction with their formal therapeutic perspectives and skills in the special character of the therapy context. Nevertheless, the latter (awareness of therapeutic perspectives and skills) is no substitute for the former (awareness of personal perspectives and skills). It is only as therapists acknowledge their shared humanity with their clients that they are in a position to acknowledge their need for and gains from learning from their clients.

The central question being raised here is what are the consequences of whether therapists accord full human status to clients. In a therapeutic interaction, the particulars of what a therapist and a client offer and gain from each other is in part defined by the nature of the relationship as therapeutic. Even so, it also embodies (or should) some interchange between two people who accord each other the status and dignity of being equally human persons living out their lives. That question is a crucial one for the client, whose sense of worth as a human is particularly shaky at the point of entering therapy. It is also a crucial question for and about the therapist. The choice by therapists to avoid the human aspect of the interaction and to adopt exclusively the role of disembodied therapist limits their ability to help clients or to grow as therapists from their own personal experiences as therapists and in their own lives. The choice to acknowledge the human aspect of the therapist–client interaction permits therapist and client to refer openly to each other's fuller life existence and potentially enrich their lives and their interchange. It also requires them to work out the relationships between these aspects of their interactions. In our view, that task is more than worth the effort, and it will be the focus of the remainder of this book.

Who Is the Therapist?

In brief, it is not just theory, rather it is the interaction between client and therapist that shapes and determines who and what the therapist is in any given instance. As in any interaction between humans, the functioning definition of that interaction consists of those characteristics mutually agreed to, whether that agreement is explicit or implicit. This definition may be reached by discussing the therapist's role as seen by both client and therapist. Both the therapist's and the client's personal, cultural, and ethnic/racial backgrounds enter into that definition. The therapist or the client, and frequently both, may retain a private definition of the therapist's role. To the extent that those private definitions do not correspond, the discrepancies provide a continuing source of divergence and conflict in their interactions. The therapist or the client, and frequently both, act to change that definition. To the extent that they do so in an open and reciprocal way, their interactions can be facilitated and become increasingly productive. If their clarified differences lead to more conflict, their interactions can become increasingly unproductive or disruptive.

The definition of the therapist as well as of the therapist's role will change from client to client. A therapist is, or should be, involved in a continuing process of keeping these definitions sorted out in treatment planning and in reviewing therapeutic processes. Therapists are also well-advised to continue to review their definitions of themselves as therapists. It seems likely that, if therapists are actively attending to their work, they will change their definitions as they accumulate more experience.

Nevertheless, therapists must start from the premise that their self-perceived definitions of themselves as therapists are the product of their respective individual experiences, ethnic ecosystems, and formal training. The primary struggle for the therapist is that of integrating a set (or sets) of traditions and values provided by formal training with his or her life experiences or values. As is inevitably the case, they involve conflicts as well as convergences. How to maintain one's own cultural continuity and personal and professional identity, and yet accommodate to new values around forming *therapeutic* relationships, is an ongoing task. In answering the question, Who is the therapist? the therapist must integrate personal characteristics, ethnic/racial legacies, community perceptions, and the client's perception of helpers. That task does not seem to us to be an impossible one. It does seem to us to be one that is likely to be more fully accomplished if it is viewed (1) as an ongoing process rather than as a question to be answered once and for all, (2) as involving the range of elements we have noted repeatedly, and (3) as a reciprocal process involving both the therapist and the client.

Who Is the Client?

Clients also enter the therapy situation as individuals with embodied ways of life and identities. They have resources and capabilities as well as limitations, senses of individuality and dignity as persons and as members of ethnic/racial ecosystems within a broader pluralistic culture. They also have conceptions of who and what therapists and clients are and what it means to be a client. (In a sense we can say that client and therapist come with similar sets of human backgrounds, e.g., a personal history, an interpersonal history, a racial/ethnic history.) Even though they may not have been in therapy before, clients have conceptions of the various ethnic ecosystems and world views that they expect therapists to manifest. They have had occasion to seek assistance from or protect themselves from the socially sanctioned actions of at least some of society's designated helpers and protectors of what is considered to be the public interest. When they begin to interact with a therapist they utilize cues from the setting, demeanor, and conduct of the therapist as guides about how to define and conduct themselves. Consequently, they may orient themselves to presenting the image or the material that they believe the therapist expects. Clients as well as therapists embody multiple realities and can potentially appeal to them or obscure them in ways that may benefit themselves and/or their therapists.

For example, a therapist of about 60 was seeing a young woman of college age at a university counseling center. Both were white, but he was Anglo and she, whom we will call Elli, was of Middle Eastern descent. Elli's many difficulties included her inability to reconcile her Americanized views with the expectations of her family, although their commitment to their Middle Eastern conception of family and marital roles had encased them in a viciously destructive family life pattern. As the therapy progressed it became more evident that she valued the therapist's age because she wanted desperately to know that older people could work out meaningful lives. Yet Elli also feared to discuss with the therapist her own sex life and her hostility toward her parents. She feared that an older person would inevitably condemn her for her behavior and her feelings.

The effectiveness of that therapeutic interaction rested to a considerable extent on the therapist's willingness to begin working with her within the framework of her definition of her role as a client and his role as a therapist. Elli saw herself as someone (a client) who needed help from someone else (a therapist) who had a set of characteristics that precluded him from helping her. The therapist, through his willingness to acknowledge his age and accept her youthful expectations that he was beyond understanding the passions and transgressions of youth, accepted her perspective as valid for her and as a basis for beginning therapy. His definition of her as client was as a person with conflicting expectations and no way to resolve them. He also defined her client role as that of his teacher, and particularly so with regard to the specific contradictions her ethnic heritage presented as she tried to build a life in the mainstream culture of the United States. Further, he was quite comfortable with the idea that his current effectiveness at coping with life's exigencies after a substantial number of years of working at it might provide her with a model. Finally, it did make sense to him that he might not understand youthful passions as she embodied them and needed to keep an open mind about that possibility. In short, both he and she were able to begin and develop their therapeutic relationship with shared (though obviously not completely verbalized and discussed) definitions and expectations of their roles and their enterprise. They both saw themselves and each other as having strengths and limitations and as embarking on a collaborative process to explore some problems that seemed intractable but that needed solving.

NATURE OF THERAPY

An Interpersonal Interaction Tool

Stripped to its essentials, psychotherapy is an interpersonal interaction tool for promoting individual and collective effectiveness or psychosocial competence. At a minimum it involves one person (a therapist) helping another (a client) grasp and manage his or her life and life circumstances in more satisfactory ways than that person was able to do at the time of seeking therapy. It can involve helping a client make a more realistic assessment of his or her capabilities and limits (from the point of view of external social reality as the therapist understands it and represents it), and that reassessment may focus on unappreciated strengths as well as limitations. It can involve helping someone to resolve life survival problems such as finding something to eat or a place to stay or needed medical care. It can involve helping someone to work out a less self-destructive interpretation of events, of relationships, and of his or her sense of self-efficacy and self-worth. It can involve helping someone to acquire intra- and interpersonal perspectives and skills at interpreting and managing desires, feelings, relationships, and interactions. Whatever combination of such possibilities psychotherapy involves, in the aggregate it does at least involve helping others to become more psychosocially capable or competent at managing their lives and the events in them by aiding them to acquire more effective skills for those tasks.

The uniqueness of psychotherapy, however, lies in its focus on our sense of being a person in the world, what that sense means for negotiating our lives, and what it means to us about ourselves. The central issue for us as clients is that there is something wrong with ourselves as persons and with our internal and external realities that we do not understand, cannot resolve, and cannot continue to live with.

Therapy is help oriented and distress relief oriented, and it seeks to produce change through interpersonal interaction, primarily of a verbal nature. Further, it is focused on helping individuals redefine a particular set of aspects of their internal and external realities and the relationships between them. Those aspects of therapy are essential and beneficial, but they are not what is unique to therapy.

What is unique to therapy is the focused attention on those intrapersonal, interpersonal, and nonpersonal relationships that we define as relevant to that sense of who we are as persons. Humans have a highly developed capability for formulating an abstract conception of themselves and their relation to their internal and external realities. We have a variety of ways to express our sense of this aspect of ourselves. We speak of making (or not making) sense to ourselves. We ask, "Am I losing my mind, my sanity?" We say that we can't get a grip on our lives. We note that we can't direct our lives in the ways that we want them to go. We can't go to sleep and we can't wake up. We can't quit worrying about something, or we can't think about it; in either case, we can't deal with it. We can't carry out the steps to accomplish a goal that is important to us, whether it be preparing for our marriage, for going on a date, for an examination, or for a holiday.

Another facet of the uniqueness of therapy is that the concepts and mechanisms at the heart of psychotherapy have their origins primarily in the behavioral and social sciences. (We realize that there are chemically based approaches to resolving these same problems. They are also called therapeutic, but they are not our concern in this discussion. Our focus is on the *psycho*therapies.) The psychotherapy fields rely primarily for their explanations and approaches on empirically based conceptions of the origins and nature of human conduct. They also appeal to those same sources as a basis for conceptualizing the nature of human understanding, the nature of self, and the nature of change, at least, change in people.

Finally, another unique aspect of conventional approaches to psychotherapy is the way in which we use that empirical knowledge. In other fields, as professionals we expect to be expert in our subject matter field and to display that expertise in our professional capacities and in our lives. We also expect that our clients or students are entitled to know our position on matters of judgment so that they can take that information into account as they learn from us.

We are usually taught to take a quite different perspective as therapists. We are taught to take the position that it is detrimental to the client for him or her to know the details of whether and how we contend with life's vicissitudes. Thus we leave it to the client to assign meaning to us. That silence can be particularly counterproductive around topic areas that are controversial or taboo. If clients are from a NCDG background and we as therapists are from a CDG background, we leave it to them to assume one of the following about us: (1) ethnic/racial issues are irrelevant in therapy, (2) we are like other CDG members who do not acknowledge the humanity or lifestyle legitimacy of NCDG people, or (3) we are not like other CDG members who acknowledge the humanity or lifestyle legitimacy of NCDG people, but we think that it is detrimental to the therapy process to say so. If our client assumes 1, we expect that the client will know or figure out that his or her concern with ethnic/racial issues is not germane to his or her problems. If our client assumes 2, we expect that he or she will know that we are trying to acknowledge the universality of their problems. If our client assumes 3, we expect that he or she will know that we are trying to preserve our impersonality in order not to interfere with the development of a therapeutic transference relationship. Other assumptions on our part lead to other conclusions, but they all seem to lead to the conclusion that we do not need to inform the client about our views or our assumptions. Unfortunately, most clients are ill-equipped to understand or appreciate any of these perspectives. Clients are more likely to believe that being helped with problems about their sense of themselves as persons and about their associated relationships includes and rests on being understood, on having their fellow humanity acknowledged, and on being shown openly that we personally and as representatives of society at large care about them.

The Therapist–Client, Client–Therapist Relationship

It is perhaps unfortunate that therapists are thought of in terms of *power* and *authority*, as those terms have connotations that can in themselves be non- or antitherapeutic. That is, it can be the lack of a sense of power and a history of being intimidated and defeated by authorities that has rendered clients ineffective at managing their lives, their life situations, and their feelings about themselves and others. The issue of confronting another powerful figure may be more threatening than therapeutic. Nevertheless, the psychosocial reality of our human ecosystems embodies those concepts and those patterns of relationships. They are likely to be part of the initial perceptions that clients have of therapists. As we noted in the above section, some of our therapeutic perspectives (e.g., our detachment and impersonality) seem likely to heighten rather than diminish our sense of power and authority as therapists and our clients' sense of powerlessness.

In an earlier and broader context, Argyris (1975) discussed at some length the distinction between two types of interactions. In a Model I interaction, a person focuses only on his or her self-interest. In a Model II interaction, a person focuses on the interests of all involved parties and assigns primacy to establishing equitable processes and outcomes in a manner that is open to all. Tyler, Pargament, & Gatz (1983) have explored in some depth the distinction between a perspective on the part of psychologists in which they see their interactions with students, research subjects, community members, and clients as unidirectional, and a perspective in which they see those relations as inherently reciprocal. In that discussion they argued for the merits of the latter position and suggested that such interactions be looked at as *resource collaborative* interchanges. In such interchanges it is openly acknowledged that all parties involved bring resources as well as needs to the interchange and that all parties contribute to as well as benefit from such interchanges.

From an ethnic validity perspective, it follows that therapy is going to be more meaningful if it involves a resource collaborative interchange. To participate in a therapy process as resource collaborators, therapists must acknowledge openly that they are going to have more power and authority than their clients and that they are going to be seen that way. Also, at the very least, they need to acknowledge that they do have some specialized skills and perspectives to offer and do assume some responsibilities that are not directly reciprocated for the well-being of the client. Therapists need to acknowledge to themselves and to their clients that their clients also bring a sense of humanity and of life experiences to the exchange from which they both will learn and be enriched. Finally, they need to aid and support the client's learning to perceive the therapeutic exchange and other exchanges as reciprocal ones.

The above statements are not consistent with most therapeutic teaching and practice. It may be, as Argyris (1968) has argued, that individuals socialized in the culture of the United States just cannot behave in a Model II fashion. Further, although Argyris has not specifically applied his generalizations to therapists, it may be that therapists cannot behave in a Model II fashion. It may be that therapists' conceptual frameworks teach them that they are being bad therapists if they acknowledge to themselves, let alone to their clients, that therapeutic exchanges are enriching to them. In any case, therapists often end up inarticulate and unaware that they are confused about their relationships with clients and clients' relationships with them. They consequently cannot help clients sort out in an enriching way the relationships those clients do have with them.

One of the aspects of the special power that we often stress as part of our role as therapists is our capability of accepting people as worthwhile quite apart from how we feel about their particular behaviors or their direct relationship to us and our own way of living. Yet, in part, we glean our enriched understanding of people from interacting with them and our sense of worth from helping them. We also may gain in our own stature as humans from our ability to be of help to them and to learn from them. We do the same with ourselves, our children, and the rest of our relatives, not to mention our neighbors and professional associates. We can facilitate those outcomes by acknowledging our involvement in them. To say "I grew up in a world in which there were no black people and I was taught that they are inferior. I don't believe that anymore, but you may have to tell me when I unwittingly act that way" is a far step from considering black clients paranoid because they are not trusting of white therapists. As a white therapist, to say "I have learned from you (my black client) about some of the problems of being black in the United States and about some of my own implicit biases about blacks" may seem like an inappropriate expression to some. It can also be seen as an honest and open acknowledgment of reciprocal gain from a therapeutic interchange. As a black therapist, to say "I have learned from you (my white client) about some of the problems of being white in the United States and about some of my implicit biases about whites" may seem like an inappropriate expression to some. But again, it can be seen as an honest and open acknowledgment of reciprocal gain from a therapeutic interchange. That is, it can be seen as shifting the therapeutic exchange from one that is power and authority oriented to one which is reciprocal and competence oriented.

The Process Dynamic

Primarily for the client but necessarily also for the therapist, the therapist and client explore and negotiate their respective social realities and other potential realities as a vehicle for potential growth. This process may also produce conflict and dysfunction in either or both.

What we are suggesting is that when a therapist and a client begin a therapeutic interaction they come together in a variety of ways. They come together as representatives of two ethnic ecosystems or as two people in different positions within a shared ecosystem. They come together as a therapist and as a client. And, they come together as two individuals meeting for the first time.

With their initial greeting, the client and the therapist begin to explore and form the nature of the social reality within which they will relate, as well as the identities they will assume and assign to each other as they do so. They also begin to define the form of their own interchange. They begin to define what they will offer to and expect from each other. They begin to identify their areas of convergence and divergence and to become aware of their areas of conflict. And, by no means least of all, they begin explicitly and implicitly to invest in each other and their relationship. They begin to draw from it sustenance for themselves and each other or to raise their protective barriers as the interaction seems to demand more of them than it offers. In reality, they do both from moment to moment and often at the same moment. They also appeal to their own problem-solving and interpersonal influence skills to shape the interaction toward their desired ends. In doing so they also exhibit dysfunctional behaviors, feelings, and reactions to themselves and each other. For example, in Tyler, Sussewell, & Williams-McCoy (1985), the following case is cited:

> A black female therapist was working with a schizophrenically disturbed young adult white female. She had been told by other staff that the client's family was bigoted and that the client had been reprimanded for racial slurs in the treatment setting. In the therapist's interactions with the client she had been called "nigger" on one occasion and had been told that the only reason she had a job was because she was black. She found that cultural/racial issues were impairing her ability to treat this client. She tried several strategies to develop a relationship with the client. They included limit setting around verbal abuse, not reacting defensively to statements implying that she lacked competence, and ventilating her anger and frustration in sessions with her supervisor.
>
> Eventually the effort that the therapist was investing in maintaining these strategies became an issue in itself. She began to ask why she should work so hard to help someone as abusive as this client. Consequently, she ceased her efforts to form a relationship with this client and with her family. She took on a role that focused primarily on managing the verbal abuse and interacting with the client around concrete tasks such as daily activities. (p. 318)

That struggle between professional commitment and understanding and personal limitations and tolerance for abuse is part of all of us. Therapists of the CDG also struggle with their commitment to reach out and help NCDG clients correct personal limitations and overcome social injustice in the face of their difficulties with the behaviors and abusiveness of those clients. Our point is that we need to acknowledge and work to transcend our own ethnic embeddedness and personal likes and dislikes when we function as therapists. To say that we will work only with people with whom we are comfortable is to abdicate our professional and personal responsibility to transcend our own biases.

Put otherwise, an important component of the process dynamic in therapy is the ecosystem imbedded in each of us, therapist or client. If we cannot acknowledge our ethnic blinders, we cannot even help others like ourselves to overcome their often self-limiting and self-defeating parochialism. Two of us (a white male in his early 60s and a black female in her 30s) conducted a workshop for a group of therapists in which we sought to sensitize the participants to their ethnic blinders. The group was racially and ethnically heterogeneous and included both men and women. We began by holding up cards indicating that the white male was the therapist and the black female the client. We asked them what was the most salient issue in that pairing for the therapist, and what for the client. We asked what the therapist would gain if the therapy is successful, and what the therapist would lose. We asked the same questions about the client.

We shifted the cards so that the black female was the therapist and the white male the client, and asked the same questions. The respondents' answers suggested that we had created a different ecosystem and that they embodied different ecosystems among themselves. For example, white women respondents focused (for both therapist and client) on gender issues as important when the therapist was the white male; on race and age issues when the therapist was the black female. In contrast, for both pairings the male respondents focused on more traditional therapeutic issues such as therapist credibility or difficulties the client would have in giving up his or her defenses or in gaining new ways of living.

This kind of exploration of perspectives needs to be pursued far more thoroughly and systematically than was possible in that particular workshop. Yet even there the differences noted and the total impact of the exercise on the participants were striking. It seems safe to say that at the very least their consciousness was raised substantially by this brief exposure. What we need is to incorporate that consciousness more systematically into our practice of psychotherapy.

The Mechanism

The therapeutic interaction is defined as one in which therapists help clients initially by reviewing with those clients their ways of going about living. Therapists differ on whether this aspect of therapy involves a retrospective exploration of a client's earlier life experiences. Some therapists focus on a client's past life experiences, some on a client's present ways of dealing with life, and some on the client's future orientation. In any case, the focus in the interaction is on bringing into the picture some samples of the client's self-views, world views, and ways of interacting with life events. Further, that material is viewed in relation to the satisfaction of the client and of significant others with those characteristics and patterns. In that process, though it is not often stressed, therapists are at least indirectly learning about their own worlds and ways of life as well as about the client's. They are also learning about their own efficacy as therapists and their reactions as persons to the client, to the events being reviewed, and to the world in which the client lives. Further, in that process the client is learning about how the therapist functions as a therapist, about how the therapist's ethnic ecosystem is brought to bear on the relationship and the process, and about the therapist as a person.

There are other interactions and learnings involved in any therapeutic interaction. The patterns mentioned here are important, but they also serve to focus attention on the complexity of the interactions involved in psychotherapy and on the ecosystem aspects of those interchanges. Therapists are presumably more skilled than clients at differentiating ecosystem from individual aspects of therapeutic interactions and at responding to those aspects in constructive ways. However, that differential does not always favor the therapist. In cross-ethnic/racial interactions, the therapist may be much less skilled, particularly if the therapist is from a CDG and the client is from a NCDG. The central focus of this book is that very complexity.

The Change Pattern

Presumably what psychotherapy provides is a context in which clients can begin to identify and change dysfunctional components of their ways of viewing themselves, viewing the world, and dealing with both. That process may seem straightforward enough, but it is more often fraught with difficulties that stem from a variety of sources. They include the reality that many of our ways of viewing our lives are not characteristics or patterns of which we are aware, nor are we aware that they are optional and subject to scrutiny. And we may not wish to change them. Nevertheless, just learning that they are changeable patterns and characteristics that we have acquired as guides for living does change how we view them and their place in our lives and relationships.

An individual's characteristics and life patterns may also be difficult to reevaluate and change because they are products of ongoing injustices, exploitations, or oppressions that their perpetrators do not wish to see changed. Such patterns and characteristics may become so controlling of our lives that we lack the skills and resources to change them effectively, yet we find ourselves unwilling to tolerate them. Such patterns may be difficult to change because we do not know what we want to become and because it is difficult to learn new ways of being and living.

It may also be difficult for a client to change because the therapist must change in order to permit the client to do so. Therapists may believe that they have complete theories and sets of answers about the nature of people in general, their clients in particular, and human change processes. In those instances therapists believe that they really have nothing to learn from their clients but the details of the clients' dysfunctional behaviors. Such a perspective makes the therapeutic tasks of clients even more difficult.

On the other hand, therapists may view their clients as human beings trying to put their lives together. Such therapists do try to understand the unique way that each client is trying to manage and negotiate the events in his or her life. Both of those tasks facilitate the progress of therapy. They also require therapists to extend their own paradigms, possibly at a cultural or ethnic ecosystem level, possibly at an interpersonal or personal level, or possibly at a level of interacting with the world of work and society at large. Such therapists open themselves to extending their personal competencies and their world views as well as those of their clients. Those tasks are demanding and difficult at best. They can also be exhilarating and fulfilling.

The Termination Pattern

Ideally the client and therapist decide that they have accomplished their mutually agreed on goals, at least to the extent feasible under the circumstances. They then undertake the task of coming to terms with that decision. It requires them to close out their working relationship and go about their separate lives in light of how they have changed, or given up on changing themselves or each other, or decided to take another approach to changing (even if that choice involves changing to be more accepting of their existing situation).

The idea suggested ideally is that termination of therapy is a mutually arranged activity. Unfortunately, in many instances that simply is not the case. Clients decide for a variety of reasons that they do not see any gain in undertaking such a conclusion to the relationship and the therapy process. Therapists may reject the possibility of any reciprocity in the termination process for theoretical reasons, or they may themselves be inept at farewells. However, if a client or therapist does decide to conclude therapy by working out termination, these activities become possible.

Both therapist and client need to evaluate and appreciate what they have given each other and gained or lost from doing so. They also need to conclude the relationship—to say goodbye—and acknowledge that they no longer will share their time and humanity with each other in this effort to work toward agreed upon common goals. Finally, they need to redefine who they now are. That is, they need to redefine how they now feel about themselves and their world and how they are now going to interact with the events in their lives. Those redefinitions may be largely personal; they may involve rethinking how each or either feels about whole groups of people and ways of life; they may fall somewhere between those extremes. Nevertheless, in our view, these termination activities are important, and both client and therapist lose important components of the therapeutic process if they omit them.

SUMMARY

In this background section about the processes and patterns of psychotherapy, we have touched briefly on the general form and nature of therapeutic relationships. We have made an effort to identify and describe the role and status of the therapist and the client as somewhat autonomous individuals and as embedded in their respective cultural and ethnic/racial frameworks. We have sought to sketch a view of therapy as involving individuals in a human interchange that has a particular therapeutic focus but that is not unrelated to our more general human discourses and interactions. Therapy relationships are special in many ways, and we need to be sensitive to those special characteristics. Nevertheless, therapists and clients are individual human beings. We need to be equally sensitive to those human characteristics as well, for they too are part of the therapeutic process.

In the next chapters we will build on this background material to develop a more elaborate and detailed presentation of the issues and complexities involved in therapeutic interactions. A more detailed presentation can highlight for all of us the complexities and difficulties involved in demythologizing and rehumanizing therapeutic interactions. It can also highlight the potential richness and rewards that are inherent in doing so. It is that richness and those rewards that we feel have been lost by ignoring or minimizing the presence of the ecological and the unique individual factors in therapeutic interactions.

6

Forming a Relationship
The Ecology of Therapy and Its Participants

Ecological systems are relatively self-contained and self-sustaining systems. They include not only living but nonliving elements in a relatively stable relationship to one another as well as with the larger context that defines the conditions of their existence. Thus, the components in an ecological system are in a dynamic balance that sustains the various elements as well as the overall balance of the system. That balance also provides the context for interrelated adaptations and changes of the components in the system.

When we discuss human ecology, we try to encompass the totality of relations between individuals and their internal and external environments, including both tangible and nontangible components. The tangible elements include climate, geography, products of nature such as foods, human products such as structural features of buildings, and human physical characteristics. The nontangible elements of our environments include those experiences and meanings created from the process of living with its necessary interactions between the tangible and nontangible aspects of our ecology.

Although our characteristics, such as size, pigmentation, facial features, and gender, are tangible physical characteristics, they do have a profound effect on the nontangibles that make up our worlds. Further, they are more difficult to change than nontangibles such as people's understandings of their significance. In other words, we are saying that we have considerably more capability for changing what our tangible attributes mean to us and to others than we have over changing the attributes themselves.

Nevertheless, whatever may be the possibilities or limits of change or the need for stability, this human ecology provides the context for our individual psychosocial realities and to some extent is also shaped by them. Adapting ourselves or adapting our external reality so that we maintain a relatively stable self-sustaining relationship with the contexts outside of ourselves is essential to our existence. We must not only maintain breathable air, drinkable water, and adequate food and shelter; we must maintain a mutually tolerable relationship with the other creatures in our relevant environment to sustain our lives. We must also maintain a world and relationship with that world (and ourselves in it) that will provide us with at least a minimally adequate desire to use our energies to stay alive rather than to destroy ourselves.

Psychotherapy is one of the nontangible processes by which we endeavor to help one another survive in both the tangible and nontangible aspects of our lives. Further, psychotherapy usually involves an interpersonal relationship that is based on a rather special form of interpersonal trust. It is the complex activity of establishing trust and forming therapeutic relationships that is the focus of this chapter.

Human Ecosystems

We are going to use the term *ecosystem* to refer to subsets of the human ecology that include relatively self-contained units, such as a community and its environment. In that sense the concept of ecosystem represents various social realities and systems and provides a means of further defining levels of human experience, abstraction, and interaction. We will use it to describe different types of individual–community–environment patterns (e.g., work ecosystem, family ecosystem, middle-class white ecosystem, culture-defining ecosystem, therapeutic ecosystem).

It is impossible to identify and describe all of the various and somewhat overlapping psychosocial ecosystems that each of us forms and abstracts to provide frames of reference for our experience. Yet it is important to acknowledge their presence and conceptualize the nature of their interrelationships. Two somewhat different schematic frameworks may be helpful as guides for formulating these interrelationships.

As we move from thinking about the formative contexts that are central to each of us toward the more peripheral contexts of our lives, one type of framework that may describe those relationships can be represented by an oyster shell or the cross-section of a tree. An oyster shell displays quite clearly the ever larger rings that have marked its growth and that extend primarily in one direction from its center. Tree rings tend to grow more evenly around the tree's center, but they also show uneven extensions with varying climatic circumstances. In either case, the newer rings (e.g., ecosystems) form around a beginning core.

On the other hand, the overlapping ecosystems of a person's life may seem more like Venn diagrams. Venn diagrams are the overlapping circles that statisticians draw to show how much statistical variance is shared between two or more characteristics. An important aspect of Venn diagrams is that they depict overlap without conveying a sense of organization among attributes. They enable us to portray interrelationship without implying organization or direction of effect.

Whether we visualize oyster shells, trees, Venn diagrams, or all three, it is important to attend to the interrelationships among our ecosystems and to their impact on our lives. People who have lived primarily in a homogeneous and relatively simple ecological context may organize their individual, family, interpersonal, community, and work ecosystems in highly overlapping ways. Not too many decades ago, many people lived on family farms in largely self-contained ecosystems. Perhaps diagrams of their lives would have been relatively undifferentiated and adequately represented by the rings of a tree growing in an open field in a stable climate. In contrast, people who have lived in heterogeneous or turbulent environments may require much more complex representations of their lives—larger and more irregular oyster shells or interlocking Venn diagrams that look like the trick ring puzzles one can buy.

Understanding, contending with, and trying to change the multiple aspects of the realities in our lives is an issue of central importance to the existence and quality of life of each of us. When we explore the domains of cross-ethnic, cross-racial, and cross-gender psychotherapy, we confront directly the possibilities and limits of potential change. As individuals, we are born with the distinctive physical characteristics of Negroid Africans, of Asians, or of Caucasians. We may find our societally defined racial identity desirable or undesirable; nevertheless, each of us has to negotiate life with that identity simply because it is almost impossible to change or disguise those characteristics. In contrast, some characteristics, such as ways of defining oneself and others, of dressing, or of behaving, stem from personal, ethnic, or culture-based experiences. They are more malleable. It is not only possible to take the boy or girl out of the country, it is also somewhat possible to take the country out of the boy or girl.

The Individual as a Psychologically Autonomous Unit in the Ecosystem

Much of the history of human civilization has involved defining the nature of individuals and their relationships to one another, to their societies, to their world, and even to the universe. Perhaps, unfortunately, far more attention has been given to the rise and fall of civilizations than to the struggles of individuals. Nevertheless, people do strive to create themselves as individuals and to form families with a sense of continuity. Small bands do strive to create communities and senses of continuity. It is the results of those efforts that comprise the forerunners of our current ethnicities and cultures.

Unfortunately, those efforts have often included defining some people as more human than others. Further, some people have defined themselves or been defined as having a subjective character (that is, they think of themselves or others think of them as having some freedom to control their destinies), while others are defined as objects controlled by their circumstances. To be thought of or to think of oneself as an object controlled by circumstances is to imagine an oyster shell or tree with no capacity to form its cohering center or of a Venn diagram whose circles do not include a self-aware and self-directing area. As noted in the previous chapter, these issues of humanness and control are central in therapy. Both therapists and clients focus on the client's self-development, self-knowledge and understanding, self–world perspective, and self-directed conduct as the primary domain of attention and change in therapy.

From our perspective it is unfortunate that in therapeutic interactions also there is often the shared implicit (if not explicit) belief that the client is, by virtue of having less self-control and understanding, in some sense less human than others, including the therapist. For example, those of us who are therapists may include in the Venn diagram of ourselves a circle that defines ourselves as having psychological difficulties or even being somewhat neurotic. Nevertheless, we do not think of our problems as the central factor in our being. In contrast, we all too often think of our clients in just that way. They become "cases" or "neurotics" or some other category, with the implication that they are flawed human beings.

The position that underlies the current presentation is that everyone is equally human. We all are shaped by our heritages and circumstances, and we all have some latitude to abstract from, reflect on, and influence our internal and external realities, human and otherwise (e.g., spiritual, material). We view individuals not just as victims of their ecosystems but also as agents capable of modifying those ecosystems and joining or forming others. In other words, our oyster, tree, or Venn diagram incorporates the view that we are at least to some extent active agents, creative forces, in our lives and in our various ecosystems. That assumption also leads us to the belief that we can understand other individuals only by interacting with them as individuals and involving them in providing accounts of their own realities. We also assume that we need to obtain external accounts of those internal and external realities and begin to put the two together. It is only then that we can even begin to approach the creation of a comprehensive account of any individual's ecosystem. For example, it is just inexcusable to assume that our therapist expectations as to what clients should think of therapists is objective and that clients' differences from that perspective are defensive or inaccurate. Their views stem from their individual experiences and from their conceptions of an ecosystem involving therapists. Those views are valid and functional. We may believe that other views will serve them better in their therapy and their future lives. It will not serve us or them better to believe that their perspectives are necessarily flawed, limited, and inadequate because of their patient or client status.

The Individual Interacting with Self and Others

When any of us begins to think about who we are, we focus on a psychosocially formed reference perspective since our knowledge of our intrapersonal being is in part interpersonal. That is, the internal reference perspective to which each of us compares ourself is formed out of our interactions with the world outside of ourselves as well as with the world inside. We can never completely sort out our unique internal attributes and our externally derived attributes; we are psychosocial beings. We do seek to understand our individual conceptions of ourselves. We also seek to understand those conceptions of ourselves that are based on the distinctive response of others, not from our own self-generated experiences. We try to separate those aspects of our ourselves that are unexamined internalized evaluations by others from those that we have formed by actively examining our role in our experiences. To understand the psychosocial nature of our self-interactions requires discussing that process in an abstract way, such as we have just done. It also needs some concrete examples. We will focus on them in the following paragraphs.

Convergence

When a person makes a judgment of satisfaction or dissatisfaction with himself or herself, he or she does so in comparison to some set of expectations and standards. If those standards are based on that person's own previous actions and experience of those actions, the resulting judgments are based on internal individual convergences. When that same individual feels satisfied or dissatisfied because of assessments by others, the resulting internal convergence has more of a social character. For example, a client, Elli, was distressed with herself because she was going on eating binges. She experienced the binges as unpleasant and knew that she had managed her eating behavior quite adequately at other times in her life. She also knew that she generally managed her life better when she controlled her eating. Her distress expressed a sense of convergence with regard to her own experience and judgment. She added the information that she felt even more distress because she has friends who have similar patterns of behavior and judge her current behavior as out of control. When she added that additional information, she conveyed a sense of social (as well as psychological) convergence. Yet her internal convergence is based in part on earlier labeling by others of her behavior, and her social convergence is based in part on her internal reactions. In short, the two, internal and external, are inextricably intertwined.

Divergence

One of the authors experiences considerable diversity within himself about reading. He loves to read and is interested in a wide range of materials. His bedside, as well as his desk, are strewn with materials that are being read. He is quite aware that different facets of himself want to read different types of material; some are interested in novels, some in psychology, some in public policy, some in art, some in travel, and on and on. His usual solution is to accept this internal diversity and respond to the most persistent voice of the moment.

In some instances, it may be more important to search out the reasons for divergent desires. It may be only by doing so that we can come to accept such desires as divergent ways of accomplishing similar purposes. One example is of a couple from a small town, each with a deep sense of loyalty to his or her family of origin. Each wanted "to go home." Their desires were similar, similarly rooted, and equally valid. They resolved their potential conflicts by accepting that their childhood homes were separate homes and going their separate ways. When they visited their home town, she stayed with her parents and he stayed with his.

Conflict

At times we are aware that our conflicts are within ourselves as well as with others. Elli, who binged on food, experienced a sense of urgency to eat and at the same time a sense of revulsion at her self-destructiveness. She even struggled within herself over which impulses were a reflection of her own nature and experience. Was she inadequate and self-destructive? Or was that aspect of her something she had come to internalize from her hostile and abusive mother? She also wondered whether she had survived and become successful in college because of the validity of her own integrity and struggles or because of the support of her father? Was her binging her only way of containing her internalized acceptance of the belief that to be too successful and self-accepting was to set off her mother's self and family destructiveness? Were her successes only her way (and her only way) of showing that she valued her father's support?

ETHNIC ECOSYSTEMS

The examples in the above paragraphs do not involve us in cultural or ethnic aspects of the way we understand ourselves and others and live our lives. Nevertheless, an understanding of the ethnic heritage of the people described could provide us (and them) a fuller understanding of them and their processing of these aspects of themselves. We need to explore the ways in which cultural and ethnic factors do become part of our self-perceptions and of our reference standards.

An ethnic ecosystem is therefore a subset and specialized ecosystem that is comprised of individuals who hold customary beliefs, history, values, and ways of relating. Ethnic ecosystems, like all ecosystems, are open systems in that they are influenced by, react to, and are shaped by other systems. Many of the realities that define one ecosystem have been developed by the interaction between ecosystems. Collectively, ethnic ecosystems and other specialized systems comprise the human ecology and build our social realities. Ecosystems are units that function together as a whole within a specified context and environment.

The Individual as a Psychologically Autonomous Unit in the Ethnic Ecosystem

We have already rejected the view that someone in a client status might be viewed as less human than others. In this section we want to reject the view that some ethnic or racial groups are more or less human than others. We cannot deny the evidence that there are groups and individuals who base their self-perceptions, self–world relationships, and means of negotiating their lives on their belief in their superiority or inferiority. We see no basis for such claims. Rather, we view such differences as historically and ecologically developed and as offering both advantages and disadvantages. None of the ethnic, racial, or cultural groups that asserts claims to superiority in the human realm is demonstrably superior on all criteria for all human circumstances and instances. Nevertheless, we do need to formulate a way consistent with our ethnic validity perspective for understanding and working with people who hold such views. That is our focus in the following paragraphs.

Convergence

As we have discussed earlier, a sense of convergence comes from a sense of commonality. We may feel that we have conducted ourselves in a way we have desired. If so, we experience convergence between our desired sense of self and our perception of our actual, or "true," self.

Our particular focus at the moment is how does ethnicity enter into a sense of convergence? We are exposed to ethnicity by the very nature of our living within any society (ecosystem) that is complex enough to include multiple ethnic/racial groups or that has occasion to be aware of various ethnic/racial groups that interact with that society. As we noted earlier, a contributing factor to the form of one's existence is being part of and being seen as a member of a culture-defining group or of a non-culture-defining group.

For example, let us look at an extremely unlikely hypothetical situation of an entering black male college student who has lived in residential areas and attended schools in which black populations predominate. To himself and to the people in his environment, his appearance is natural and in general acceptable and desirable. He can come to define the convergence between himself and the black people in his world as an ethnic/racial convergence only when people from his background or from other backgrounds tell him or react to him in ways that indicate that their responses to him are based on his racial/ethnic identity. Even so, the decision to designate that convergence as of an ethnic/racial nature is a decision within himself.

Divergence

To continue with our example, this young black man will begin to have a sense that his blackness and his life in a black ecosystem are divergent from those in white ecosystems at the same time as he comes to understand that his convergence with other black people is in part ethnically/racially based. He will begin to see others as different, not just because they are different individuals but because of their nonblackness. Their identity also is in part ethnically/racially based. It is under those circumstances that he begins to see these issues of divergence and conflict as ethnic/racial in nature. Let us look first at divergence.

Suppose that this young man has been reared in an environment in which he was exposed indirectly by parents and others to the reality that there are many different kinds of people in the world and their ways of living are all respectworthy. That is, he can come to experience himself and others as ethnically/racially different and to accept their differences in a nonevaluative way. He can experience their behavior and their responses to him as unique, as objects of curiosity, and as areas for exploration. He can share his own experiences as unique and as respectworthy. He can interact with a sense of optimistic trust and with directness. In that context, the reality and legitimacy of ethnic/racial divergence assumes an internal legitimacy. (That is, there are different ways one can live that are valid, and his is acceptable as the one that he has chosen and that is sustaining and enriching for him.) That divergence also has a social legitimacy. (The people he observes and with whom he interacts are different from him and from one another. Their ways are valid for them as his are valid for him. Those differences may even enrich them.)

Conflict

Difference, heterogeneity, and hierarchical inequities may also lead to quite different outcomes and all too often have done so. Our young black man may have entered a predominantly white college in an atmosphere in which he and his ethnicity are devalued. Thus, he faces conflict about the relative worth of ethnic/racial concepts and of particular ethnic/racial ecosystems. He must decide whether it is fair for others to discriminate against him and unfair for him to expect equal treatment for himself. In other words, he may come to believe as his own reference point that his ethnicity marks him in ways that he cannot overcome. At that point he does not need others to devalue him because of his ethnic/racial identity; he will do it himself. He may even come to shape his world in a way that keeps him in an inferior position. If he responds that way, he has moved back from conflict to convergence at the cost of limiting of his worth, possibilities, and efforts to sustain and enrich his life and relationships. He has acquired a way of reconciling his expectations with those of his environment and thereby avoiding (or minimizing) external conflict.

On the other hand, this same young black man may respond to his denigrating college atmosphere by continuing to believe and acting to assert and validate that he and his ethnicity are valid and not inferior to the ethnicity of whites. In other words, he may adopt a stance of distrust and conflict with powerful elements in his broader social framework. That stance and struggle may lead him to feel a lowered sense of self-efficacy and of the efficacy of his ethnic ecosystem. It may also provide him a means of validating and sustaining his sense of self-worth and the psychosocial worth of his ethnic group's existence. In any case, it exemplifies a conflict-oriented stance to the college ecosystem.

We have viewed the situation of this young black man in a white college setting as illustrative of ethnic ecosystem issues. It is also illustrative of racially based ecosystem reality with one important difference added. This young man's racial appearance usually identifies him immediately, he has no way of avoiding that aspect of his reality. He has some latitude about how he interprets himself and others, and about how he does conduct himself. He may accept their view (convergence) and redefine himself. He may maintain his own view and search for ways to pursue his own course (divergence). He may confront the whites' incompatible and denigrating views and seek to change them or at least change their impact on him (conflict).

The Individual Interacting with Others

What we sketched out in the preceding paragraphs was the situation of individuals living in a multi-ethnic environment. We focused on their self-definitions and self-defined expectations as they formed them on the basis of internal and external feedback. We need also to look at the impact of their interactions with others that grow out of their ethnicity.

Convergence

Individuals may converge on their expectations of themselves and others because they have a shared sense of the meaning of their own and each other's ethnicity. Their interactions are unlikely to involve any direct attention to their ethnic heritages. It is more likely to be that only as they have discordant experiences will they focus on their ethnicities. Let us look at another hypothetical example.

A white professional couple, one Jewish and the other Protestant, bore one son and within 6 months adopted a second child, a black boy. Thus they completed their family. Within their home they actively sought convergence of perspectives and experiences. To a considerable extent they accomplished their goals. Nearly two decades later their family is close knit and functioning. Yet their lives present different challenges to that convergence when they leave home to interact with the world outside and when they return. The most obvious is the situation of the black son. Each time he interacts with a race-conscious world his race is brought to his attention. When he returns home, he and the family must deal with the consequences of the discrepancy between their functioning coherence at home and the divergence and conflict that he experiences in the larger world. When he is troubled by his away-from-home experiences, he cannot be certain whether they are an expression of racial bias or of his behavior as an individual. His family may not even know of his discordant experiences, so they may not know whether to respond to his discomfort as a racial issue or as a personal one.

The three white members also leave their common environment and confront their ethnicity as personally experienced and as the world defines it in interactions with them. In their daily lives their ethnicity is not ordinarily as visible, yet the parents are in helping professions and work daily with people from diverse backgrounds. In responding to those people, their own socialized perspectives influence their responses. When they interact with people different from themselves but similar ethnically to someone else in the family they confront their own real and potential divergent and conflicting expectations. They also confront the biases toward themselves and toward others like them of individuals from those other ethnicities. The husband encounters negative reactions to Jews and must sort out whether his wife shares those perspectives and feelings. She encounters negative reactions to Protestants and must sort out whether her husband shares them. Each must in turn sort out whether he or she harbors the prejudices that are encountered regularly about the ethnic group of his or her marriage partner.

The biological son is also caught up in this matrix. His grandparents represent divergent ancestries and hold conflicting views about each other's ethnic world view. He and his brother are racially different. Is he more valued because of his racial and genetic similarity to his parents or less valued as evidenced by their choice of another son who is racially and genetically different?

The possibilities for confusion and conflict in this family unit are myriad and can be elaborated far beyond what we have noted. The central point is that maintaining a sense of convergence (of family unity and identity) takes on ethnic/racial as well as personal dimensions for the members of this family. Even in ideal circumstances, creating and maintaining enough convergence to build a stable, supportive, and gratifying family ecosystem is an achievement. Achieving convergences becomes more of a task as the network becomes more heterogeneous and as that heterogeneity introduces real and potential conflicts in the respective life views and life realities of the people involved.

Divergence

Perhaps one of the most crucial aspects of any ethnic perspective is its position with regard to diversity. Each of us acquires a set of standards about ranges of acceptable behaviors and beliefs from our own enculturation and socialization experiences. Those standards include guidelines about forms of response to conduct that does not conform to our standards and beliefs.

My ethnic/cultural background may have been one in which people relate informally; yours may have been one in which people follow prescribed guidelines for formal interactions. For us to socialize with each other we must both accept that our different approaches are simply conventions with somewhat similar meanings, and we must be willing to adapt to those differences in each other. If we cannot make those adaptations, then we must go separate ways or engage in conflict until at least the ethnic validity, if not the existence, of one of us is sacrificed.

For instance, a couple who were no longer religious in a conventional belief sense spoke of being pleased that they both had a Jewish heritage and upbringing. They converged on both expecting to have a big dinner on Friday night and relaxing on Saturday. Their example points to another potential conflict of the family we spoke of earlier. If the father prefers the Jewish pattern of rest on Saturday and the mother prefers the Christian one of rest on Sunday, they have a potential conflict unless they have worked out a weekly rhythm in their lives that respects their divergent heritages.

There are numerous divergences in the psychosocial ecosystems of blacks and whites in the United States, with its particular history of racism. Those divergences become important in understanding individuals socialized in each of these traditions. For example, blacks in the United States tend to relate to one another along lines more often associated with traditional cultures. They tend to have and expect more respect for age and the wisdom that comes from experience. Whites have become more modernized. They relate more in terms of people's extrinsic status and role relationships. Yet, paradoxically, whites are more trusting and self-disclosing; blacks are more likely to test relationships before they can feel trusting. Their experiences have led them to focus more on the dangers of unwarranted trust and self-disclosure; whites may be more focused on the benefits of openness. These statements are broad generalizations and may sound like stereotyping, but we are trying to emphasize that people can and do form divergent styles of living and relating to others and to themselves. Those styles are frequently based in the collective experience of their ethnic/racial heritage. It is important to be sensitive to them to find areas of convergence and acceptance of divergences. If we are not, we foster conflict and misunderstanding. It is such conflict that we focus on in the next section.

Conflict

We are ordinarily most attuned to the issues of interpersonal conflict based on disparate and incompatible ethnic/racial/cultural heritages. The ethnically/racially/culturally unique child often confronts the harsh reality of the insensitivity of dominant ethnic/racial/cultural mores. The individual who does not fit or choose to accept the reality imposed because of others' expectations gets caught in a very tangled web. If those expectations are associated with physical characteristics (racial, sex) that cannot be changed or hidden, the individual's difficulties are even further compounded.

For instance, a talented young black woman sought acceptance in her university's honors program. She was admitted because she was well qualified, but she quickly found herself alone. There were no other black honors students with whom she could share her experiences or expectations. She sought out faculty to find out about support for talented black students. They referred her to programs for marginal black students or left it up to her to work out her identity issues on her own or with talented white students if she wished. When she turned to her black peers or they became aware of her, they accused her of being an "Oreo," of being black on the outside and white on the inside. She found herself struggling to develop her superlative talents while retaining her black ethnic/racial identity, but faced ethnic/racial conflict from blacks and whites. Black students who were less talented pushed her toward ethnic/racial conformity through abandonment of her talents and identity as talented. Whites pushed her toward abandonment of her ethnic/racial identity. Both groups fought with her over her desire to define herself as a person with an atypical set of individual and psychosocial characteristics. In short, they fought her challenge to their ethnic/racial conceptions of people and of the world.

Likewise, the psychologist Ezekiel (1984) provides us with a personal example of the internal and external conflict that arises from being ethnically or racially different. He has cited his experiences as the only Jewish child in a school system in the predominantly Christian southwest United States. He remembers vividly his own discomfort at being confronted with the school-based Christian-oriented activities at Christmastime. He could participate, at least in form, in the singing of hymns and other activities at the expense of his own sense of personal and ethnic validity and worth. He could openly indicate his difference and confront the consequent expected rejection and ridicule of his peers.

It was his memory of those internal struggles and the utter insensitivity of his classmates and teachers to those struggles that he felt provided him the most basic personal sense of the struggles he later encountered when he spent 2 years among black residents of the Detroit slums. He found himself returning to his own earlier experiences as a means of trying to understand the conflict that these black individuals lived with and tried to express to him on a daily basis.

Those earlier conflict-laden experiences also provided him with a basis for understanding the insensitivity of the white culture-defining group to blacks in America. Here are some highlights:

> Despite denial and despite inattention, one central truth of American society is that it is a society in which the whites dominate the blacks. Whites and blacks live in two separate worlds; whites and blacks fear and hate each other; not all whites have power, but the power that exists is held almost entirely by whites and is used, consciously or unconsciously, in a way that is sensitive to race. (pp. 214–215)
>
> The ultimate lesson of this sojourn among the black poor is separation. I express the lesson in several phrases: "us and them," "the invisible blacks," and "whitey is cold." These phrases refer to ways that blacks and whites think about themselves and each other. (p. 216)
>
> Since whites seldom notice themselves creating the separation, they seldom think about it. Since blacks live within the effects of the separation, they think of it often. (p. 218)

What Ezekiel has expressed so powerfully is the depth of the conflict between ethnic/racial ecosystems as played out collectively and, consequently, individually. In doing so he highlights how the individual and thus collective denial by whites of their self-interests that conflict with those of blacks protects whites and perpetuates those conflicts. In turn he notes how blacks get caught up in perpetuating the stereotypes and the conflict.

Blacks even get caught up in conflicts among themselves about the meaning of their ethnic/racial heritage in their own lives. An example of this occurred in a graduate program in which one of the authors has taught. There were two black students who related quite differently to their common African American heritage (ecosystem) and who were enrolled during the same period of time. One of them asserted that he was a human first and only secondarily black. He identified himself in that way, defined his ecosystem that way, and demanded that others interact with him in that way. The other asserted that she was a black woman who was a human. She insisted that others interact with her by first acknowledging her black and female reality. Their self-defined ecosystems were incompatible and they quickly found themselves unable to find any areas of convergence or divergence as a basis for interaction. Others could interact with them separately and find areas of convergence and divergence with either or both of them and build patterns of relationships on those agreements. If they were both in the same situation it was not possible to interact with them or pursue any course. To endeavor to do so activated the conflict they saw between their ecosystems. If everyone was treated in the same way, one of them found it unacceptable. If blacks were treated deferentially, the other found that unacceptable. They had apparently convergent backgrounds in an African American ecosystem, but as individuals they interpreted their experiences in divergent and totally conflicting ways.

The choices those two students made face each of us. That is, each of us has some latitude to decide which aspects of his or her ethnicity to identify as defining his or her sense of self-efficacy and self–world relationships. As the behaviors of these two students so aptly illustrate, how we choose to deal with that latitude can create conflicts with others who share our ethnic/racial heritage as well as between ourselves and those with other heritages.

THERAPIST AND CLIENT AS ECOSYSTEMS

Therapists have roots in their own ethnic ecosystems and so do clients. Both can become entrapped in those ecosystems and not be able to understand or transcend them. The ethnic validity model describes exchanges as including these ecosystem-related patterns and provides a basis for bridging such differences. We assume that both the therapist and the client bring to their interactions the histories of their ethnic ecosystems and the historical ways in which their systems have related. The historically framed character of these initial interactions helps to define and establish their initial way of relating, including the power relationship that is initially set up in therapy.

The Individual as a Psychologically Autonomous Unit in the Ethnic Ecosystem

When therapeutic interactions have been examined, the focus on the adequacy of the therapist has usually been on his or her adequacy to fulfill a role defined and sanctioned by therapists. That examination has usually been based on the twin assumptions that the therapist could and should have transcended his or her *individual* psychological conflicts and that the therapist role is context free. The therapist presumably embodies an unbiased conception of normality and of the context in which lives are lived. It is important to challenge that set of enculturated or socialized assumptions. Rather, just as anyone else embodies to some extent an ethnic identity, so does the therapist. The three authors of this book are therapists. We share many values and perspectives on the nature of effective therapy. Nevertheless, one of the authors is a white male who grew up in a lower-middle-class family in the rural Midwest; one is a black female who grew up in a middle-class family in the suburbs of a large east coast city; and one is a black female who grew up in a working-class family in a small southern town. Each of us is in many ways an autonomous individual, yet each of us has as a background a distinctively different ecosystem, and each of us has a distinctively different position in our present ecosystem. Those unique identities and distinctive ethnic/racial attributes are not and cannot be left outside the therapy room.

Similarly, a client entering therapy is to some extent an autonomous individual. It is the capacity for some autonomous choice that underlies that individual's decision to seek therapeutic help. Nevertheless, the individual enters the therapy room as an autonomous white, black, Latin, or Asian male or female; as an autonomous rural or urban individual; or as an autonomous troubled college student or adult in a midlife crisis.

The Individual Interacting with Others

The point that follows as we focus on ourselves as autonomous individuals within our ecosystems is that all aspects of ourselves are involved in interactions. When a white female college student seeks therapy and enters a therapeutic room with an older white female therapist, their interaction involves both their individual ways of functioning and their ecosystem perspectives. The therapist has a sense of her own college experience, and she also has a sense of her current view of college-age women. Both of these perspectives shape her perspective as a therapist. The young woman has a view shaped by her own upbringing of what undertaking therapy involves and implies. She also has a sense of her generation's view of older women.

Convergence

The reality that people from different ecosystems have different perspectives does not preclude interaction, communication, understanding, or common purpose. Possibly a nearly universal example of convergence across fundamental differences is evident in all of our lives as we try to communicate with, relate to, and understand one another across gender differences. We can argue that males and females simply occupy different places in a larger ecosystem, and in some ways they do. Yet in many ways their lives and world views are shaped by their gender-based ecosystems. In short, to some extent our physiology has generated a humanity marked by two distinct ecosystems, one of females and one of males. We never completely transcend that aspect of our nature and perceive life through the eyes of the other sex. Yet we do manage to find convergence in many ways. At least one basis for that convergence is a shared interest in common outcomes, such as the procreating and rearing of children or experiencing the satisfactions of heterosexual relationships. Another basis for male–female convergence is the enrichment that comes from sharing different and at times complementary perspectives on many of life's activities, such as music and art. Those different perspectives are not necessarily gender linked, but often differences in socialization make them so.

In therapy, convergence may come from an asymmetrical reciprocal investment parallel to that which a parent and child may share. Each in his or her respective ecosystem must incorporate a legitimate role that permits and may even value such an overlap. The older therapist working in a college counseling setting must see legitimacy and fulfillment in being helpful to men and women of a younger generation. Their clients must be able to view seeking help in a trusting relationship with older adults as a legitimate way of negotiating their own life issues.

Finding that cross-generational convergence may also require the therapist and client to transcend their ethnic ecosystems in unexpected ways. For example, a young white woman attending a predominantly black college may be overwhelmed with issues and go to the counseling center. She is likely to find that her therapist is an older black woman, perhaps someone who looks like a woman who worked as a domestic in her parents' home. The ecosystem in which she is enshrouded may present particular difficulties for her as she tries to relate to her therapist as a professional, with the status which that role implies. The therapist may have experienced discrimination from young white women when she was in college. Her ecosystem may embody viewing young white female college students as unsympathetic figures. For her to find a basis for convergence with this young woman, she must be able to transcend that inhibiting perspective. For the young woman to find a basis for convergence with this therapist, she must be able to transcend her inhibiting perspective. Each of them must find within herself a way of viewing a therapeutic relationship between them as personally and professionally legitimate and gratifying.

Divergence

Another important facet of the ethnic ecosystem of a therapist and a client is the potential of each for accepting divergence in ways of life. In college situations, a topic that often challenges therapists' acceptance of diversity is the norms for sexual cohabitation between college-age men and women. They have changed drastically in little more than a generation and can pose major problems for therapist–client pairs. Perhaps a good illustration is the situation of a white male student who seeks therapy because of the difficulties of his relationship with a black female student with whom he is living. He may feel that their relationship is legitimate and that interracial dating is an acceptable part of the peer group norms he shares. He may encounter an older white male therapist whose ecosystem expectations are negative about premarital sex as well as cross-racial dating. When they begin to interact, each confronts evidence of his and the other's ecosystem perspectives. Some indications of their different perspectives will be quickly evident; other cues may be subtle but they are likely to become evident. Their potential for interacting at all rests on their capacity to find a way of identifying and respecting their different perspectives on these and other variables.

This therapist has begun to respect their diversity when he can say that he does not approve of premarital relations or of cross-racial dating, but that he will work to understand and respect the client's perspective. The young man has begun to respect their diversity when he can say that he will try to understand the therapist's view as well as the legitimacy of the therapist's effort to transcend their disparate views. As they learn to respect their differences they can both come to have more respect for themselves and for their capacity to work together. In sum, they both enrich their intrapersonal autonomy to the extent that they accept and transcend their interpersonal differences.

Conflict

The above example rather graphically sketches out the potential for conflicts in world views on the basis of generational differences and often related changes in ethnic world views. The older therapist may find no way to incorporate into his ecosystem acceptance of the young man's world view with regard to premarital sexual relations and cross-sexual dating. He may insist that the young man's personal issues involve guilt over moral and societal transactions. Nevertheless, the young man may feel that the therapist must be understanding and accepting since the university counseling center has represented its services as being nonjudgmental. He may also feel that his relationship with his girlfriend is basically legitimate, but troubled. He must struggle with the therapist to verify his self-worth, his trust of society's institutionalized helpers, and his approach to life and to seeking help. Unless they can find some grounds for convergence, the two of them cannot develop a relationship in which either feels true to himself, to his internal assessment of his integrity. Unless they can at least agree to respect each other's right to part ways, their interaction will of necessity be destructive to each one's sense of integrity.

THERAPIST–CLIENT INTERACTIONS AS THE INTERACTION OF TWO ECOSYSTEMS

In this initial encounter of two people from different ecosystems, the power and authority issues that arise derive largely from their historical sense of the interactions between those ecosystems. If the historical power, authority, or other dimensions of the relationship was one of domination and of oppression (or any other defining pattern), then the initial encounter should be assumed to have that as a barrier. As a consequence, there are ecosystem aspects to forming a therapeutic relationship that require attention. They include the creation of a new ecosystem, of two new identities, and of a new power/authority relationship.

Specifically, within the confines of the therapist's office a new ecosystem is created that will bring with it a reality that either challenges or confirms the historical relationship of the therapist and client as representatives of their respective ecosystems and as individuals. The first step in that process is acknowledging that the ecosystems exist and that a power relationship exists between them. The processes of converging, diverging, and conflicting are crucial aspects of the renegotiation process. To renegotiate, the therapist must be open to the idea of a multiplicity of realities and ways of being. The therapist must search his or her ecosystem for ways of being that are both different from and similar to those of the client. The therapist must also learn from and educate the client about his or her awareness of the client's ecosystem and how to decipher, understand, and use it in problem solving. Once the client has competencies in understanding his or her ecosystem and ways of living within it, issues pertaining to power/authority can be more easily negotiated. It is in this process that both the client and the therapist grow.

If the client and therapist share the same ethnic ecosystem, the power relationship to be negotiated pertains to the therapist's and the client's authority as defined in that ecosystem. The therapist is seen as an individual whom the community has recognized as being the bearer of skills and knowledge pertaining to effective functioning.

If client and therapist are from different historical ethnic ecosystems, the power relationship to be negotiated involves the relationships between those systems as well as relationships within them. Further, the two participants are less likely to have an accurate knowledge of each other's histories and expectations about self–world and individual–systems relationships. They must negotiate how to inform each other. For them the task of defining a mutually agreeable ecosystem for interacting is a complex and potentially perilous task.

In either case, the traditional assumption is that the therapist's understanding of these issues, in general, represents the competencies and social realities of the ecosystem within which the client must work out his or her difficulties. Further, it is ordinarily assumed that the therapist is an effectively functioning person who holds as basic values the tenets of the ethnic ecosystem. As a consequence it is assumed that the therapist can and will to some extent educate the client about appropriate self, self–world, and coping styles. Nevertheless, when a client begins to examine self, self–world relationships, and coping styles in terms of the principles of the ethnic ecosystem, those conceptions of authority and power must be renegotiated, and the therapist must begin to learn from the client. In fact, if he or she does not, the interaction will break down as it will not permit resolving conflicts between their respective ecosystems.

The Individual as a Psychologically Autonomous Unit in the Ecosystem

As we focus directly on the interaction between a client and a therapist as embodiments of two distinct ecosystems, it may seem contradictory to focus on the autonomy of each individual in his or her ecosystem. We think not. Let us illustrate with a rather farfetched example from a different realm. There are a variety of ways to drive an automobile, but there are certain general requirements that must be met to drive successfully. Even so, those basic requirements may vary depending on the construction of the car and the nature of the environment in which one is driving. If a person who is trying to teach another how to drive is seated in the same car during this process, the major constraints on effective interaction are their different styles of complex skill acquisition and the compatibility of the teacher–student interaction. But, if the teacher is driving an automatic shift, rear-wheel drive Buick and the student is driving a manual shift, front-wheel drive Toyota, then the ecosystem of each is somewhat different. If we add to these complications that the teacher is in Great Britain communicating by telephone with a student in the United States, then the ecosystem characteristics become even more different. The control mechanisms of one car will be a mirror image of those in the other. One driver will be oriented to driving on the left side of the road, the other to driving on the right side of the road. For our illustration to be even more appropriate we need to assume that these ecological realities are not visibly evident nor are both parties necessarily aware of them. The psychosocial ecosystem that each of us embodies usually is not directly visible. We may not know just what the other person's ecosystem is like; in fact, in most instances we have only a vague notion of its character. We often do not even know how our own ecosystem is embodied in us. In other words, our respective ecosystems may well be as different as those represented in this example.

As a more directly relevant example, let us consider the situation of a young white man whose childhood traumas had been orchestrated by his overcontrolling, unpredictable, and harshly judgmental father. He was assigned to a slightly older white male therapist. The therapist's childhood traumas had been orchestrated by his overcontrolling, unpredictable, and harshly judgmental mother. They were from similar lower-middle-class backgrounds. The therapist had survived and escaped by immersing himself in his schoolwork. The client had retreated into himself to the extent of social withdrawal and an increasingly uncertain sense of his own identity. The therapist sought to help this client understand himself in relation to his family life. The success of that task rested to a great extent on the client forming a clear "reality-based" picture of his family. He had to make some decisions about the nature of that family ecosystem that he was willing to accept as a basis for defining and eventually redefining his own life. He had to exercise some psychosocial autonomy about the nature of that ecosystem, his role in it, and its impact on him.

The therapist recalled his own family ecosystem as a way of beginning to understand the client's struggles. Some of his experiences served as a valuable guide, but the shift from thinking in terms of the dynamics of a destructive mother to the dynamics of a destructive father is complex. The therapist of necessity drew on his own experiences in trying to understand this young man and help him create a coherent sense of his (the client's) history and psychosocial nature. That task required him to reexamine the picture he had of his own psychosocial nature and ecosystem and reconsider its adequacy.

The Individual Interacting with Others

As we have already noted, when we interact with others our ecosystems and theirs become part of that interaction. Gibbs (1980) has pointed out a vital dimension on which black and white ecosystems may differ in ways that can make a crucial difference in efforts to form a therapeutic relationship. She has noted that within the dominant (white) culture, the formation of a professional relationship traditionally rests on the mutual acceptance by the therapist and the client of the therapist's professional credentials validating his or her competence. In contrast, the black client, particularly if that client does not associate himself or herself with middle-class values, may be more inclined to see professional credentials as weapons of unresponsive power and privilege. Such a client is looking for informal indicators of empathy and concern, of warmth and genuineness. It is those indicators that convey to the black client that this therapist will not use his or her formal ecosystem characteristics to deny that client's reality and its expression even when it is hostile and angry toward whites and white oppression. It is vital that the therapist conveys that he or she accepts the black client and that client's view of the ecology. Only then can the client begin to form a new ecosystem in which the therapist can be seen as potentially benign and trustworthy.

Yet even that first step may not provide a sufficient basis for interacting. For example, some black clients live in ecosystems in which their senses of self-efficacy and trustworthiness rest on demonstrating a shared distrust of whites. A black student may feel that he or she could trust a white therapist yet say, "If my friends find out that I have gone to a white therapist, they will swear that I have sold out and will reject me." That same student may feel and say, "I know that I can trust you, but I can't afford to do that. If I trust you I might be tempted to trust another white person and that's too dangerous." The therapist who responds to those concerns as personal deficits of the client or as manifestations of interpersonal conflict, rather than as part of the client's psychosocial reality, is conveying that he or she endorses an ecosystem that ignores or denies the psychosocial reality of the black student.

In an earlier section, mention was made of Elli, a Middle Eastern woman. Her approach to the therapist was characterized by repeated testing, and it eventually became clear that part of her motivation for doing so grew out of the conflicts in her family's ecosystem. She was a college student in a university in the United States who was a third-generation descendant of a Middle Eastern family. Her therapist was one of the authors. Elli's life experience in her family and ethnic group reflected excessively demanding personal compromises, disillusionment, unhappiness, and hypocrisy among the older generations. Her community's elders disliked, lied, and cheated on each other in the service of maintaining an appearance of ethnic solidarity. Her parents seemed particular embodiments of this type of life pattern.

She approached therapy with deep ambivalence. She was also approaching graduation and was frightened that she would ruin her college career at the last moment by some self-destructive act as she had ruined previous undertakings. She felt strongly the need for some protection from her self-destructive impulses. At the same time she believed that all older people were untrustworthy.

The characteristics of the therapist that were both frightening and important to her were his sex, his age, his ethnicity as an Anglo member of society, his openness about his own imperfections, and his belief that his life had some integrity to it. Once she began to decide that the therapist was somewhat genuine, she began to test whether he as an individual and a representative of his ecosystem was going to condemn her as an unworthy human because of her ethnic group membership, her frustration and conflict as she sought to relate to the different worlds of her past heritage and of the future she wanted, her self-destructive behavior, or her active heterosexuality.

One of those perspectives that was particularly relevant in the building of this relationship was the age discrepancy. In more traditional societies such as those in the Middle East, high value is placed on the wisdom of older members of the community. In modern U.S. society, people, including therapists, are accustomed to seeing their perspectives devalued as they grow older. Thus, a convergent ecosystem in which this pair could work required accepting that divergence and turning it to therapeutic purposes.

Convergence

Ecosystem convergence can occur along many dimensions, but it is inherently going to be incomplete even in the lives of identical twins. Besides, one twin is not likely to be a therapist for the other. The reality of approaching a therapist–client relationship itself creates a picture of diverse realities, that of the helper and that of the helpee. Yet, on other dimensions, the realities of the therapist and of the client may be quite similar or quite different. Convergence and the grounds for easy convergence seem most likely in circumstances in which the two people involved do have common ethnic/racial backgrounds.

The prototypical pair in the history of psychotherapy in the United States has involved two white people with middle- or upper-middle-class backgrounds or aspirations. The client may even have read about therapy and heard others talk about therapy. Thus he or she is socialized into a perspective of expecting a particular type of relationship. When the client walks into the therapy room or is greeted in the waiting room, the person who says "I am your therapist" is someone who looks and acts like the people in the client's ecosystem. A young woman going to a campus counseling center may be greeted by a middle-aged woman who dresses like, looks like, and acts like that young woman's mother and her mother's friends and acquaintances. She has reason to feel she is still in a familiar world whose rules she knows. In reality a major aspect of her therapy may be learning that the therapist does not embody that familiar ecosystem, that underneath those superficial similarities the therapist embodies a quite different ecosystem and view of the world.

A young black woman coming to that same counseling center and being greeted by that therapist may find a more limited basis for convergence. Perhaps the primary ecosystem convergences will stem from her experience that older women have proven to be warm and supportive figures and guidance counselors have been helpful in the school systems she has known. Her conduct is likely, perhaps even without her awareness, to be guided by those cues. If the therapist's conduct confirms those expectations, then a basis of a convergent ecosystem (American middle class) can function to guide their interactions.

Another client who comes to that counseling center and is referred to that same therapist may be a young white male. As with the young white woman his ethnic/racial background provides him many ecosystem similarities with the therapist. She may represent the manners and modes of his mother and other middle-aged women from his home town, including teachers and counselors. However conflicted he may feel about that ecosystem, it is familiar to him. It provides a basis for convergence.

If the client who comes into that center is a young black male, then he and the therapist are not going to find ecosystem convergence on racial grounds. Nevertheless, as was the situation with the young black woman, he may share with the therapist a sense of being a middle-class American and of having had middle-aged women as supportive teachers and counselors.

Divergence

People's ecosystems also differ on many dimensions. Those differences also are factors in our interactions whether we are conscious of them or not. For example, the four young people we just described who were referred to the white middle-aged female therapist at the counseling center had divergent as well as convergent ecosystem relationships to that therapist. The young white female client had a quite divergent view of appropriate dating styles from that of the therapist, divergences reflecting a generation gap within an otherwise homogeneous white middle-class ecosystem. The young black female client had a markedly divergent view from that of the therapist of the benevolence and trustworthiness of white female professionals. The young white male client had a divergent view from that of the therapist of the benevolence and trustworthiness of white females—professional or not. The young black male client had a divergent view from that of the therapist of the competence of whites and of females. The point is that whether the issues are those of competence, benevolence, or trustworthiness, those issues guide the discrepant bases of interaction for the therapist and client. They diverge on grounds that may have little to do with their personal characteristics, but which are products of their ethnic heritages and the attributes characteristically associated with their heritages. Those divergences can be considered to be prejudices only if they are not open to new evidence. Even so, it behooves therapists to keep in mind that it is not enough that they may have transcended some of the limitations of their own ethnic heritage. They must also be sensitive to the reality that others, clients in particular, do not know that. Further, the burden of understanding and accommodating to that reality can more properly fall primarily on the therapist than on the client.

Conflict

It is in the realm of the conflicts between ethnic ecosystems that most has been written. The underlying theme expressed is that enculturation and socialization within nonoverlapping and/or conflicting racial or ethnic realities or ecosystems produce people whose realities must conflict and be mutually incomprehensible. It is only from a perspective such as that of transcendism that it becomes believable that people can both be products of incompatible ecosystems and find areas of convergence. However, before looking at the possibilities of convergence, we must first look at the realities of conflict.

Again, let us provide an example to illustrate our point. The young black woman who walks into the counseling center and finds herself facing a middle-aged white female therapist may well be confronting a conflicting ecosystem. Her therapist may view black females as academically inferior, impolite, lazy, and demanding. She may feel that it is her obligation to work with this young woman and help her accept her limitations. The student may have been socialized and enculturated to feel that her personal conflicts stem from the prejudices of whites such as the therapist and that there is no way she can expect to sort out her feelings and identity by talking with a white woman, therapist or not.

The young white woman may have been socialized in a context in which women did not assume professional roles and in which those women who did so were assumed to be sexless and ineffectual. Her goal in coming to therapy has been her desire to understand her inability to form warm emotional relationships with men. The therapist may have struggled under hostile conditions to establish her professional competence and believe that young college women who assign highest priority to their capability of forming warm emotional heterosexual relationships are betraying their own integrity. From her perspective the young woman's goal is self-defeating, not self-fulfilling.

The young black man may be seeking some support in his struggle to define for himself a sense of positive self-worth and self-efficacy. He may have a past in which it was categorically asserted that white women can see nothing positive in black men. As he looks at the woman who is saying she is going to be his therapist, he is looking at the embodied conviction that his search must fail. Here is a woman who can only see his inadequacies and confirm his worst fears. The white woman therapist may have been socialized in the tradition that blacks, particularly black men, expect women to support them while they indulge themselves. In her ecosystem, black men are not inferior, they are lazy, and they need to stand up for themselves.

These different patterns require different resolutions. They also need further elaborations of how they become part of the process of forming therapeutic relationships. What has been developed up to this point just touches on that process. The focus in the next section is on the process of forming a therapeutic relationship.

Forming a Therapeutic Relationship

Forming a therapeutic relationship involves creating a new shared ecosystem within which the two people involved can form a professional/personal relationship that they can use therapeutically. The therapeutic use of that relationship is going to be tested and extended (or contracted) by the way in which the therapist and the client negotiate the issues that arise in therapy. For the moment though our focus is on the forming of a relationship that will enable them to meet with the shared thought that "We can use some of our time and energy to explore other issues. Our primary concern is no longer the task of establishing a basis for working together."

The Individual as a Psychologically Autonomous Unit in the Ecosystem

It may seem strange to begin a section on forming relationships by reasserting the autonomy of each individual, but we think it is important to keep that perspective in mind.

One of the authors worked with a black female graduate student whom we will call Anita. He and the students working with him thought it would be difficult for him to establish a trusting relationship with her. In the first session he structured therapy in a fairly typical manner. He began the process of creating a therapeutic ecosystem within which he and the client would build a working relationship. She very quickly responded with amazing frankness, describing details of her sexual life and of participation in illegal activities. The therapist's reaction was that her manner of response signalled something other than the formation of a relationship within which such disclosures are appropriate. In other words, he exercised his autonomy within the new therapeutic ecosystem he had just described as an essential component of their working together successfully. He reacted by thinking that neither her previous cultural, institutional, and personal experiences, nor her 30 minutes of interaction with him, provided adequate grounds for sharing these particular aspects of her life so quickly.

Rather, the therapist formed some alternative hypotheses about how Anita functioned in relationship to herself as well as in relation to others. Specifically, each of us sorts or categorizes our experiences and thoughts into those we consider to be personal and private and those we consider to be in some sense social and potentially shareable with others. No matter how intimate our relationship is with someone (how extensive our shared ecosystem is), we retain a domain of privacy and autonomy. We count on others doing the same. We reject the idea that we can assume full responsibility for another person's existence. We even say to others, "I can't live your life for you." In this instance the therapist began to hypothesize that this client had not learned how to form a constructive and sustaining sense of her autonomy. What she seemed to be saying was the following: "When I am with someone else, I assign to that person total responsibility for defining who I am and for providing for my welfare."

The therapist decided that an important therapeutic goal in working with this client was one of encouraging her to develop a sense of responsibility for her autonomy. For example, if she would disagree with him about a suggested interpretation of some thought or action on her part or the part of someone else, that would be an indication that she felt capable of asserting her independent existence in the therapeutic relationship. If she would indicate that she took an independent stance in some other situation, that too would be an indication of her capability of acting autonomously to define and sustain herself.

He supported her continuing to talk about the issues that concerned her. However, in his responses to that material he paid particular attention to asking about her role in taking responsibility for her decisions. It was some 2 months later that the client first described taking responsibility for her role in a relationship. She began a therapy session by announcing that she had been shopping during the past week and had found the salesman to be pleasant and friendly. She noted that he was a recent high-school graduate and consequently at least 6 years younger than she. She then described how she had decided that she would like to become better acquainted with him, become his friend, and encourage him to go to college. She told him so, indicated the kind of relationship she wanted, gave him her telephone number, and encouraged him to call her.

The therapist had also been encouraging her to put his (the therapist's) comments in perspective. When he offered a possible interpretation to her, he was careful to stress that she needed to decide whether it rang true for her. After the incident reported above and a number of others in which she reported assuming a similar kind of responsibility for herself, the therapist asked her to begin exploring the nature of her relationship with him. He asked again how their race, sex, and age differences influenced their interaction. (He had asked in the first session whether his being white, male, and somewhat older presented problems for her in working with him as her therapist. At that time she had simply said that it made no difference.) At this later point she talked about race, sex, and age as relevant characteristics in herself and in those she interacted with in her life.

The therapist now began to feel that they could build a relationship. They could begin to create a shared ecosystem. He was now recognized by her as a person with certain ethnic and personal characteristics. She had acknowledged herself and him as people who had both a personal identity and an ethnic identity.

In contrast, in working with Elli, the young Middle Eastern woman mentioned earlier, the same therapist felt a different set of constraints in forming a shared ecosystem with her. To her it was important that he was an older white male who lived with some integrity and had some positive and genuine relationships. To him that meant that the only identity he could have in a shared ecosystem was one of idealized perfect fantasy figure. In short, he could not be a real human being. A turning point came one day when she was caught up in her distress over a fight between her parents. She asked her therapist whether he ever had arguments with his wife and he said yes. That response was not followed by distance or further testing on her part. Rather it was followed by her exploring further what had been genuine in her previous relationships. She had always abandoned such relationships under parental pressure when her parents learned about them, out of fear that they would find out about them, or out of fear that those relationships would succeed and she would have to continue them. She also began speculating about how to form genuine relationships, what they are like, and how to sustain them. At this point the therapist began to believe that he could be a person in a shared ecosystem with her. He could now believe that they had a basis for a therapeutic relationship and, in fact, had established one.

The Individual Interacting with Others

At some point a therapist or client begins to believe that his or her identity, personal and ethnic, is at least somewhat acceptable within the ethnic ecosystem of the other member of the therapeutic dyad. Or perhaps that person merely begins to wonder whether he or she is acceptable. In either case, at that point the question becomes part of the therapeutic interaction.

Convergence

The conception of convergence, which we believe is important to explore and understand, is different from more traditional perspectives concerning the nature of a desirable therapeutic relationship. More traditionally it is asserted that the therapeutic relationship should be established devoid of any considerations about the feelings of the two participants toward each other and their respective psychosocial realities. In particular the therapist is admonished to avoid forming any kind of countertransference feelings toward the client. From an EVM perspective, we believe that destructive countertransference elements can be avoided only by acknowledging the presence of bases for them. It is essential to acknowledge with a client that, for example, we are both black or white or Asian, both male or female, or as a male and female we have in common our interest in and frustrations about ever understanding the opposite sex, or as a black and a white we are both desirous of relating to others on some basis other than race.

At the risk of being repetitive, we think it is important to emphasize that we encounter each other as representatives of ethnic ecosystems. We then proceed to explore the ways in which we can relate. We seek to find areas of convergence of a kind that assures us that we can place some trust in each other, feel some hope that our relationship can produce benign outcomes, and have some expectation that we can work together productively. As therapists we may speak of our search for convergence as the determination of how much ego strength the client has. We may articulate only our assessment of the strength of the client's defenses. In either case we seem to be focusing on finding out how much and in what ways we can trust our clients. Our clients are engaged in asking a comparable set of questions about the strengths, limitations, and trustworthiness of us, their therapists.

Again, let us turn to an example to illustrate the ecosystem and individual factors involved in the interactive process of establishing a convergent basis for a therapeutic relationship. Meagan, a white woman graduate student in her early thirties was referred to a white male therapist in his early sixties who was working in a counseling center. She was completing her Ph.D. while employed as a social science teacher in a nearby high school. She sought therapy because of her inability to study for her graduate courses and because of her more general depression, which had been precipitated in part by the recent breakup of a close friendship.

In their first session the therapist inquired whether she felt comfortable working with him as an older male therapist and what, if any, particular issues their age and sex differences might present for her. She indicated that she did not see those differences as a problem, and that she was totally immobilized and did not know what to do about it. She also said that she was not optimistic about the possibility that therapy could help but that it was the only recourse she could think of. She asked if the therapist believed that therapy would help her. He indicated that he could not guarantee a positive outcome but thought there was that possibility and was indeed willing to work with her toward that end.

The therapist decided that enabling her to find some way of functioning competently, no matter how limited, was the best way of building a relationship and increasing her hopes that she could begin to deal with her own life again. He asked what she would like to work on, and she focused quickly on her sense of immobilization on weekends. She was living by herself in an apartment. Her mother and two siblings lived in the same metropolitan area,. She had been reared as a Catholic but was no longer active in the church. She spent her summers with her personal friends, most of whom were members of a semiprofessional softball team on which she was a player, but they lived (and the team played) in a city about 600 miles away where she had previously taught and gone to college. The recent friendship rupture had occurred when one of those teammate friends had stopped for a visit while passing through the metropolitan area. The client had very ambivalent relationships with her family and no close personal ties on her job, in her graduate program, or in the area. She was indeed alone and was feeling her loneliness quite acutely. She discussed all of these ties when asked about the emptiness of her weekends but did not see in them any hope or potential for lifting her assessment of hopelessness, her assessment that she was totally inefficacious.

The therapist suggested that the client describe a day on a weekend, a day at school, or an evening in classes at the university. He would respond to those descriptions by indicating their value in helping her and him to have a basis for considering the nature of their significance, other meanings they might have, and other options they might offer. After several sessions and considerable probing by the therapist, she began to explore the possibility of finding some favorable prospects in her life at school. As it turned out, very tentative efforts on her part such as speaking to her colleagues produced warm friendly responses.

She began to arrive at her therapy appointments somewhat less overtly depressed. Nevertheless, she retained her dominant orientation that her situation remained essentially hopeless. The therapist kept to his focus of engaging her in a collaborative exploration of any topic, incident, or interaction she mentioned.

She began to talk about her childhood, her family, her socialization in parochial schools, and her relation to the church. Her parents had espoused strict Catholic morality for their children but drank heavily every evening and fought constantly. The client was a good student, a good athlete, and a good daughter. Nevertheless, she was harshly criticized, while a brother near her age was indulged. Her parents, particularly her mother, were concerned about her interest in athletics as not sexually appropriate and also concerned that her daughter might not be a good girl if she dated boys. These concerns were echoed by the nuns in the school setting.

As we discussed these topics, we explored particular incidents and the question of whether she could have met the conflicting standards imposed on her. We also talked about whether it was all right for her to feel angry, resentful, and confused. The therapist consistently refused to endorse their condemnation of her and her consequent condemnation of herself. Rather, the therapist continued to accept her and even suggest that she had as much right as they to set up standards for judging her and her conduct. Those discussions led to consideration of the possibility that she could even use her own standards as a guide for leading her life.

It was at about this point in her therapy sessions that she began to report having good days in her life. She began also to take a more active role in the sessions and in managing her own life on a day-to-day basis. She later reported that it was at about this time that she began to believe that the approach we were taking in therapy was being useful and she even began to want to come to therapy. She began to want to talk about her problems and try to work them out.

What had happened? We had built at least a tentative relationship. What were the factors on which we had converged? In retrospect and with the knowledge of the issues she subsequently explored, it seems more evident what her central concern was. She had feared initially that the therapist would condemn her or judge her as inadequate as others had done. She slowly came to believe that he would accept her as she was and help her understand and live with herself as well as with the world. As her trust in the relationship began to grow, she began to discuss more central (and frightening) issues. She was neither rejected nor condemned. Consequently she moved on to other issues and began to feel more hope than dread about facing her conflicts and working out ways to deal with them. She had formed a convergent base for a relationship by interacting with the therapist and testing out its possibilities.

Divergence

One aspect of relating to another person is the acceptance of differences and the capacity to put them into perspective. An instance of the importance of identifying and accepting diversity arose in the therapy of Meagan, the female graduate student mentioned above. She presented to her therapist a problem area in which it was necessary for the therapist to work within a framework of diversity. The client's orientation to life was firmly imbedded in her religious heritage. It was not one that the therapist endorsed; in fact, he disagreed with some of its beliefs. Yet he did not believe that it was appropriate to require the client to accept his value stances. He did think that it was important to inform her that he was not a Catholic and so did not necessarily endorse those views. He also indicated that he did not consider it his right to impose his values on her. The therapist indicated, for example, that it seemed appropriate to him that she or anyone could take some personal responsibility for and exercise some latitude in formulating a personal code of morality. From that perspective he said that what he could and would do was to help her clarify her views and explore options with her for thinking about relevant value issues, then she could decide for herself and he would respect her decision. In this way the therapist's modeling of a way to deal with divergence provided Meagan a way to work out her own difficulties with others in her life.

Conflict

Often in interactions between a therapist and a client there are simply incompatible views. For a productive therapeutic relationship to be established, the members of that dyad must work out a way to disagree and accept that reality without that reality disrupting their relationship. One of the authors was the therapist for a first-generation Chinese woman, Li, who was a graduate student. Her grades were not high enough for her to be granted the degree she sought, and she was having trouble concentrating on her studies. In addition, she was dating and wanted to marry a Chinese man of lower status than that of her family. They disapproved. Li was in conflict with her teachers and her parents. She felt her academic performance was adequate overall and she was being unfairly penalized. She did acknowledge that some of her performances had been substandard. Her father, who had a Ph.D., was unhappy with her grades; her mother was unhappy because her daughter was not an obedient daughter. In the client's eyes, her boyfriend was her only ally.

In the first session the therapist indicated that he could not tell her what her feelings were, nor could he be the judge of the validity of her point of view. He could suggest and explore alternatives with her and help her sort out the potential costs and benefits to various courses of action she might take. He asked whether their racial, ethnic, age, and sex differences posed any problems for her in establishing a therapeutic relationship. She dismissed those differences as irrelevant but insisted that she needed some answers from the therapist and asked whether she should return for additional sessions. The therapist explained that he could not make that decision for her but felt there was a possibility that therapy could be of value to her. She repeated her question and the session finally ended with the understanding that the therapist would keep the appointment open for her for a week while she decided whether to return. At that point the therapist could see no substantial grounds for thinking that Li could take substantial steps to build a shared ecosystem with him or to define either him or her in relation to each other in that framework.

She did return the next week and for several weeks thereafter with little appreciable change in the pattern of interaction. She would explode and spew forth her frustrations of the week and her overall fury that neither her parents nor her teachers would bend to her will and validate her and everything about her. She would demand validation for her perspectives or answers as to what she should do. The therapist would reiterate that he could provide neither, and would then ask whether she could consider other perspectives in regard to the behavior of her parents or her teachers, or other alternatives to her own conduct. She would then announce her angry convictions that nothing would work anyway so there was no point in trying. He would ask about her feelings and she would deny having any. She would demand to know whether she should return the next week. He would repeat his position, the hour would be left open, and she would return.

Despite this surface stalemate, Li did begin to respond selectively to the content of the therapeutic interactions. She remained in therapy for a semester. During that time she traveled with her family to a neighboring state to visit with her father's brother and her terminally ill grandmother who was living with him. She was given her grandmother's blessing for her forthcoming wedding and encouraged by her uncle to accept the way her parents were changing, allow them more time to change, and quit fighting with them. She got into a fight with them on the return trip but did not completely destroy the gains that had been made. She also held her academic performance together satisfactorily during that semester and maintained constructive relations with her graduate faculty.

By the final therapy session she had come to acknowledge that she now had a somewhat limited shared relationship with her parents and that it might endure without a complete rupture. She had come to believe that she might be able to build and sustain a relationship with them by accepting that they had and would continue to have a different world view from hers. She was also coming to believe that they might accept her and her life view, though they would never endorse it as superior to their own. She was beginning to have some disagreements with her boyfriend, but thought that her emerging acceptance of diversity might also provide a basis for continuing their relationship. She even acknowledged that the therapy sessions had been of some value but saw no reason to continue them, given that her life now had some positive direction to it.

Did this client and therapist ever form a relationship? The answer to that question is *no* if your criteria include overt expressions of any positive ties or validation by the client of the humanity, identity, or perspective of the therapist. Yet at some point the client came to trust the therapist and his perspectives and to act on that trust. She came to trust that the therapist could function without (and would not demand of her that she make) a permanent commitment to a course of therapy. She came to trust that she could blame the therapist for anything and everything and he would not get angry or fight back. She came to accept that the therapist would not take the responsibility for her life nor would he pass judgment on her, her parents, or the others in her life. She came to accept that the therapist could accept conflict in a relationship and build beyond that conflict. He could also accept that conflict and still accept himself. Whether she attributed any of those characteristics to the therapist's ethnicity, age, sex, professional training, or personal qualities she never said. In fact, she never even acknowledged, at least to the therapist, that she trusted the therapist or those characteristics. For that matter, she may not have acknowledged it to herself. Nevertheless, at some point during the course of the therapy she began to act on that trust. The therapist became aware of that trust because she kept coming to her appointments and she began to change in accordance with her changing views. It would be nice to report that the therapist knew when those changes began to take place. Unfortunately he does not; he saw no obvious signs. Yet, in retrospect, it seems evident that out of the conflicts between them they built a relationship and it was therapeutic, even though it may have led only to limited gains in the client's capacity to deal with her life and relationships.

7

Sustaining and Utilizing a Relationship

The Ecology of Therapy and Its Participants

Background

In the previous chapter we noted that when we think in terms of human ecology we are trying to encompass the totality of relations between people and their environments, internal and external. Our central theme throughout this chapter will be that ecosystem realities continue as part of the interaction between the individuals involved in sustaining and using a therapeutic relationship. The therapist and the client form a new, somewhat unique ecosystem as the basis for having a constructive therapeutic exchange. Nevertheless, their new relationship will exist in and embody the context of their own ethnic ecosystems and the relationship between those systems. For that reason we begin this chapter by sketching out the general nature of our involvement in sustaining and using relationships in our lives quite independently of the therapeutic context.

The Individual as a Psychologically Autonomous Unit in the Ecosystem

Each of us possesses at least some capability of changing our relationship to our ecosystem or changing that ecosystem. We may change that relationship by changing our understanding of it, that is, by changing our internal reality. We may also change it by changing our pattern of interaction with it, that is, by changing the reality of our self–world relationships. We may also change our external reality itself. We may change that ecosystem by modifying it physically, as when we remodel our home or move the furniture around in a room. We may also change it by influencing people in it. We may inform someone that we wish to be treated differently or to have a different relationship with that person. To the extent that we are persuasive and they change their way of relating to us we have changed our ecosystem. These possibilities and realities of changing the internal and external characteristics of our ecosystems are relevant during ongoing relationships as well as in the forming and dissolving of relationships. Nevertheless, we are more likely to be inattentive to them while we are in a relationship. In other words, we tend to assume that once a relationship is formed it stays formed in some unchanging fashion. We do not think of it as constantly being strengthened, weakened, or just modified. Yet it is.

The Individual Interacting with Self and Others

As we live our lives, we continue to affirm or change our selves and our reality by the ways in which we interpret self-mediated events in our lives. We also reinterpret and restructure our internal interpreting and mediating structures and processes. At the same time we are reinterpreting and restructuring ourselves as a function of our interactions with others. We acknowledge our psychosocial nature by continuing to sort out which parts of it are psychological (coming from us uniquely) and which parts are social (coming of necessity from the nature of our external world and our interactions with it).

Convergence

Convergence is an interactive process even when it occurs within an individual. Each of us has a history of experiences involving relationships with others. Further, each of us has expectations and standards concerning our own way of thinking about, guiding, and judging our feelings and conduct in a relationship. Consequently, during a relationship each of us can and does assess our contribution to that relationship and its meaning to us. That is an internal process whose nature stems from our past history with ourselves and others.

In a dyadic relationship we also monitor ourselves, the other participant, and the relationship in terms of what we see as the perspective and contribution of the other participant. For example, in the preceding chapter we mentioned Elli, a young woman who went on food binges. She learned from a friend during her freshman year in college to induce vomiting after an eating binge to control her weight. That behavior confirmed her internal sense of herself as lacking self-discipline, but it also provided her with verification that she could continue to escape the consequences of her behavior. Interpersonally, the convergent outcomes were also mixed. The sharing by her friend strengthened her feeling that she and her friend could accept each others' limitations. It confirmed her fear that her friend would not protect her from her self-destructiveness, but rather would aid and abet it. In other words, in this instance convergence for Elli involved her confirmation of her own internal nature, of her friend's nature, and of her sense of her relationship with her friend. That convergence included confirming some negative as well as some positive aspects of herself, her friend, and their relationship. Finally, all of those convergences stemmed from an *interactive* process of comparing experiences with expectations about herself or about her friend.

Divergence

The central issue of divergence in interactions is that the participants may want and take different things from a relationship for themselves. For example, two men may form a friendship because they both enjoy watching sports, reminiscing about earlier common military experiences, and talking about psychology. Each of them will have a sense of the relative importance in his life of those activities and of the satisfactions he gains from them. Each also has a sense of how completely his friend fulfills his expectations with regard to those activities. They may maintain their friendship while it satisfies those various expectations, as it changes in the extent to which it satisfies them, or as one man, or both, changes in the extent to which those expectations are important to him. If they change in different ways, what they invest in the relationship and take from it may become more diverse. They may continue the relationship but come to value it in increasingly different ways. Yet that process involves primarily the internal reality of each unless one or the other of them brings it to their joint attention.

However, either of these friends may begin to change his interests or his view of the way his friend relates to him, to their friendship, or to the interests they share. In that case, they are becoming more diverse in their self-perceptions, self–world perspectives, and patterns of interaction through an *interactive* process. For example, one of them may base his changes on his observation that his friend seems to be sinking into nostalgia and becoming boring. Consequently, he may decide to enlarge his focus on personal and professional growth, but retain the friendship for old times' sake.

Conflict

As noted before, convergences and divergences often command our attention less readily than do conflicts. For example, we tend to be less attentive to the kinds of divergences mentioned above unless they pass a threshold and become conflicts. That is, most of us probably dream of and hope for completely symmetrical relationships, but we know and accept that our relationships often contain asymmetrical aspects. Each and every one of us is all too familiar with what we call "the honeymoon" period of new relationships. The end of such a period, particularly in romantic relationships, can be distressing in part because it is so unexpected. It is unexpected because we are less likely during such a period to think about the changes in our symmetries and our asymmetries and in their impact on our relationships.

Let us look at a hypothetical, though probably fairly typical, example among young adult couples. The man may be interested in sports because he enjoys them, they offer relief from tension, and they provide a means of demonstrating his masculine prowess to young women. The young woman in the couple may be interested in sports because they provide a forum for witnessing and/or demonstrating to others the masculine prowess of her male partner, because they offer a chance for mixed male and female group socialization, or because they offer an opportunity for her to confirm her attractiveness to others. As long as their divergent needs are met, the reality that they are divergent and asymmetrical may not command their attention. Yet as their relationship continues, his pattern of sports involvement may become more sedentary and spectator oriented so that he spends numerous evenings and weekends watching sports on television. Sports now provide him recreation and a vicarious sense of participation but no longer involve any social component. Her interest wanes since that social component was far more central to her interest in sports. Sports have become a source of conflict rather than a shared interest that had met divergent needs for the two of them.

Each of them may have changed in their interest in sports and see those changes as a function of their own changing view of themselves. To the extent that they do so, their changes and resulting conflicts stem from primarily internal changes. On the other hand, the couple may have changed as a function of their changing view of their relationship. She may have come to see sports as an appropriate socializing medium for young adults but as immature for people in middle adulthood. He may increasingly have come to see sports as his only vehicle of relief from stress as he is overly committed in his work in a very competitive situation in which he can't relax with his colleagues. She now wants him to continue to meet her expectations as someone she respects and admires by changing in ways she considers more appropriate. He now wants her to continue to meet his expectations as someone who supports him and admires him in the ways he chooses to relax as well as demonstrate his prowess.

ETHNIC ECOSYSTEMS

The examples mentioned in the previous section are based on widespread human experiences. They involve the same issues that we have discussed in previous chapters. What is different is that we are now focusing on the interplay of these factors in relationships once they have been established, once the people involved have committed themselves to an ongoing tie of some kind for some set of satisfactions or purposes. The forms of these issues are not unique to any particular ethnic or cultural groups. Yet relationships become further complicated in both general and particular ways as they involve cultural and ethnic factors. In the next section we will give consideration to some of those additional factors.

The Individual as a Psychologically Autonomous Unit in the Ethnic Ecosystem

The implicit and explicit culturally and ethnically based patterns that are part of all of us continue to impact on ways in which we try to maintain, enjoy, and use relationships for any purpose. Further, each of us is continually involved in making judgments about those factors during our relationships. In this section we focus again on that autonomy.

Convergence

In this section we are going to look at the convergence of perspectives in sustaining and utilizing relationships that are formed across the gap of ethnic difference. We are going to use a hypothetical example of a relationship involving a person from a culture-defining group and a person from a non-culture-defining group to illustrate the role of ethnicities in sustaining relationships. Specifically, how do two such people relate to each other in a human egalitarian way when the heritage of one is domination and the heritage of the other is deference?

In our earlier discussion we wrote of the black male college student who had lived in a predominantly black environment. To himself, he and his environment are natural and embody issues of superiority–inferiority only as they relate to the way his world is defined by the dominant white ethnic group. We now enter into the picture a white male college student who has been reared in a predominantly white environment. He has not had to explore directly the issues of the ethnicity-based nature of his existence. He may have absorbed or rejected the ethnocentrism of others in his milieu out of his own internal reflections, out of his interactions with particular black and white people, and/or out of his unreflective immersion in the dominant society and its culture. Let us suppose that events bring these two young men together, they span the ethnic gap between them, and they form a friendship. We then face the question of how their ethnic differences will impact on how they maintain and utilize their sense of convergence, their sense of common concern for and shared life with each other.

As these two young men pursue their friendship, the young white man may do so with the expectation that his personal willingness to transcend their ethnic differences means that they can have a relationship just like he would have with another young white man. The willingness of the young black man to form a relationship may have a similar personal basis, but it has a different ethnic component. He knows that forming personal relationships across ethnic differences exposes him to rejection, not just as a person but as a non-culture-defining ethnic group member. The young white man can bring down on him the culture's sanctioned denigration of him as black as well as personal rejection.

As they continue their friendship, both will experience ethnically based sanctions. The young white man will be scorned by whites and blacks, the young black man by blacks and whites. Both of them will have to create new cross-ethnic conceptions of themselves as well as of their friendship. They may very well find their friendship rewarding and want to maintain it and extend it to involve sharing more and more of their lives. In doing so each can build on his sense of their shared caring for each other, their shared world views, their pleasant experiences together. For each of them those aspects of their interactions embody individual as well as shared convergences. In fact, one consequence of those impacts is that each of them may develop a convergent sense of sharing the slings and arrows of ethnic prejudice.

Divergence

Nevertheless, as we continue with our above example we need to attend to other facets of it as well. The young black man in that friendship will continue to have an ethnically based struggle against the external world and his own historical reservations as the friendship becomes more rewarding and fulfilling and also more risky. He has more and more to lose. For the young white man there are similar kinds of risks, but that struggle is different for the two of them.

If the relationship fails, the young white man has lost a personal friendship and perhaps little more. He retains the potential of retreating into his culturally defined superior status as a way of defending against any sense of loss if the friendship fails. On the other hand, he may have begun to define himself and his self–world relationships in terms of ethnic/racial dimensions. Thus he may come to redefine himself in terms of his perceived failure to sustain a cross-race relationship. Of course in this latter type of instance, his losses are different and do involve a sense of loss in his capacity to form cross-ethnic relationships.

The young black man, as noted above, knows that he is exposing himself to negative sanctions as a non-culture-defining ethnic group member and as an individual. He may also resort to reaffirming negative stereotypes about whites if the relationship fails. Yet that solution offers less protection to him. It can strengthen his feelings of being oppressed (of lacking the capability of self-determination) and being a victim of an oppressive group (that is, as needing to be even less trusting and hopeful about the world in which he lives). It may also add a sense of personal failure from his ineffectiveness at overcoming ethnic/racial barriers to sustain a friendship. In that sense there is divergence in how they approach, understand, and develop their friendship. There is divergence in what they can and wish to gain from that friendship, in what they have to do to sustain it, and in what they lose if their friendship founders. Further, much of that divergence is linked to their respective ethnic/racial identities and heritages.

Conflict

After the friendship of these two young men is established, it is inevitable that differences will develop. Each of them will change in different ways. Each will also have different experiences with the other's friends and families, and with the world at large. Those experiences will have explicit and implicit ethnic/racial connotations. The interpretations that each of them assigns to those experiences and his resulting responses to them will also have implicit, if not explicit, ethnic/racial elements in them. Consequently, each of them must confront those issues if their friendship is to survive and to evolve. At some point one will say something to the other that conveys the message, "you think (or did) that because you are white, (black)." That statement will signal that their ethnicity is an element in their conflict. They must then use their friendship to explore and arrive at a new understanding of their own ethnic imbeddedness for their friendship to develop. Their friendship has become a resource on which to base other changes in themselves. In this case it has become a resource that is of sufficient value that they will undertake some potentially painful explorations about their views of themselves, each other, their friendship, and the ethnic group to which each belongs. One aspect of those explorations will be largely intrapersonal. Each of them will need to undertake for himself an analysis of his own ethnicity and views of those from other ethnic backgrounds.

The Individual Interacting with Others

In the paragraphs above, the primary focus was on the contributions of and changes in the autonomous self and self–world perspectives of each of the two persons in a friendship as they maintained and used that friendship. In the following paragraphs we turn our attention to how the ethnic/racial aspects of their interactions with each other and those around them contributed to their reshaping of the ethnic/racial aspects of their self and self–world perspectives and ways of interacting.

Convergence

Let us return to the two young men, one black and one white, whose friendship we have been considering. They may have been brought together by being assigned to be roommates in a college dormitory because neither of them had indicated a preference for a roommate on his application form. To the extent that each sees himself as a person of integrity who treats others as individuals, he will react to the ethnically based surprise of their first meeting with an effort to respond to the other as an individual, not as a representative of an ethnic group. Thus they will approach each other with an interest in getting acquainted and arranging mutually satisfactory living arrangements, and with a sense of personal openness to becoming agreeable roommates and possibly friends. They will converge around those goals and expectations. To the extent that both are relatively comfortable with themselves and open to new experiences and to forming new relationships, their interactions are likely to be fairly active and direct. They can talk out living arrangements, planning for school, finding facilities and resources, and other matters in a relatively open and task-oriented manner. Those interactions will begin to build expectations that they can be friends—people with compatible lifestyles and orientations who can and do care about each other and want to share their pleasant and unpleasant experiences with life. In sum, their interacting will provide an interpersonal convergence element to their interactions and thus to the creation of an interpersonal sense of convergence and to an interpersonal rapport.

That convergence will be challenged personally and ethnically when their interacting as friends becomes evident to others. Others will respond by asking each of them how he can form a friendship with someone who is ethnically different and whether he isn't betraying his own identity by betraying his own ethnic heritage and identity. They may even be told that a choice must be made: "You can't be my friend and his too."

For these two men to remain friends and build their friendship, they must begin to acknowledge that they must confront the ethnic ecosystem aspects of their friendship. They must work out a way of maintaining their personal convergence, and they must evolve a way of converging around a shared sense of the impact of these ethnically based assaults on their relationship. Those interactions contribute directly to the interpersonal (psychosocial) aspects of their own senses of self-efficacy, self–world perspectives, and approaches to dealing with their lives.

Divergence

Each of these young men has some sense from his own observations that his ethnic heritage, black or white, and that of his friend, are different. Yet that sense of divergence has not been formed out of having experienced a cross-ethnic friendship. As they live out the experiences of their friendship, their differences of and about their ethnicity become part of their lives, their interactions, and their friendship in a new interpersonal way. Each of them is confronted with evidence that the experience of their friendship is different for his friend than it is for him.

When the family of either of them visits, it is the son's responsibility to mediate between friend and family. The family of the young black man has its own heritage of discrimination and oppression at the hands of white people. It has its own mixed feelings about the son and brother's excursion into a predominantly white university. It has its ways of relating to the young man's friends. The family of the young white man has its own heritage of ignoring, oppressing, avoiding, or interrelating with black people.

To maintain and develop their friendship, the two friends will have to understand and accept that the family-defined ethnic contexts of and goals for their friendship are distinctively different. They will both have to accept that the young black man is investing in the friendship in spite of family opposition; the young white man is investing in it with family support. They will also have to accept that the black family considers ethnic differences all important; the white family considers them to be secondary or of little or no consequence. The two friends will need to accommodate to each other's perspectives and work out a shared one, even an agreement that they will continue to assign different importances to ethnicity and respect each other's perspectives. These accommodations are interpersonally arrived at; they are psychosocial.

Conflict

As we have noted before, the potential of conflict is much more likely to command our attention. As they live together, the friends will go to their classes, relax together, form other friendships, begin dating, and otherwise immerse themselves in their college lives. They will do so in ways and with rhythms that they have formed, often unknowingly—some with personal roots and some with ethnic roots. In any case, their different paths are inevitably going to create conflicts. Those conflicts may be about such matters as when and how loud to play music in the room or what music to play. Soon the conflict over music becomes one over who personally and ethnically really understands music and what it expresses, and what that understanding (or lack of it) says about the worth of the friend and the friendship. Beyond that there are personally and ethnically conflicting styles of arguing.

For the friendship to survive, it must contain substantial mutual value and trust plus a way of coping with conflict and negotiating solutions to differences. Those intrapersonally, interpersonally, and cross-ethnically (psychosocially) based attributes will of necessity be reexamined and reshaped as a product of the friends struggling with their frustrations about their own and each other's limits and biases. In short, they will form newly based senses of self, self–world perspectives, and ways of negotiating the events in their lives. Those new perspectives will in turn change the nature of their friendship. If their resolutions extend their capacities for relating constructively to more and different kinds of experiences, then they can strengthen and extend their friendship in a variety of ways. If their resolutions restrict their capacities for dealing with diversity, they are likely to restrict and even end their friendship.

Comment

In this section we have emphasized the racial/ethnic and ecosystem aspects of relationships between individuals. It is not our intent to suggest that interpersonal relationships have no direct personal and interpersonal style elements. Of course they do. It is our intent to say that they also of necessity involve ecosystem aspects. Even if the two (or few) people involved in such a relationship want to transcend ethnic/racial concerns, the world around them will continue to intrude those concerns. Thus individuals need to be attentive to the racial/ethnic aspects of themselves and others as they maintain and participate in those relationships. They need to be more sensitive to those various levels of their identity and their lifestyle than is ordinarily the case in homogeneous ethnic/racial relationships. They also need to be more aware of the roles played by those various levels of their relationship.

Awareness of our nestedness in ethnic/racial ecosystems is essential to cross-ethnic/racial relationships. It also contributes to the quality of our lives, whether or not we are involved in such relationships. It provides us a perspective on the possibility that we and our relationships have a history and meaning and can be better understood in that context. It also provides us with the perspective that all of those "realities" can be examined and potentially we and our perception of them can be revised. The availability of different ethnic/racial ecosystems in that sense provides us with ready-made alternative ecosystems with their own meanings, forms, and strengths and limitations. Thus living in a heterogeneous society can enrich the potentialities of all of us by improving the quality of our lives and relationships. Realizing those possibilities requires an openness to self-scrutiny and a willingness to acknowledge that not only are there many realities, there are virtues and limitations in all realities—our own as well as those of others. The quality of relationships grows from how well we understand our respective strengths and limitations and negotiate the possibilities and problems they offer. Those same considerations are relevant to our understanding of therapeutic relationships, as we seek to illustrate in the following sections.

THERAPIST AND CLIENT SUSTAINING AND USING A RELATIONSHIP—A THERAPEUTIC ECOSYSTEM

A traditional assumption in the therapeutic literature is that when a therapeutic relationship has been formed or "rapport" established, that relationship is fairly pristine in its character and uncontaminated by ethnic, racial, gender, or other characteristics of the therapist. Further, to the extent that those same characteristics are seen by the client as relevant to the therapeutic interaction, they are assumed to be a function of neurotic (i.e., destructive/pathological) aspects of the client. It is not commonly assumed that the world as lived in is part of the therapeutic context or that the therapist and client embody their own worldly identities in that context. In contrast, our point of emphasis is that even within the context of an established therapeutic relationship, the therapist and client continue to embody their respective ethnic ecosystems and their roles as representatives of those systems.

The Individual as a Psychologically Autonomous Unit in the Ethnic Ecosystem

The therapist and the client embody their ethnic ecosystems and cannot completely escape them. Yet they do have some autonomy in how they identify with, survive in, or extricate themselves from that ecosystem. They have some autonomy in regard to how they shape their individual identity, their ways of relating to the world, and their ways of negotiating their life's events.

For example, one of the authors grew up in a small town in the rural Midwest in which it was customary to express oneself openly and directly (to be plain spoken) and inappropriate to impose one's lifestyle on others. Even today, after many years away from that context, after substantial advanced education and training, and after living and teaching in several cultures, he is viewed by others as relatively plain spoken. In teaching and in consulting with therapists in Colombia and in India, he experienced a substantial disjunction of perspectives. In both of those cultures, direct confrontation (plain spokenness) is considered quite inappropriate. Issues are dealt with indirectly in ordinary life and in therapy. (As he has struggled to learn to speak Spanish, the author has been quite struck by the realization that Spanish speakers use the subjunctive mood far more than do English speakers. English speakers more often couch their sentences, and thus their communications, in a declarative mood. In short, the very form of the Spanish language seems more to emphasize speaking indirectly.) On the other hand, in both Colombia and India it is expected that senior established individuals, including therapists, will provide more structure and guidance (relative to patterns in the USA) concerning how others should conduct themselves. Consequently, therapist trainees from those cultures expect more direction from this teacher/supervisor than he is willing to give.

The stylistic differences just described have held up over several years and in spite of numerous formal and informal exchanges. In short, we are not forming working relationships, we have formed them. The author continues (though not unbendingly) to be relatively more plain spoken about issues and less structuring about how others should work out solutions than his colleagues in those countries. His Colombian and Indian colleagues continue to be (though not unbendingly) less direct about issues and more structuring about how others should work out solutions. We have accommodated to each other's cultural and personal styles, but we are all still recognizable as products of the ecosystems in which we were socialized and with which we identify. Further, we retain those characteristics that distinguish us because to some extent we want to. We could change more than we do or less than we do or in different ways than we do. We select with some degree of autonomy and with the skills we have available to change or to retain aspects of ourselves.

In a similar fashion, clients utilize some discretionary choice in the therapeutic relationships they form. They are likely to shape their therapeutic relationships to suit their personal styles, after other helping relationships they have had, or in the manner of their own cultural or ethnic background expectations. For example, Li, the young Chinese American woman mentioned earlier persisted in expecting the therapist to act like a benign authority figure, but she also kept checking to see whether he was going to require that she be obedient to his expectations (e.g., that she make a long-term commitment to therapy).

Convergence

We approach working in a therapeutic relationship from our personal perspectives, from our historical ecosystem perspectives, and from our perspectives about what is legitimately involved in personal and therapeutic role relationships. Yet across all of those interlocking and interdependent layers of perspective we find converging threads for accomplishing our therapeutic tasks as a function of our relationship. We have established that we, therapist and client, have some common grounds for resolving a set of problems that beset the client.

In an earlier section we introduced the hypothetical situation of a young white woman at a predominantly black college who goes to the counseling center and is assigned to a therapist who is an older black woman who looks like her mother's housekeeper. Further, the client reminds the therapist of the young white women who discriminated against her in college. For them to establish a therapeutic relationship, the client must come to respect the therapist as a capable professional as well as the individual she is. The therapist must come to accept the client as a troubled young woman seeking help as well as a representative of white oppressive ethnicity. In other words, both of them must take some responsibility as individuals and as members of their particular racial/ethnic ecosystem to transcend their preconceived perspectives. They must work to perceive the other partner as a person with a certain identity and history who is seeking to relate to them as an individual with a certain identity and history. We often relieve the client of any such responsibility by depersonalizing the therapist and the relationship and by assigning to some diagnostic stereotype the client's unwillingness to assume the role of a responsible individual. We often relieve the therapist of responsibility by depersonalizing the relationship through labeling the client's conduct as transference and warning the therapist against countertransference.

Divergence

People do have different ways of dealing with their lives, and some of those ways are more characteristic of particular ethnic heritages and even become ways of identifying oneself. Conversely, peoples' imbeddedness in a particular ethnic heritage becomes itself a justification for particular ways of relating to events. It is difficult for most of us to accept, let alone understand, that there are very few aspects of life that need to be understood or dealt with in only one way. Nevertheless, the potential for utilizing an established relationship to influence another person rests on a capacity to understand and respect such divergences.

For example, a 17-year-old girl who had lived on the streets for some time and had a very ambivalent relationship with her parents expressed her anger over their unwillingness to accept divergence. She said, "They just say I'm immoral; they don't say that my morality is different from theirs." She also said of her own room at home, "It's not my home or my space; it's their home." Her parents would not respect her right to organize her own living space. When she tried to return home they would intrude on her space as well as on her sense of how she should define herself.

Conflict

Ecosystems incorporate quite different views about many issues, and at times they conflict. One example emerges in the turmoil of a U.S.-socialized feminist therapist confronted with a female graduate student client from Puerto Rico who was married to a Puerto Rican male. The client was struggling with her task of defining herself as a graduate student in social work in a liberally oriented university in New York City and of working out her relationship to her husband. He did not have any higher education but had, somewhat atypically for men of his cultural heritage, supported her going to graduate school. He did insist that she call home if she planned to stay for evening classes or library work. This expectation was difficult to meet at times and was also a source of conflict for the wife. She thought that his demand might be unwarranted, but she was not sure. She did not want to create more trouble and face a crumbling marriage or a demand that she leave school so she sought guidance about how to cope with her own future as well as with her marriage.

The therapist saw her own life view as a universal one, so she could not accept that there might be ethnically valid cultural divergences in marriage relationships. Rather, she was convinced beyond doubt that the requirement was utterly inappropriate and simply an expression of his "macho Latin" demands. She responded that way to the client and added a further conflict to the client's worries.

The Individual Interacting with Others

All of our vignettes in the preceding section have involved people interacting with one another. However, in them we have been focused on the autonomy of each of the people involved. We have stressed that each of them had latitude in how he or she interpreted and dealt with that situation. In the following sections we want to pick up on how the people involved interact with each other. Our focus shifts now to the potentials of and problems inherent in those interactions and particularly to the role of the ethnic characteristics and perspectives of the participants in shaping those interactions and their outcomes.

Convergence

When the young white female client and the older black female counselor have formed a relationship at even a minimal level, then they can begin to use it. The client can begin to rely on it as a basis for hearing what the therapist has to offer as insights into her conflicts and into different ways of thinking about her own role in those conflicts. She can also begin to rely on it as a basis for considering the value of trying out other approaches to her life situation.

The therapist can rely on the relationship to accomplish her focal counseling goal, that of helping the client to work out a better life for herself. She can also begin to rely on the client's expressed and exhibited respect and trust as a means of rethinking some of her own preconceptions about young white women. Further, she can rely on that relationship as evidence of her own capabilities for transcending in her professional capacity.

Divergence

Working with the young street girl to help her make sense of her life rested on respecting her space. In fact, she defined "home" as a space into which her parents could not intrude. In order for anyone to help her define how to retain her autonomy and also have relationships with people, it was first necessary that a would-be helper respect her autonomy and how she defined it. That definition (a space into which others cannot intrude) might seem to provide an untenable base for any kind of relationship, but she was going to modify it only if others could accept and respect her perspective. Further, she was going to let us enter into her space only to the extent that we could understand and adapt to what it meant to her to open that space to us and adapt to how she would go about doing so. Street youth do define their autonomy and space differently from people who have stayed within the confines of the larger society. Their bluntness, abruptness, and arbitrariness are useful survival characteristics in that ecosystem. We can ask that they respect us and our right to deal with life our way once we have demonstrated that we accept theirs. Then we can ask them to consider alternatives and even get them to try ours. We need in turn to be open to rethinking our own perspectives.

Conflict

The American feminist therapist and her Puerto Rican female client were confronted with a conflict in world views. The therapist had developed a productive therapeutic relationship with this client, but they had become stuck on this point of the client's autonomy as she attended graduate school. The therapist sought consultation because she wanted to know how to convince the client to accept the therapist's view of what was right and therefore take a stand for her autonomy as the therapist defined it.

The essential thrust of the consultative response was that several issues seemed to be involved. First, the therapist needed to examine the cultural roots of her own definition of female autonomy and her own conception of an acceptable marital relation. Second, she and the consultants might have quite different concepts from the client, from her husband, and from each other of what constitutes minimally acceptable criteria of female autonomy. That gives them no grounds for imposing their standards on this young woman. Rather, trying to do so would more likely erode the relationship the therapist had established with her client. Third, the client's husband is entitled to understanding and respect also. By the norms of his culture and his immediate reference group he has taken substantial steps to accept and support his wife's extending of her role beyond their shared cultural expectations. Fourth, the therapist may want to, and probably should, try to outline the several different perspectives that they all bring to this situation. She should also note her views and her respect for the client's and for the husband's. In effect she should convey and demonstrate that she can accept and be supportive of their agreeing to disagree and still work together. If she cannot do that then she should state her requirements for continuing to work together and be prepared to accept the dissolution of the relationship. If she can accept their conflict and work out a solution with her client that would be acceptable to the client even though not acceptable to the therapist, then they can continue to build on their relationship. Further, the client can be increasingly receptive to listening to the therapist's perspectives and possibly, though not necessarily, modifying her own. In the long run it may be that this client's marriage will not last, or that this therapeutic relationship will not last. In either case it should be because the client has arrived at those choices from her own explorations and developments, not from a forced choice brought on by the therapist's ecosystem limits.

Therapist–Client Interactions as the Interaction of Two Ecosystems

We have been describing the ecosystem aspects of interactions. We have also been highlighting how they become salient in therapy. We have been referring to examples that demonstrate the ecosystem aspects of therapeutic interactions. In this section we continue developing that theme by bringing into the picture the role of the shared ecosystem that the therapist and client form. It is that shared ecosystem that provides an essential basis for them to work together as they pursue their common goal of helping the client to find a better way of negotiating his or her life.

The Individual as a Psychologically Autonomous Unit in the Ethnic Ecosystem

Again we return to the theme that no matter what the nature or extent of a relationship, each of the participants is to some extent acting autonomously. We continue to maintain some discretion and choice about how we respond within that ecosystem.

In an earlier section we discussed Elli, the young Middle Eastern woman and her forming of a therapeutic relationship with her older white male therapist. We noted that the clearest indication that that relationship had been established was the marked shift in the client's behavior in therapy after the therapist had acknowledged that he indeed had quarrels with his wife. Elli had apparently decided that this therapy relationship provided her with an ecosystem in which it was possible to explore her behavior, her feelings, and her questions about the conduct of others in a nonjudgmental atmosphere of acceptance and respect. From then on she focused less on testing the therapist and began to focus on her role in her own conduct. She explored how she had built up responsible roles for herself in activities or on jobs and then destroyed them. She explored how she had established relationships with men whom she knew would be disapproved of by her parents and then vacillated between informing her parents and breaking off the relationships before they found out. She talked about how at times she had followed both courses of action.

The therapist also began to reevaluate their relationship and deal with it differently since it had become a somewhat shared ecosystem. He could now rely more fully on her presentations of her cultural heritage as complete and as devoid of distortions; he too turned somewhat away from testing the nature of the relationship. He decided that he could more comfortably express his thoughts, express his uncertainties concerning her culture's customs, and even probe for more background material. He could feel less trepidation about questioning the meaning of her behaviors, her explanations, or other issues. In short, they had decided to trust each other so that each could explore new perspectives, doubts, and uncertainties.

In this section we have tried to emphasize how a therapist and a client are each making choices about how to use their relationship. Each is choosing topics to discuss, ways of discussing them, and objectives to achieve by accomplishing them. Further, each of them is doing so in a nested framework of personal, interpersonal, and ethnic considerations. Finally, each of them is making those choices in a somewhat autonomous way, even though they are made in the context of an established relationship. In fact, that element of autonomy within a relationship is an essential component to its vitality and capability to be of help to the client or, for that matter, to the therapist.

The Individual Interacting with Others

In this section we look at the input into the relationship that results from therapist–client interchanges. The process of interacting has a psychosocial impact on the participants' sense of the relationship and of who they are as individuals. It is that facet of their interacting that becomes the focus in the following paragraphs.

Convergence

At this point in the previous chapter, as we talked about convergence in forming relationships, we introduced Meagan, a young white woman who was a Ph.D. student in her thirties, who was teaching high school, and who had come to the counseling center because she was depressed, disorganized, and immobilized. A central factor for her in the development of a therapeutic relationship grew from her pattern of revealing aspects of herself that she had been condemned for. Eventually she came to believe the therapist's statement that he would accept her as she was and help her live with herself and the world.

As she became more trusting she began to believe that coming to therapy was of value. She and the therapist had developed a working relationship so she was beginning to reinvest some energy in her life as teacher and student. The question was what to do with that relationship since therapeutic progress seemed limited at best. She began to turn to exploring interpersonal relations within her family, particularly male and female roles.

Eventually she began to talk about being in her early thirties, being single, and not being certain what her future life would be. Needless to say this issue was also of concern to her family. Finally she began to talk about her limited heterosexual experience. Then she acknowledged that she had been involved in a long-term lesbian relationship with a friend who was a roommate and member of the same softball team. After that relationship broke up she had become sexually involved with another woman and team member who did not want an exclusive relationship. That second woman had rejected the possibility of an exclusive relationship with this client shortly before therapy began. In fact it was that rejection that had precipitated the depression that brought the client to therapy. So finally she asked her underlying questions. Was she a lesbian? Was she condemned here as well as in the hereafter to loneliness and rejection?

It was as these issues emerged that the basis of and the commitment to the relationship became focal to whether and how she and the therapist continued to work together. The therapist had participated in stating and supporting that she had a right to define herself and how she chose to live. She had a right to question others' imposed judgments of her. The therapist believed what he had said and stayed with that position. He did not define her. He explored with her the nature of her sexual involvements and what they meant to her. She did not find men unattractive but had had only one heterosexual experience in college and that occurred when she had been drinking. She felt that she did not know whether she could form an enduring heterosexual relationship with a man. But, she was not sure that she could form personal relationships with anyone anyway.

While the exploration of these issues continued, the client did not lapse into depression again. Rather, she continued to maintain her improved pattern of functioning and to reach out to form friendships at the school where she was employed. Even so, the therapist was aware of some of their ethnically based differences in thinking about issues and how to approach them. His own heritage was that of fundamentalist Protestantism with its emphasis on self-definition and personal responsibility for one's conduct. Her Roman Catholic background had placed greater emphasis on definition of self by empowered others and on mediating judgments and consequences through them. It also seemed to emphasize duty more than choice. (These differences may seem to some to be more a function of the therapist's and the client's world views than of the ecological styles of these differing religious groups. That may be the case, but in this instance the therapist and client were at least approaching the therapy process with these different perspectives and believed them to relate to their different heritages.) As she explored alternatives she seemed to be more focused on what would be the sanctions of various courses, and the therapist on what her choices were and how she wanted to deal with handling them and their consequent outcomes.

When she returned again to the question of whether she was fatally flawed and condemned as a person, the therapist reiterated that it was up to her to decide how she wanted to think about and judge herself and explore relating to others. In essence he stayed with the position that he could accept her as she was and see her as an acceptable person the way she was.

She explored those ideas and continued to explore her own behavior. She eventually noted that society would condemn her if she publicly announced that she had lesbian sexual relations. The therapist agreed but noted that the issue was public sanction. Was it essential to her to have public sanction for everything she did? He noted that many people live with personal sexual adaptations that do not meet society's, or some segment of society's, norms. She could certainly bring down those sanctions on herself if she wished. If she did not, she could and would have a chance to work out personally and interpersonally satisfying relations with another person or a range of people. In any case, it was up to her to work out what she wanted to do and how to make sense of it.

This pattern of interaction provided a basis for convergence between Meagan and her therapist that strengthened their therapeutic relationship. It also provided a framework in which she began to widen her circle of interpersonal interactions at work and at school. She noted that she could now look forward to returning to her ball team for the summer, as she could see herself as a whole person who could both deal with her past relations with the members of the team and free herself from her fears about trying to find out what kind of life she really wanted. She could now go ahead with her life.

Divergence

In working through any series of issues with a client, it is inevitable that ecosystem differences will arise. Let us illustrate from the interactions of a black male graduate student who established a relationship with a white male therapist after much struggle and ambivalence. The student had been socialized to be totally self-contained in his relations with teachers. In graduate school he would not talk with them or ask them questions. He grasped his work assignments as well as he could, then went off to do them by himself. If he could not complete them satisfactorily he simply did not hand them in to the professor. He seldom even worked with his fellow students, most of whom were neither black nor from a blue-collar family, or fundamentalist religion.

The therapist finally felt that a working relationship had been established with the client after he angrily confronted the client with failure to keep a commitment made to the therapist. The therapist indicated that he simply could not continue to work with the client under these circumstances and would discontinue doing so if the client broke another commitment. In their next meeting the client acknowledged the legitimacy of the therapist's complaint, then indicated that he did trust the therapist and would act accordingly.

As they continued to work together the client continued to have difficulties with professors, but not with the therapist. When his unwillingness to be more direct with professors was explored, he justified it on the twin grounds that he did need to be self-sufficient and that he did not trust them. The therapist indicated that he differed with the client's justification on both counts. Namely, he challenged the validity and utility of the client's particular definition of self-sufficiency. He also questioned whether the real or perceived deficiencies in trustworthiness of professors was best handled by complete avoidance of interaction with them. The client stayed firm in his views. The therapist suggested that, since they could not agree, he would work with the client to help him develop and pursue his strategy as effectively as possible.

Unfortunately, the student's strategy was not effective, and he was dropped from his graduate program. He did maintain his relationship with his therapist and struggled with and agonized over his failure in that program. It was only then that he was willing to begin confronting his own involvement in that failure and turn to working with the therapist on changing his views as he sought to work out other career and personal alternatives.

The ongoing process nature of therapy and its flow through convergence, divergence, and conflict is important to acknowledge. Further, it is particularly evident in this example. At a critical juncture for the student, they could not have continued without the therapist offering to accept their divergence and work with it. When that approach was not successful, it was the student's convergence with the therapist on accepting the trustworthiness of their relationship that enabled him to stay in therapy and work out some of his dysfunctional behavioral style.

Conflict

Turning to the issue of conflict brings us back to the reality that there often is incompatibility between the views of the therapist and those of the client. In the example above of the black male graduate student, the therapist did get angry and confront the client with incompatibilities about their relationship. He also challenged the student's views of appropriate ways of resolving some of the client's difficulties with his professors. Their resolutions of those issues involved both convergence and divergence.

The relationship between the older white male therapist and Li, the young Chinese–American female graduate student, offers another example. As we described in the preceding chapter, their interactions involved conflicting expectations from the beginning. The client wanted answers and support of her views. Was she reflecting her Chinese ethnic heritage or her Chinese–American amalgam of two heritages? The therapist thought it was a mixture of both, plus a pattern of parent–child conflict, which she had been told had characterized her life since her preschool days.

The therapist steadfastly stuck to his position that he could only listen, suggest possibilities, and try to help her understand and work out issues and that he could not ally himself with her against others. The one issue on which the therapist was willing to work with divergent beliefs concerned her desire to see him on a meeting-to-meeting basis since she was unwilling to make a longer-term commitment to therapy. Was he reflecting his Anglo heritage, his own distinctive lifestyle, his training as a therapist, or all of the above?

Would they have had a more or less productive relationship if the therapist had been willing to adopt a therapeutic role more compatible with Chinese cultural expectations? Would they have had a more or less productive relationship if Li had been willing to make a long-term commitment to therapy? There is no way to know; we can only speculate about those possibilities. The bases for their conflicts also lie in the realm of speculation. It seems probable that there were ethnic and personal style elements in the ways both Li and her therapist interacted and interpreted the meanings of those interactions. Nevertheless, as noted earlier, their relationship did come to embody a pattern of compatible disagreements followed by compatible discussions about how to work out ways of solving problems, sorting out feelings about self and others, and maintaining or adjusting ways of trusting each other. Further, her behavior in and out of therapy did finally begin to change, and she did begin to approach issues in a less self-defeating way. This therapeutic relationship never became an idyllic one, but it became strong enough that Li and therapist could turn the hostility and conflict she expressed about therapy as well as other issues to constructive therapeutic purposes.

SUMMARY

In this chapter we have sought to write about sustaining and utilizing therapeutic relationships. We have tried to fit this discussion into a broad ethnic validity perspective. We have also sought to illustrate that the interval between forming a therapeutic relationship and terminating it is neither empty nor does it follow some automatic course. During this intermediate period both therapist and client are contributing to sustaining and/or modifying the relationship itself. They are also utilizing that relationship as a source of hope, trust, affirmation, and challenge. It provides them with an ecosystem that is a source of energy, insights, skills, practice opportunities, and other factors essential to any joint therapeutic endeavor.

Their interactions are complex, complicated, and open-ended. At least in our view it seems unjustified and inappropriate to operate on the assumption that there is a single specifiable outcome that can be known at the beginning of therapy or when a therapeutic relationship is formed. The client is not just understanding himself or herself from new perspectives; the client is in part creating as well as recreating himself or herself, his or her world, and ways of negotiating events. The therapist is not just fitting everything into a closed theoretical and procedural framework; the therapist is also creating as well as recreating perspectives and understandings at many levels. Further, the two of them are creating and recreating their relationship as they also work together, work independently, and work against each other to accomplish some of their objectives.

In sum, we need to keep in mind that therapy takes place as part of our ongoing lives, whether we are therapists or clients. And, like our ongoing lives, therapy needs continuing attention to its nested ecosystem and individual complexities, and to its survival and implementation in the service of our objectives in undertaking it. It also needs our careful and considered attention to working toward those objectives and to reviewing them as we do so.

8

Terminating a Relationship
The Ecology of Therapy and Its Participants

Background

In the preceding two chapters, we discussed the new and somewhat unique shared ecosystem that the therapist and the client form. Further, they utilize their therapeutic relationship as a way of working together to help the client resolve some personal and interpersonal confusions, difficulties, and conflicts. In the present chapter we turn to the task of concluding our therapeutic relationships. We have emphasized that we bring our ethnic ecosystems into therapy with us and that we transcend them as we build and utilize a shared ecosystem. We have been stressing that in doing so the therapist and the client are changing as individuals in a variety of ways. Now we need to look at how they have changed and how they leave each other and go ahead with their lives. Specifically, how do they return to their respective worlds? What has therapy meant to them? What does their relationship mean to them? Personally? Ethnically? What new understandings and feelings do they carry back to their own separate worlds about others from their own ecosystem and others from different ethnic/racial ecosystems?

To answer those questions we need to ask more generally what the ecosystem aspects of relationships, particularly therapeutic relationships, mean to us. Finally, we need to ask what it means to add to these considerations the reality that this particular relationship has been therapeutic in its focus. Overall, we need to ask who and what we are saying goodbye to and what doing so means to us. We need to look as well at what we are taking with us. In other contexts, Tyler (1978) has written of the importance of conceptualizing the termination of any activity as involving culminating, concluding, and redefining. Those facets of termination are central to this discussion. When we finish an activity, it is important, indeed essential, that we culminate and "celebrate our success or suffer our failure" (Tyler & Pargament, 1982). It is only by doing so that we can fully complete that activity. Simply completing it in an instrumental sense is *in*completing it. I may finish reading a book, but I am not through with it and it is not through with me until I deal with the experience of it, the feelings it has led me to—the laughing, the crying, the dreaming, the thoughts it has generated or terminated, the exhilaration or disappointment of my experience with it. Once I have culminated, then I can conclude. I can say goodbye to that book and put it on the shelf of my past experience, even if I do not want to keep it on my bookshelf. Finally, I can turn to redefining myself. Who am I now that I have completed that activity, that book? We have all read books that profoundly moved and changed us, that led us to a new place with ourselves and the world. We have redefined who we are. We have said, "If that person can do that, I can do what I want." We have said, "That's how I want to live my life," and committed ourselves to doing so. We have said, "No way," and turned from a path that previously had seemed possible and even attractive.

Those are the kinds of issues to which we attend in this chapter. We try to look at and ask about how we culminate, conclude, and redefine ourselves and our lives as we complete and move beyond therapeutic relationships. However, before asking those questions about therapeutic relationships, we are going to look at them briefly as a part of all relationships.

Terminating a Relationship

The Individual as a Psychologically Autonomous Unit in the Ecosystem

Each of us has some range of capabilities for terminating or severing our relationships with other individuals, with our families, with our communities, with our country, or with our ethnic group. We may discontinue a friendship entirely or reduce the level of closeness within it. We may seek a total separation or we may wish to terminate a particular part or aspect of a relationship. We may even wish to terminate our relationship with our nation, ethnic group, or race. However, the world at large has developed broad race-related categories that are based on physical appearance. As a consequence, physical appearance limits our possibilities for terminating our ties with at least parts of our identities, those parts that are based on physical appearance. They do so because we need to substitute another externally believable identity to gain the world's acceptance of our new self-definition as a guide to and justification of our conduct. To some extent, our autonomy with respect to defining ourselves is limited by the necessity of gaining some external validation of that new identity as well as some external validation that we have given up the old identity.

In other words, one aspect of terminating one's relationship to one's ecosystem is to establish another one. Both internally and externally we need to have a sense of who we are. We need to be able to guide and respond to ourselves within that framework, and we need to be able to communicate and sustain that sense of relationship to maintain a sense of order and direction in our own lives. A young woman, for instance, told of having just become engaged and returning with her fiancee to her home for a visit. She spoke of the "strangeness" she felt. That strangeness included her personal experience of wearing a ring and reacting to it herself. It extended outward to puzzlement and confusion over how to deal with the vastly different (from her previous visits) ways in which people reacted to her. She was simultaneously caught up in concluding her old identity and redefining herself in a new one. When she could do neither she felt very strange and confused, as we all do.

There is another facet to the activity of terminating a relationship. That facet is the meaning of the relationship. Perhaps it should be the first facet to command our attention, but it usually is not. At times, it commands very little of our attention, usually to our detriment. We often come to take relationships for granted and lose sight of their value. When their cost becomes excessive, we leave them without assessing what positive characteristics we are also losing. We have overlooked the questions of what it means to us, why we formed it, what we are using it for, how it is enriching or sustaining us, and what we have gained or lost from our investment in it. Finally, there are the questions of how we celebrate or suffer what it has added up to and how we conclude it internally as well as externally. How do we celebrate its richness? How do we mourn its pain? To some extent these questions are part of the termination of any relationship. To some extent our manner of dealing with them is shaped by our internalized sense of our ecosystem; to some extent it is also shaped by our unique individuality.

Convergence

When any of us consider terminating a relationship, we confront our individualized internal sense of who we are, what we want to do with the relationship, how we relate to the other person or persons in that relationship, and how we want to carry out the closing of this particular relationship. We also confront our internalized sense of what is expected of us and what is right and proper of us as an individual who is from, and part of, a particular ecosystem. To the extent that those perspectives converge, we have a clear and coherent perspective and set of guidelines, a relatively clearly marked map to follow in carrying out that change. In rapidly changing societies such as that of the United States in recent years, there is often a substantial discrepancy between what young people want to do in terminating romantic relationships that they have validated through marriage or some alternative ritual and what they feel is expected of them by society. More traditionally oriented young people find more convergence between their internalized personal reservations and what they know is expected. For them, there is much convergence. For young people who are breaking away from traditional conceptions of "till death do us part," there is less convergence. They know what society expects of them and they know that those expectations do not conform to their desires to terminate a currently unrewarding relationship and get on with their lives. For them, there is much less internal convergence.

Divergence

In contrast, we may find that our individualized feelings and those embodied out of our ecosystem membership are divergent. We want to hold on to the relationship a little longer or let go a little faster than our internalized conventions would advise. Perhaps we want to be more forceful or less direct than those conventions would advise. The point is that we eventually must come to terms with that discrepancy between our personalized individualized selves and our selves as guided by our ecosystem socialization and identification. That reconciliation is not necessarily a glib or superficial process. It can be a deep and difficult struggle, but it is an internal process. What we must come to terms with and tolerate, if not accept or even value, is the divergence within us. That divergence embodies the differences between what we have become and are and the ideal or norm that our ecosystem has shaped within us as to what we ought to be. There are young career women who are enjoying their lifestyle and yet face their internalized sense that it is important to become a mother before it is too late. Each of them faces divergence within herself about how she wants to deal with her various selves. She faces divergent urges about which self she wishes to say goodbye to. Further, she faces divergent urges about how she wants to say goodbye to those ways of relating to her ecosystem.

Conflict

Those various aspects of ourselves may not just have different perspectives, they may have incompatible perspectives, especially when any one of us considers terminating a relationship. There is the part of the individual that has personally completed, finished, lost interest in, given up on, or gotten furious or disgusted with the relationship. Ranged against this part of the person is the one who wants to be true to her/his ethnic self. That part is saying, for example, "This is my marriage partner, with whom I as a member of my ethnic group have an indissoluble bond. I must maintain this relationship and make it work."

Each of us has to resolve such conflicts to manage a meaningful termination of a relationship. If we are unable to resolve that internal conflict, we are trapped and will be in conflict until we can reconcile our warring internal perspectives and impulses. What we must keep in mind is that the conflict is an internal one and must be resolved there. Others may contribute to our struggle, but they can't resolve it for us. We must do that ourselves.

The Individual Interacting with Self and Others

In the preceding sections, we have been talking about the autonomy each of us has and must deal with in resolving why, whether, and how to terminate relationships. Now we move to looking at the interpersonal aspects involved in resolving those same questions. We not only have our internal dynamics as guides, monitors, and consequences of our conduct, we also have the dynamics of our interactions with others. In a relationship, the major *others* include the person or persons in the relationship with us. They also include other people in our lives and even bystanders. Nevertheless, in this section, we are going to focus primarily on the other central person(s) in the relationship. In addition, we are going to look again at our point that there are no clear delineating boundaries between our psychological selves and our social selves. We are, in inextricable ways, psychosocial, though we differentiate those components of ourselves and of our reality. In doing so we define our psychological selves and our social selves in part as a function of our own responses. We also define them as a function of the responses of others, and it is this latter perspective that is also our concern in the following section.

Convergence

In seeking to conclude a relationship with someone else we may ideally want to establish that our objective and our rationale for it are mutually shared and understood. We would like to feel that the meaning of the relationship, its benefits and costs, its forms and feelings, and the desire for, meanings of, and procedures for terminating it have been reciprocated, or at least mutually judged to be equitable. That ideal may seldom be realized or even approached. However, it is not likely to be realized at all unless there is some shared psychosocial reality and communication between the individuals involved.

For example, in the United States, we engage each spring in graduation rituals as indicators of the completion of specified educational tasks. Those rituals involve the termination of relationships between students and teachers. For most students though, what is most central to them is the termination of relationships with their classmates. The nature and forms of those student–student terminations vary at different points in their developmental and educational progression. At the time of high school graduation, many students expect to continue their lives in their home communities and consequently expect to continue their ties. At college graduation, most students know that they will not see many of their fellow students again. In either case, even among those who will see each other, their present relationship will be gone. They may sign each other's yearbooks, wish each other well, say goodbyes, or otherwise acknowledge that they are parting. They may even affirm a new bond as fellow graduates, but in doing so they know that their new relationship may never be realized. In any case, there are generally shared personal and social norms for carrying out these transitions. To the extent that two people converge on their understanding of those norms and of their relationship to each other, they can conclude their relationship and redefine themselves in a positive way. They can not only feel good about the relationship, they can feel good about who they are or who they have become in part because of it.

Divergence

The central issue of divergence is again that two of us in a relationship may want to deal with it differently. We may want to terminate it at different times or in different ways. We may differ on what we feel it has meant. We may even shape and form that divergence out of interacting with each other. The nature of the bond may be unclear to us. It is as we come to its termination, perhaps for reasons external to ourselves such as graduation and the pursuit of different careers in different places, that we bring to our shared awareness our mutual desire to define the relationship so that we can part from it. As we do, and directly or indirectly exchange thoughts, we are likely to encounter meanings that were not formed before or that were understood differently. As we do that we shape our own psychosocial sense of the relationship's meaning and perhaps crystallize that it has different meanings for the two of us. We may even come to see that we need to say goodbye in different ways and for different reasons. We come to know that we will carry different memories with us as we go different ways.

It is in the tolerance, the acceptance, perhaps even the celebration of these differences that divergence has its meaning in our relationships. It is here too that divergence has its significance in leading us to define our relationships as meaningfully asymmetrical in many ways. Here, we find the social complexity of our being and our intertwining with other people. We can come perhaps to see our separateness as part of us and of our relationships. Then, we can see that partings have their values as well as their costs. We can also see that the divergent significances that our relationships have for us and our partners are an inevitable part of our relationships and our partings.

Conflict

Again we come to the all too evident point that we are more often aware of our conflicts than our commonalities. As in the forming of relationships, we struggle to iron out conflicts so that in their termination, we struggle to seek a final triumph, sidestep a final struggle, or avoid a final defeat.

Students completing an academic career may make one final effort to be heard and affirmed as competent by professors who have steadfastly reminded them of the professors' superiority and their inadequacy. "You're still just a student" is conveyed by body language as well as words and tone of voice. Those same students may be beset from another quarter by family members who want to insert one last reminder that they could not have made it without parental genes, good will, and support. Those struggles may turn an otherwise potentially enriching and fulfilling termination of a long and difficult passage into a mutually hostile and embittering redefinition of any of these kinds of relationships. Beyond that, they may even lead to a redefinition of the entire educational process and experience as more characterized by conflict than by support.

Ethnic Ecosystems

The issues and vignettes sketched out above are quite generic. They are part and parcel of relationships in one form or another across ethnic groups and cultures. As we have stressed before, relationships inherently take on other complicating facets as they involve our efforts to relate across ethnic ecosystems. Further, those ethnically imbedded factors become particularly salient as we terminate relationships. It is at that time that we confront the possibility that "You didn't mean it after all. See, you're going back to your own." We now want to turn our attention to that issue and others associated with termination as they are contributed to by ethnic ecosystem considerations.

The Individual as a Psychologically Autonomous Unit in the Ethnic Ecosystem

Just as we develop an identity at the individual level and establish some sense of control over our identity, we do the same at the ethnic level. That ethnicity shapes how we leave relationships, and our individual way of expressing it affects our processes of terminating relationships. In this section, we are going to return again briefly to looking at the role our own autonomy plays in charting the course we take in terminating relationships.

Convergence

Here too we confront our relationships to our individual and ethnic understandings of ourselves. To cite a hypothetical example, a white male reared in the "tough" American male tradition, which prohibits the expressing of feelings or the revealing of weaknesses, has an internalized sense of how to deal personally and ethnically with his departure from a friend whom he knows he may never see again. He knows that they may joke about their good times and adventures together; they can insult each other and swear at each other; they can have a mutually and jovially aggressive party together, then they must shake hands, look each other in the eye concealing their sense of pain and impending loss, wish each other well, then turn and walk away nonchalantly.

Each of them can feel a sense of convergence within himself to the extent that he can reconcile that personal and ethnic sense within himself and manage the parting accordingly. And, as is more pertinent in the next section about interpersonal relations, to the extent that they can both manage together that pattern of parting, they will have converged psychosocially within and between themselves on their personal validity, their ethnic validity, and the validity of their relationship as an expression of their personal and ethnic heritages.

Divergence

Each of us has a sense of what is the "natural" way to part from a friendship, an intimate relationship, a business relationship, a mentor–student relationship, or a casual conversation. It is the way we and our reference group (be it our ethnic group or some other) have parted throughout our life experience. It just seems right. Then we form a relationship with someone who has a different sense of what is natural about parting. Therein lie the seeds of divergence or conflict.

One of the two young males that we mentioned in the previous section moves on to form a friendship with a South American friend he has met on his new job. They are both relatively outgoing and come to enjoy spending their free time together. They enjoy sports, like to work on cars, and spending leisurely evenings drinking and talking. They come to think of each other as good friends and even say that to each other. Then, the South American learns of family responsibilities and decides he must leave his job and life in the United States and return to his home country. Each of them responds by wanting to get together for a final farewell. The one from the United States wants to go out for an evening drinking and have a "blast" but not discuss their feelings—for him it is over. The South American wants to go out for an evening too, but he wants to talk about their friendship, even express his affection with a parting hug, and share the conviction that they will be friends for life. What they are lacking is a shared way to incorporate their different expectations into the evening. If they can each understand in himself as well as his companion that they express farewell differently and can each accept what the other's rituals convey, then they can accept their divergence. Each can in his own way feel validated.

Conflict

There may be incompatible elements in ethnic ways of saying good-bye. The above mentioned North American and South American cannot both talk about what their friendship means and not talk about it. At least, they cannot do both at the same time. The North American can say to himself and feel that the South American was a true friend only if they say farewell in the North American way. That means that the South American must transcend his ethnic limits. In contrast, the South American can return to his country feeling that the friendship was valid only if they had an expressive outpouring of their affection and agreed to be friends forever. That validation would come from the North American transcending his ethnic limits. If they clash over these differences and cannot resolve them, then each in himself will conclude the relationship with a sense of disappointment, and redefine in a more restrictive way his feelings about himself and the kinds of relationships he can have and wants to have. Further, in redefining himself he will do so in relation to his ethnic identity as well as his personal identity.

The Individual Interacting with Others

Now we turn again to the reality of how these ethnic orientations to saying farewell are affected by interactions with others. First, by interacting with others who are different, we become aware of varied orientations. Through interactions our ways progress from being *natural* to being a matter of awareness and choice. In that manner, others' acceptance or rejection verifies or invalidates our ethnicity, its worth, and ultimately our worth.

Convergence

The two young white males mentioned in the preceding section on convergence had little occasion to think about the ethnicity evident in their farewell. Yet each implicitly, if not explicitly, had his ethnicity verified and validated by the ritual of their parting. They parted with a sense of themselves as validated members of a society that was also validated as inherently good and proper.

More complexities are involved for the North American and the South American to establish convergence about their parting. Probably the first awareness that they do not *naturally* converge on how to say farewell arises when they discuss planning a farewell occasion. Since their natural rituals are not the same, they must become aware that their preferred rituals are just that, preferred rituals. They may achieve convergence by taking a collaborative approach and deciding to have a Latin-style party and a North American-style party. At a more personal level, they may part with both a handshake and an affectionate embrace. All in all, what they converge on is the realization and shared acceptance that what is central is the meaning of their parting, not the symbols of that meaning. In some sense, they both become transcultural or transethnic. In doing so they can cherish their friendship, go their separate ways, and respect their own and each other's ethnicity as well as individuality.

Divergence

Ethnic differences lead to different patterns of departure, yet even within an ethnic heritage there are differences and varying degrees of tolerance or acceptance of that diversity by each individual. A typical example of the differences within an ethnic heritage can serve to illustrate the issues of cross-ethnic divergence. A white male college senior from a rural blue-collar background who has been successful academically, in campus leadership, and interpersonally may feel he has validated his own adequacy among people and in contexts that have held him and his heritage in contempt. Yet he may retain his identity with his heritage and his home community and know he wants to return there without feeling he has violated himself or his heritage.

As he completes his college career, he faces parting from his college friends. When it becomes time to arrange for a farewell ritual, he may discover that their conception of how to close off their college years and culminate their mutual friendships is to make a public display expressing their contempt for the college's traditional values. They know that such a symbolic act will be looked on with bemusement in the world from which they come and to which they wish to return—it represents the culmination of "sowing their wild oats." He knows that to act that way seems to him to be a mark of personal and ethnic presumptuousness. He also knows that the people in his home community will see it the same way. He must confront within himself the diversity between his standards and those of his college friends and decide how to seek with them convergence on a way to culminate and conclude their relationship. He must seek to work out with them a way of celebrating the termination of their college careers by arranging a less flagrant demonstration of their resentment about their enforced dependency in college. If he is successful, then both he and they will redefine themselves and what their relationship has meant in a fashion that is more sensitive to their own and each other's ethnic backgrounds.

Conflict

Mutually unacceptable means of resolving how to manage divergences become conflicts. In the above instance the young man may express his views that his friends' proposed celebration is unacceptable to him, and that he can neither agree to participate nor does he want to condone their celebrating in that way. If his friends question his perspectives, particularly on grounds of the validity of his ethnic perspective, then he and they are in conflict. Depending on its resolution, that struggle may diminish or enrich their friendship and their parting. Whatever the outcome, it is shaped by and shapes further the ethnic imbeddedness of their self and world views and their ways of dealing with their lives and relationships.

Therapist and Client Terminating a Relationship: Exit from a Therapeutic Ecosystem

We have just emphasized attention to the ethnic elements of our identity and to their imbeddedness in the ways we say goodbye. However, as we have noted in our earlier chapters, the traditional assumption in the therapeutic literature is that the therapeutic relationship is (or should be) uncontaminated by ethnic, racial, gender, or other characteristics of the therapist or the client as persons behaving in that context. At this point it is essential to remind ourselves that similar assumptions are applied to the termination of therapy. It is these assumptions that we are challenging.

We have proposed that the therapist and the client have formed a many-faceted relationship. In some ways they have formed a therapeutic ecosystem. That ecosystem contains their senses of themselves, their relationships, the goals they have accomplished, the issues they have avoided, the struggles they have surmounted, the differences they have accepted, the still remaining conflicts they have. Those aspects of the relationship have individual, interpersonal, and ethnic facets. They both may acknowledge, desire, and accept that their relationship has been a special kind of relationship. They may agree that they want to conclude it and get on with other activities and aspects of their lives. Yet even to accomplish that much, they need to understand the relationship and resolve their involvement in it and in each other. They need a way to go back to what they were about before they met and what they are about now. Therapists need to be able to incorporate the meaning of each relationship in the broader framework of their own lives. They need redefinition and renewal to continue their work with others and their life as individuals and as members of their own ethnic groups. Clients have similar needs to fulfill in order to rejoin life without therapy and without encapsulating in that therapeutic ecosystem.

The Individual as a Psychologically Autonomous Unit in the Ethnic Ecosystem

As we have said before, we possess some latitude in how we embody our ethnic ecosystems. That latitude includes our capacity to shape in an internally satisfying fashion how we terminate relationships and what that process means to us. One of the authors grew up in a small town in the Midwest. When he was a child, everyone in that town of 300 knew everyone else, and everyone with a role in the community was involved in everyone else's life. Everyone was white and protestant, but there were ethnic differences related to the cultures of the countries in Europe from which their ancestors came. Yet everyone was in some sense personally involved with everyone else. Relationships never really terminated in the sense that people simply disappeared from one another's lives. Perhaps that is why he is troubled by the notion that therapists and clients should interact for a limited time and a defined purpose then simply write that relationship off as an essentially impersonal transaction.

In a more general sense, we can ask what bases any client has for defining the nature of a therapeutic relationship. Presumably, those bases lie in that person's experiences and most likely, in previous helping relationships that have had to do with that individual's life as a person. Often those relationships have been with a teacher, a member of the clergy, a member of the medical profession, or a member of a social service profession. In a small community those relationships tend to be a mix of professional, friend or acquaintance, and concerned community member. Roles may or may not be carefully delineated. The same may be said of homogeneous ethnic communities from common immigrant backgrounds.

The expectation of depersonalized and clearly delineated professional–client relationships has an ethnic origin also and seems natural to people who have been socialized in that way. Thus, in part what each of us expects as a comfortable termination of a relationship stems from our individual history in an ethnic tradition and includes both personal and ethnic elements. How each of us feels about the form that termination takes and how it is defined by the other participant also comes from our personal and ethnic roots.

Convergence

For a therapist and a client to converge in terminating a therapeutic relationship and go on with their separate lives they must create a shared set of expectations. Further, that sharing must take into account their past ethnic and personal expectations as well as those they have formed in their therapeutic interactions. For example, we mentioned earlier the young white woman at a predominantly black college who had an older black woman as a therapist. The relationship involved confronting troubling past experiences for both of them. As they approach taking leave of each other, they both need to conclude their shared experience and assign significance to it. Its central reality is that somehow they bridged their ethnic/racial as well as personal differences and formed a productive therapeutic relationship. To go on with their respective lives, each of them must acknowledge that reality to herself—to her internal reality as well as to her external reality. Doing so requires that each review a whole set of previously arrived at beliefs about cross-ethnic/racial relationships and about individuals from their two ethnic groups. Nevertheless, termination will be incomplete for each of them unless each redefines her own ethnically/racially based view of her own and the other's racial group.

Divergence

We have just noted that two ethnically different people can share a common positive view of their relationship and deal with that reality, no matter how skeptical they may have been of its possible occurrence. We also want to note that they will do so in somewhat different ways. Each of these women will turn to her past personal and ethnic history to interpret and incorporate this experience.

The young woman must deal with her sense of self and its ethnic bases. She must acknowledge (or deny) that she has been benefited by this therapist whose ethnic heritage is one that she (or at least those like her) has devalued, exploited, and mistrusted. Thus, she must reevaluate the meaning of who she is and of what her relationship to others of her own ethnic background means.

The therapist, though she may be more experienced with such terminations, is nevertheless confronted with similar questions. Even so, she confronts them from a personally and ethnically different perspective. She is a survivor of discrimination and is thus aware of the potential dangers of misplaced trust. She is probably also more aware that empathizing with the difficulties of whites, even students, and relating to them is likely to produce distance from her black colleagues and friends.

These two women not only begin in different personal and ecological places as they focus on terminating their relationship, they may very well end in different places. One of them may make drastic changes in her conception of and relationship to individuals belonging to the other's racial group, and the other may make few or none. The young woman may negotiate her personal difficulties and her difficulties in coping with her college education because she has changed how she feels about and relates to black people and to being in a predominantly black school. The older woman may feel good about her work with this young woman but remain skeptical of the integrity and possibilities for change in young white women in general.

Conflict

A recurring theme throughout a therapeutic relationship is that of the personal and ethnic conflicts between therapist and client. Those conflicts arise around termination also. The black therapist–white client pair we have been discussing may serve to highlight such conflicts. For example, the white student may want very much in parting to communicate that it is not just the personal help that she appreciates. She also appreciates the therapist as a role model in teaching the client about her previous unvoiced conceptions of black people as inferior. The black therapist, on the other hand, may want to define the values of the relationship as a colorblind professional one. For the issue of race differences to be brought up at this point is to diminish her significance as a therapist. She does not want to be seen as an "enriching experience" for white students. Thus as they meet for a final time, they are going to confront that conflict. Further, they may even part without resolving it.

THERAPIST–CLIENT INTERACTIONS AS THE INTERACTION OF TWO ECOSYSTEMS AND THE FORMATION OF A SHARED ECOSYSTEM

We have just noted that a client and a therapist may terminate on a note of unresolved ethnic conflict in perspective. Now we want to turn to a facet of their relationship that may be of service in resolving that conflict. Namely, they have formed a relationship and have been using it as a basis for the client to work out some of his or her problems in living. We have already dealt with their individual ecosystems; now we are going to look at their shared one and its impact.

The Individual as a Psychologically Autonomous Unit in the Ethnic Ecosystem

Even though we have formed a shared therapeutic ecosystem, each of us retains some autonomy. Thus as we confront parting, we bring different expectations to it and different ways of coping with it, even though we have shared much of ourselves and perhaps even pledged ourselves to a shared identity during that relationship. That autonomy in part includes our ethnicity regardless of the defined nature of our relationship. Thus, when the older black woman therapist and the young white female terminated their therapeutic relationship, they did so within a somewhat shared meaning because of their therapeutic relationship. Each brought her ethnic/racial heritage to interpreting what the relationship meant, but they also brought their shared experience in that relationship. To the extent that it was different from their previous relationships, that shared ecosystem provided another perspective that contributed to how they could, and wanted to, part and redefine themselves.

Further, we would like to think that terminations are complete when they are formalized, but they ordinarily are not. Each of us continues to mine that experience as we have newer ones that relate to it or as we want to understand more of its significance. Let us turn to another example to illustrate this point. One author once had a client who was a doctoral graduate student in English. She was attractive, vivacious, talented (she was a singer with a popular music combo), and filled with self-doubts. Our therapeutic work focused primarily on her inner turmoil and her related self-defeating behaviors, including her unwillingness or inability to take any stand in her own behalf. Although circumstances prevented the therapeutic relationship from continuing at great length, she did exhibit substantial changes. At the time of termination, she reported herself to be less than problem free but making progress and quite prepared to forge ahead on her own.

A year after that termination she was included by happenstance in a sample chosen for a followup evaluation of the agency's effectiveness. She reported that she still felt good about her gains and was continuing to move along a more constructive path of self-development. Nevertheless, in retrospect she felt some disappointment that her therapist had never discussed with her the "true" nature of her disorder in classical psychopathological terms. She did not know whether she had a personality disorder, was a neurotic, or just how to classify herself. It became clear from her response that she was still working on assimilating that experience into her life. Perhaps she had never culminated and concluded that experience. Perhaps she had but was continuing the process of redefining herself. There is no way of knowing.

There is, however, a way of knowing how the therapist reacted to that new information. It stimulated him to rethink his role in not attending to the issue of labels. In his own view, the existing diagnostic system does more harm than good. It reifies human difficulties and tends to diminish the people who get labeled. However, he now asked himself whether he should have tried to inoculate her, and his clients more generally, against the potentially harmful effects of ill-considered diagnostic labeling. Thus for this therapist there was also a reculmination, reconclusion, and redefinition of a relationship that had been terminated some time before. He is now more sensitive to the labeling issue and inclined to work it through more carefully than he would have before getting this feedback.

The Individual Interacting with Others

Now we want to focus on the particular character the therapist and client give to their parting because of their relationship, because they have been able to come to know each other and work together. For example, to Elli, the young Middle Eastern woman client, it was important that she have older role models who had managed to maintain personal integrity while being successful in the world as well as to their families and their ethnic heritage. She had come to see her older Anglo therapist as embodying some of these characteristics so that she could believe in such a future. She was less sure about individuals with her ethnic heritage until she learned through a class on feminism that her aunt was active in the feminist movement. She already knew that her aunt had a marriage that seemed genuine. Thus she came to believe through her interactions with her therapist and through her classwork that she could accomplish her goals either in the Anglo culture or within her own ethnic heritage.

Convergence

Part of the value of shared ecosystems such as those we develop in psychotherapy is that they provide a shared framework within which the client and therapist can identity and work with the nature and consequences of their ethnic and individual convergences, divergences, and conflicts. As a consequence it was possible for Elli and her therapist to identify some additional issues and find bases for convergence in working them through.

It was important to her in terminating the relationship to find out whether the therapist really believed in her capabilities and whether he cared about people or was just doing his job. To her it was important that his caring transcend his therapeutic obligations since in her ethnic heritage personal involvement is a significant component of a professional relationship. She and her therapist explored these questions as well as their personal and ethnic bases. The therapist conveyed that he did like her as a person and think she was indeed a likeable, capable, and resourceful person. He also pointed out that it would be inappropriate for her to take his acknowledgment as support for her not taking full responsibility for herself and her life, but continuing to indulge her self-destructive behaviors. She responded by indicating that she saw his remarks as an unbiased, nonmanipulative statement that she did have before her the possibility of continuing to develop command of her own feelings and behavior as she made a meaningful life and career for herself. In brief, their termination sessions served to validate the constructiveness of their relationship, their respect and caring for each other as persons, and their mutual respect for each other's ethnic as well as personal ecosystems. For them the process of culminating, concluding, and redefining themselves and the work they had done together was a mutually positive one.

The convergence that this same therapist and Meagan (the graduate student whose central identity concerns centered around her involvement in some homosexual relationships) had developed during her therapy sessions was more limited, but equally relevant in the terminating of their relationship. The therapist's acceptance and support while she talked about the issues that troubled her had led to a convergent relationship in which the client came to feel comfortable and enabled to reevaluate her life and herself. When she and her therapist sat down to discuss termination she continued to express a sense of convergence. The therapeutic relationship had been a good one for her and she felt that she could now build on her own strengths. She expressed her appreciation for the opportunity to work with her therapist and valued what she had gained from it. The warmth and equanimity that she had developed seemed to the therapist to have led her to be better equipped to manage her life and to be a more pleasant person to work with and interact with. They parted on cordial terms. As the tenor of these remarks may show, she had not become a notably warm, outgoing, and effusive person. The therapist thought she showed glimpses of more warmth, but he continued to converge with her on her right to decide how far she wanted to go in that direction.

Divergence

We approach parting in terms of our history and our internalized sense of what is right. In fact, we may have higher expectations about the validity of our manner of farewell than about other aspects of our relationships. We have struggled to form a relationship, and we have built on it—surely we can share how to say goodbye. Unfortunately, it does not work that way. Therapists, as any self-reflective therapist or therapist supervisor knows, have their own doubts and idiosyncracies. As therapists we think we know the correct way to do this part of the ritual, but we do not necessarily know how much of that presumed knowledge is the ethnic person that each of us is. Clients have even less to go on. Clients may want a last affirmation that their therapists have not seen it all as a waste of time, but rather see their respective clients as of intrinsic merit. They may also want a kind of termination that will be consistent with their ethnic history.

For that matter, the therapist and the client may just differ on how to terminate or on what courses make sense after they do. For example, the black male graduate student and his white male therapist were confronting their parting of ways as the student accepted his termination from his graduate program. The therapist felt that the most constructive solution for the client was to salvage what he could of his educational experience, build on his newer understanding of his own role in negotiating systems, and focus on the next steps in his life. The student wanted to get on with his life, but he felt that to vindicate himself he wanted to make a final protest citing the injustices in the system. The therapist explored with him what he hoped to accomplish and how he could best approach doing so while refraining from endorsing that course of action. It was the therapist's view that challenging the student's choice would potentially alienate him from the therapist. Supporting him to work out the dynamics of a constructive protest would serve to underscore the therapist's support of the student as capable of acting in his own behalf. It would also provide the student with an exercise in confronting authorities within a system. It seemed to the therapist that these factors outweighed his view that a better course would be for the student to get on with his life. Perhaps the therapist was more persuaded by his own heritage in the ethnic Anglo mainstream and a more pragmatic view of protest as worth the effort only if it was likely to succeed; the client by his in the black minority group that protest was important as a form of defiance and self-assertion regardless of the outcome. Whatever the underlying reasons for their divergence in perspective, the therapist felt it was essential to respect the client's view. He shared his own view and reviewed the consequences of the alternatives with the client. He then indicated that it was the client's decision, he would respect the client's right to make it, and finally that he would support the client in whatever course he chose.

Conflict

Even in closing we may face further conflict and need to resolve it. We noted that the older black female therapist and her young white female client were going to face such a conflict in their task of saying farewell. The client wanted to express her particular appreciation of the therapist as a black woman; the therapist wanted to part on terms of therapist–client, not black–white. The client was asked about her closing thoughts and brought up her issue. The therapist tried to accept the expressed positive feelings but then noted that she wondered if the client had resolved all of her feelings about their cross-race pairing. The client responded that she had gone even further than seeing their relationship as a black person and a white person interacting. She felt she had gotten beyond the particular therapeutic rapport and was able to see the broader social context that she had unwittingly endorsed before. The therapist, still uncomfortable, asked whether the client was not rather saying that she was still devaluing blacks as a group by seeing the therapist as extraordinary. At this point the client, who was beginning to feel somewhat uncertain of her own ground, said that she did not mean it that way. Now the therapist began to respond to her own insistence that their relationship be seen as just individually based, not representative of any larger frame of reference. She too felt unsure but did not want to change her view of how their relationship should be seen. She decided to ask about other aspects of their relationship. The client felt relieved to turn to the topic of gains she had made in her openness to others and to interpersonal skills she had acquired. They discussed those, reviewed the other qualities of their relationship, and parted. They couldn't find convergent grounds for culminating the experience of their relationship and their work together. They could not find divergent grounds, and they did not work through their conflict. Neither of them was able to culminate, to celebrate or suffer fully with what their relationship and their work had meant. Consequently, neither of them was able to conclude, to resolve completely the meaning of their interactions. They each felt a little less fulfilled than might have been the case had they been able to resolve their final conflict. As a consequence, they were unable to redefine themselves and their possibilities clearly.

SUMMARY

At this juncture we want to sum up what we have been trying to say about termination, about saying good-bye and what that involves. First, it is important to note that we have just called attention to some considerations. We do not believe that we have in any way exhausted this subject. Nor have we provided specific answers for anyone as to how to handle termination. What we have tried to say is that the issues and examples here provide some important topics to think about and some ways to begin doing so. We hope that it is evident by now that in this chapter we have tried to touch on examples of the complexity of the steps we need to take to move out of therapy and back into our world without it. Because we are now different, that world is also different. We see ourselves differently as individuals and as members of our various social and ethnic realities; we see our individual and group memberships differently; we see others differently.

We have elaborated on the conception of endings of the phases of living as three-faceted, as involving culmination, conclusion, and redefinition. We have suggested that we need to celebrate our successes, suffer our failures; conclude or close off our involvements with the activities in which we are engaged; and redefine ourselves, our relation to our world, and our ways of experiencing and negotiating our life events. When we have moved through all three of those phases of termination we can move on. We have also emphasized that those activities have ethnic as well as individual aspects to them.

We are not suggesting that people in therapy necessarily change their perspectives on all facets of their life as a function of therapy. They may, for instance, reduce their willingness to explore alternatives or relate to people of a different ethnic identity than their own. Those are not outcomes that we would ordinarily hope for, but they may occur, and if they do they will indeed shape the lives and future of the people who change in those ways. If for no other reason than to minimize the possibility of such outcomes, it is important to be sensitive to how we interact with people in terminating our therapeutic relationships with them. After all, we see those relationships as helpful and in our other interactions we see the closing—the departure—as a significant component that confirms their character. In ordinary parlance, we want to leave "with a good taste in our mouth." So, too, with therapy we want to leave it with a good taste about it.

To have a good taste about it, we need as clients to feel that our personhood has indeed been and will continue to be respected. We want to be remembered and remember ourselves as a person, not just as a patient or as a label assigned by a therapist.

On the other side, we have similar concerns as therapists. To put together our memories "with a good taste in our mouths," we too need to relate the experience to our individual and our collective—be it ethnic or whatever—humanness. We have tried to touch on some of the issues that must be sorted through to accomplish that kind of objective. We have done so to provide stimulation for thought and exploration, not as a set of final answers. We too are groping through largely uncharted human territory.

9

Case Examples of Racial Dyads

In the preceding chapters, we have discussed how one's membership in either the culture-defining group (CDG) or in the non-culture-defining group (NCDG) provides an ecological framework for understanding the dynamics of interpersonal relationships. In exploring these dynamics within the context of psychotherapy, we have made four critical points. The first was that ethnicity is always a variable to be accounted for and processed in analyzing any therapeutic relationship, even when two people from the same ethnic/racial group have formed a therapist–client relationship. The second point was that NCDG and CDG statuses are ascribed and denote one's ecology and connote one's level of power and influence in society. In any heterogeneous society, one group tends to set the standards for that society. These standards do not typically reflect the diversity of that society or culture, but rather the values, attitudes, beliefs, and meanings of the more powerful group. The third point was that the legacy of slavery continues to shape enculturated messages concerning the power base, intellect, and humanness of America's NCDGs. Furthermore, these messages have significantly contributed to the nature of relationships between blacks, between blacks and whites, between whites, and between members of other groups. The fourth critical point was that there are therapeutic gains and losses associated with all dyadic patterns. In any relationship, there is something that one can potentially gain from that interaction and something that one is at risk of losing. The gain or the loss can refer to self-esteem, sense of confidence, affirmation of coping skills, or other attributes.

In the present chapter we will continue to explore these ethnic validity model (EVM) principles by way of case examples that are prototypical of racial dyads: white–white, black–black, white–black, black–white. We will try to highlight EVM principles by examining the gains and losses, and the convergent, divergent, and conflicting processes or aspects in each therapeutic relationship. No one case will embody all of the issues that we have discussed in the previous chapters. Instead, each case will provide concrete examples of some relevant EVM principles.

WHITE THERAPIST–WHITE CLIENT DYAD

Background Factors

Client Background

Mary is a 46-year-old Irish-American Catholic woman who resides with her two daughters in a two-bedroom apartment in a major city. She lives in a community comprised mainly of working-class, white Irish Catholics, most of whom have generational ties within that community.

Mary's parents, who are both dead, immigrated to America from Ireland prior to her birth and settled in a community of other Irish immigrants. They were devout Catholics and consequently Catholicism played a prominent role in shaping the values taught in her home. Mary has fond memories of her childhood, including a strong sense of family, a commitment to home, and growing up with two older brothers and two younger sisters. She was not interested in school, was a "C" student, and went to work in a factory after she graduated from high school.

Mary married at age 20. She was expected to manage the family affairs, teach her son and three daughters their religious values, and maintain the home. Her husband drank heavily, but she did not consider him an alcoholic. He was a truck driver and provided the sole economic support for his family. The children had difficulty adjusting to their father's death in a car accident, which had occurred 10 years previous to Mary entering therapy. Mary attempted to date 3 years after her husband's death. Her two youngest children protested, feeling that she was abandoning them and the memory of their father. Mary did not feel she had the energy to fight them on these issues, so she abandoned the idea of dating since she was not "that interested in the gentleman."

Mary entered therapy on the recommendation of her daughter's social worker. Her youngest daughter, Kathy, age 17, had for 2 years been dating a 20-year-old man who lived in their neighborhood. Since she had been dating him, Kathy had been missing school, performing poorly in school, and had become sexually active. Mary learned from her eldest daughter that Kathy had gotten pregnant and had had an abortion. Mary, who did not believe in abortion, was outraged. She confronted Kathy and during the confrontation slapped Kathy's face several times. Kathy, who had rarely been hit by Mary, called the Department of Social Service and reported her mother for abuse. As a result of the subsequent investigation, both Mary and Kathy were referred to individual therapy. Mother–daughter sessions were to be conducted by Kathy's therapist every 6 weeks.

Therapist Background

Sarah is a 34-year-old single, white, Anglo-Saxon Protestant, who was reared in an upper-income New England family. She is the youngest of three children. She received her Ph.D. at age 29 and had been working as a clinician in a community health center since that time.

She has a close relationship with her parents and visits them on holidays. She is closer to her brother, age 37, than to her sister, age 44. Sarah has recently experienced a love loss. She and her boyfriend of 2 years recently parted because he did not feel he wanted to make a commitment to a marital relationship.

Forming a Relationship

Mary was quite surprised when she met Sarah, who was petite and looked very young. Sarah began the initial session by asking Mary what brought her to therapy. Mary appeared hesitant in answering this question but explained that her youngest daughter Kathy had been "giving her trouble" over the past 4 years. "When I found out about her abortion, I was angry and had enough. So, I slapped her. She ran away and reported me. I got blamed for being abusive and am told that I need help. I think you all are sick. And society is sick when a parent is blamed for flying off the handle once. I am responsible for my daughter. Furthermore, it is wrong for any place to give her an abortion without my knowledge and permission. Abortion is murder and a sin. These agencies have no right to dismiss my beliefs as the head of the family and let her do this. They have all of you people with no values trying to tell the rest of us what to do."

Sarah sat and listened. She heard it all before from other irate parents who felt victimized and did not want to deal with their daughters' autonomy. She allowed Mary to express her anger at the system and at the process that brought her to therapy, then she asked Mary how she was coping. Mary then began to talk about her needs and wants over the years. Sarah ended this initial session by suggesting that possibly she could be of assistance to Mary in dealing with the pressures and stresses around her family and personal life. Mary accepted this as their task and said that she would return.

Mary attended future appointments on time and seemed to make good use of her therapy time focusing on issues of control, feelings of self-worth, and her depression. She struggled to quit feeling responsible for Kathy's moral life and accept Kathy's rebelliousness as Kathy's need to establish her autonomy. However, Mary had spoken with her parish priest, who was sympathetic to her concerns about Kathy's abortion and supported Mary's need to help Kathy get control of her moral and spiritual life. Mary had also enlisted the support of various family members and friends to talk to Kathy to convince her that her boyfriend was not a good person. Kathy was in therapy and continued to miss school. It was clear that she would not graduate from high school due to her absences. As things did not improve with Kathy, Mary appeared to seek the support of a larger network of people.

Sarah felt that Mary was either not being honest about her feelings about therapy or not truly in touch with her feelings. Mary was enlisting the support of various individuals in her network, yet telling Sarah that therapy was helping her to cope with her circumstances. Sarah's notion was that if Mary was in control and coping better then she would not be utilizing a core group of about seven people as confidants and collaborators.

Sarah addressed the issue of Mary's use of her extended network to seek advice and guidance by asking Mary two questions. The first was whether therapy was meeting her expectations and the second was what were Mary's expectations of therapy. Mary indicated that therapy was meeting her expectation of getting help with her stress. Sarah told Mary that when one involves many people in attacking a problem, that approach can increase stress and that Mary should be careful not to burden herself in listening to multiple solutions and strategies. Mary, however, continued to utilize her network for advice as well as for support.

Mary's pattern continued to trouble Sarah, who began to experience what she called countertransference feelings toward Mary. Sarah began to feel tired before her sessions with Mary and found it difficult to listen to Mary's reports of collaboration with others around her troubles. She also began to wonder whether she had truly established rapport with Mary and whether Mary was being "passive–aggressive" (i.e., was Mary still feeling angry about being required to come to therapy)? From an EVM framework, Sarah was experiencing conflict in this relationship because her role as helper was not being affirmed in the manner to which she was accustomed.

Another troublesome part of the therapy for Sarah was Mary's devotion to Catholicism and the role it played in her life. Sarah did not understand how religion could play such a central role in Mary's life, and she did not know anything about the tenets of Catholicism. A third area arose because Sarah's concept of competence was tied to her idea of control. To the extent that her input was given high priority by others or influenced them, Sarah felt in control. Her model of competence and control was hierarchical. That is, it appeared to be based on a traditional perspective of control and competence in which the therapist's place of importance is based on having a "solitary" voice with the client.

In order to break the cycle of conflict, Sarah had to ask the question, "How can I learn about Mary's ecology and how can Mary and I build a relationship on my ecology and on hers?" To address these conflicts Sarah needed to know more about Mary's ecology. Who were the significant people in her life and how did they relate to her and to each other? How long had this network been together? To what extent were Mary's relationships reflective of an ethnic or cultural tradition? Also, how did Mary view Catholicism? How was it integrated into her daily life and relationships?

What is important about these questions is the frame of reference from which they are asked. At this point, their thirteenth session, Sarah turned to Mary as the *knower* and expert on her world. Sarah was asking to learn about Mary's world through Mary's eyes.

Over the next several sessions, Mary described a closely knit network of about seven Irish Catholic women who had been friends since early adolescence. What emerged for Sarah was that Mary had a network of seven core women who nurtured and mirrored one another's reality and identity. What Sarah had thought was passive–aggressive or resistant behavior was Mary's normal pattern of interacting and behaving within her ecosystem. The women in this group shared everything, even the insights from Mary's therapy sessions. Sarah had unofficially become a member of that group and, as such, her opinions, like those of the other women, were subject to scrutiny. It was a sisterhood, and Sarah was an honorary member. Sarah also learned that Catholicism played a crucial role in framing the moral codes and value system for these women. Was this sisterhood an aspect particular to the Irish Catholic culture? Sarah asked Mary this question. Mary did not know and she commented that she had never thought about it.

With this information from Mary, Sarah learned about Mary's relationships and her ecosystems. Through Sarah's questions, Mary experienced being a *knower.* In teaching Sarah about herself she became more aware of the strengths of her coping patterns and relationships as well as some of the limitations of those relationships. In addition, with this understanding, Mary and Sarah finally formed a collaborative relationship and an area of convergence. Their relationship incorporated both attributes of the hierarchy and of the collective. Mary continued to share aspects of her therapy with the group. However, she now shared her strategies for growth and her accomplishments rather than just the details of her sessions. With Sarah she learned to keep some things private and separate and to maintain closeness with the group while doing so. Also, she began to develop a sense of autonomy and a capability of being difficult.

Sustaining the Relationship

Mary and Sarah continued to clarify and refine the meanings and parameters of their relationship. Sarah refined her understanding of Mary's network and her role in that part of Mary's life. Sarah also gained additional knowledge about female support systems and about the strengths and weaknesses of networks like Mary's. Mary continued to struggle with learning autonomous modes of problem solving within her network or group context. Part of that struggle was discerning what was part of her core versus group beliefs.

A major hurdle that emerged in the course of treatment was Sarah's and Mary's views on a woman's right to choose to have an abortion. The context within which the issue arose was a discussion of Kathy's autonomy. Mary felt quite strongly that Kathy had some obligation to obey her and to do the right thing as Mary defined it. More importantly, she felt that Kathy's actions had influenced how she was evaluated as a parent. For Mary, Kathy's abortion was a major indictment of her failure as a parent, as well as of Kathy's lack of basic morals.

In an attempt to stay away from the abortion question, Sarah attempted to reframe the issue of Kathy's abortion as Kathy's right to be a separate person and to make choices for herself, even when those choices are contrary to Mary's beliefs. Mary responded by saying that abortion was wrong and that even though it was legal to have an abortion, it was illegal within the context of the church. Then Mary asked Sarah whether she felt abortion was wrong. Sarah responded by saying, "If my opinion and moral beliefs about abortion are similar to yours, what does that mean for our relationship? And if my opinion or moral beliefs about abortion are different from yours, what does that mean for our relationship?" Mary first responded by saying that she did not know. Then she added that if Sarah agreed with her, then of course she would feel good; and if Sarah disagreed with her, then she would feel upset. It was difficult for Mary to think that a person whom she trusted could hold fundamental beliefs very different from hers. Sarah began to work through with her the notion of how different Sarah could be, yet have a relationship around which there was mutual respect and trust. In tackling this issue they began to develop a model for dealing with conflict and divergence.

Over the course of two additional sessions, Mary and Sarah grappled with the issue of sameness and difference. Finally Mary concluded that their therapeutic relationship was not contingent on Sarah possessing the same concepts of right and wrong on every issue, and that Sarah had provided a great deal of support to her and had been helpful.

Mary also noted that Sarah had never given an answer to her question. Further, she decided that she did not want to hear Sarah's views on the abortion question. Sarah asked whether Mary's decision to withdraw the question indicated that a negative answer would indeed disrupt the relationship. Mary said that was possible, but that she had made up her mind that it was not important so she did not want to know.

Sarah accepted Mary's response as a constructive step within the context of the relationship and within the context of their similarities and differences. In this case, the dyad agreed to incorporate a major divergence as part of their relationship, even though that divergence was never firmly established. This change shifted the focus of the divergence from a moral issue to a therapy relationship issue. It also represented a new way for Mary to view a close, sisterhood-type relationship. That experience also stimulated her thinking about Kathy. Mary actively began to think about the range of acceptable similarities and differences between herself and her daughter.

Terminating the Relationship

Termination was discussed when Mary and Kathy had achieved several months of therapeutic working time in the context of their newly formed ecologically compatible relationship. This time included enjoyable activities as well as disagreements that were resolved to their satisfaction. When Sarah brought up termination, Mary found it very difficult to discuss. In Mary's network, women do not terminate relationships. Once a bond has been established and sustained, contact is always maintained.

What the dyad faced was a divergence in the meaning of termination. For Sarah, it meant the end of regular contact with Mary around Mary's life hurdles. Termination did not mean Sarah was unavailable for a future crisis. It also did not mean that she had not valued her relationship with Mary. But termination did mean Sarah had assisted Mary in meeting her goals and that her therapeutic task was completed. For Mary, termination meant severing ties. It also brought forth images of abandonment and of being alone. Also, in thinking about termination, Mary began to question Sarah's bond to her. Did Sarah only view Mary as her work? If she did not view her in that way how could she initiate a discussion of termination without some sense of sadness?

In discussing their feelings about and understanding of termination, Sarah shared with Mary that when she enters into a therapy relationship to assist an individual with a particular life puzzle, it is her understanding that when the puzzle is solved the relationship ends. When a therapy relationship ends, it means that there is no ongoing contact with the client. However, clients often keep in periodic contact with Sarah, and in some cases she makes follow-up calls.

Mary appeared to understand Sarah's perspective on termination. Mary made the analogy that being a therapist is much like mothering. Mothers nurture their children knowing that they must leave. She is always preparing for their leaving. A therapist does the same. They were able to converge on their meanings around termination and to come up with a plan to terminate that felt comfortable for Sarah and Mary.

Commentary

From an EVM perspective, Mary and Sarah did not address several important characteristics of their dyadic relationship that were influencing their patterns of gains and losses. The first issue was their race. Because they were both white, race did not appear to be a salient therapy variable. Yet, their *whiteness* did influence how they related to one another since it provided a context for convergence around their shared enculturated values and cultural expectations and norms.

One issue that characterizes the white–white or CDG–CDG relationship is the meaning and the use of power as denoting one's status within the CDG structure. In the present case, Mary and Sarah had similar enculturated values in their shared belief that one's power is measured by society's yardsticks of education, income, profession, family origin, and social class.

For Sarah and Mary, this aspect of their culture arose through Mary being told to enter therapy by CDG authorities. Mary was seen as incompetent and not living according to CDG expectations. Sarah represented these CDG values and was charged with assisting with Mary's resocialization. Within an EVM framework, a major task they confronted in their relationship was the balance of power. Since Mary and Sarah's therapeutic relationship was initiated by outside authorities, the personal power experienced by Mary was less than what it could have been if she had sought therapy on her own. Mary had been labeled in need of help and referred to a therapist of a higher socioeconomic status background than her own. More importantly, she had been labeled incompetent at the one task that she thought she knew best, childrearing.

Furthermore, her religious beliefs and values were being questioned by CDG authorities. Overall, Mary and Sarah constituted the typical hierarchical, power relationship between therapist and client and had to confront that asymmetry to establish and maintain a therapy relationship.

The second issue not discussed that shaped the meanings they attached to their relationship and to their understanding of power within the CDG framework was their gender. There is a growing conviction among some women and men that women possess a world view and perspective different from that of men. That is, women tend more to define themselves in relationship to other people, rather than as separate from other people. Sarah and Mary had to discover how each of them understood her voice as a woman and what coping strategy each used to negotiate that voice. Simultaneously, they had to create a mutual voice that would define their ecosystem and relationship. They did so when they converged on their understanding of the *sisterhood*. However, they never defined themselves as such or addressed how the nature of their relationship or of Mary's relationship with her friends was a part of their gender identity. Nor did they deal with it in terms of how it influenced the termination process or their notion of power and control.

The third issue not discussed but also shaping their dyadic relationship was age. Age connotes different things according to one's ethnicity, gender, and personal experiences. It also frames our interpretation of reality given the historical times in which we live and experience the world. As a first generation Irish-American, Mary had been reared in a time in which academic competencies were not valued in a woman as much as her competencies to hold her family together. Her ethnic legacy and her ecology had reinforced that aspect of herself and had supported that role as had her self–world relationships.

In Mary's eyes she had been referred to therapy because the younger generation did not deem her to be competent at what she had assumed was her role, that of keeping her family together. However, from her friends she received validation of her self-perception, world view, and self–world relationships. For her to cope with the conflicts experienced in her life, she needed that kind of validation. A discussion of age differences and what they mean in terms of ethnicity and gender could have provided her with that validation from Sarah. It could also have helped Sarah, as the age variable was also an issue for her. She was often seen as being younger than she actually was, and she often operated as if it was not an issue in her attempt to assert her authority.

Mary and Sarah did not have a point of convergence around the role Sarah would play in therapy. In Mary's experience women hold family wisdom and support each other; men hold the authority. Mary could connect with Sarah's supportive role in the therapy relationship because that's how women relate—that's what a good mother–daughter relationship is like. However, this point of convergence was not enough by itself to solidify the relationship and establish trust.

In summary, these three variables, race, gender, and age, had significantly shaped the lives of Sarah and Mary. They conducted their sessions in terms of specific issues, but these broader ecologically and ethnically shaped issues had set limits on the possibilities of their resolving those specific life issues in more constructive ways. Their abilities to grow beyond their particular visions or to stay confined to their world views were related to the extent to which these characteristics were addressed.

Sarah's gains as a therapist grew out of her ability to begin to incorporate another world view into her way of viewing support networks. She became open to the idea of culture as an influence on how people organize their lives. Sarah's losses were lost opportunities. Specifically, she lost the opportunity to explore gender concepts and identity from another person's perspective and the opportunity to look at her CDG issues of power and control.

Mary's psychosocial gains in her therapy relationship with Sarah included her ability to see herself as both autonomous and yet connected to others, and her ability to recognize divergence as part of being human and of human relationships. She was also able to generalize her understanding of divergence and conflict management to other relationships. Her losses included (1) her inability to recognize the world from a perspective other than that of women or to understand the role of gender in shaping her perspective, and (2) her inability to expand her knowledge of her ecology beyond her racial group.

Black Client–Black Therapist Dyad

Background Factors

Client Background

Ebony is a 32-year-old single black female who works in an upper-level management position for a large corporation on the East Coast. She has lived most of her life on the West Coast, where she grew up in a predominantly black middle-income community. Her parents are Southerners who migrated to the West Coast when Ebony was 1 year old. Her father is a bricklayer and her mother is an elementary school teacher. Ebony's closest sibling is her 40-year-old sister, who has a graduate degree in business. She also has a 37-year-old brother, who is an attorney, and a 29-year-old brother, who recently finished college and works in sales for a high-tech company.

Ebony had a good relationship with her parents. Her father often stressed what a "dog-eat-dog" world it can be and that if you are black you have to be the best to deal effectively with it. Her parental and adult world had encouraged her independence and respected her talents, but she and her siblings were expected to achieve and to do well in life. She enjoyed school sports, dance, and music. She and her siblings, known as "good children" and "very bright students," were given much attention because of their academic abilities. Ebony was proud of this family reputation.

Throughout her childhood and adolescence she was seen as a leader in both school and church activities. Ebony was bused to a predominantly white school for her junior high and high school years. She was an achiever in both her segregated and integrated school settings. In her integrated environment, she was one of the few blacks tracked in honors courses. Ebony saw herself and felt that others viewed her as a superstar. She felt that, unlike some of her black peers, she was able to maintain her superstar identity in the transition from a segregated to an integrated environment. From her perspective, her self-image and concept had remained intact in the transition, whereas those of some of her friends had not. Her success in the academic world continued through her undergraduate education and work experiences. During those years her confidence was high, bordering on conceit.

Ebony's level of confidence was severely jarred when she left her home and a familiar environment to attend a highly competitive graduate program in business at a predominantly white institution. She entered an environment in which everyone was considered a superstar and in which she had no history or legacy. Her fellow white students and her instructors judged her based on her race, and did not appear to entertain the thought that she was as special and as bright as the other students or as she thought she was. Their comments, which were most disturbing to her, were filled with assumptions about the nature of the black intellect and her presumed academic inferiority.

Ebony was equally troubled by her relationship with her fellow black students, as she did not receive the esteem from them that she had received from the community where she grew up. She perceived them as being either too radical in their views toward whites or too weak and lacking pride, integrity, and self-confidence.

Ebony struggled to reestablish the same power base and place of prestige that she had felt at home. To her, being aligned with powerful others and being known were equated with emotional and interpersonal security. In a predominantly white institution, the power base is white, so she aligned herself with the white faculty and students. Most of her active friendships were with whites and she dated white men. She encountered instances in which she felt "stabbed in the back" by white women, especially in terms of how they responded to her dating white men. She did not interpret these incidents as having racial overtones, but as representing life in a competitive world. She cultivated the attitude that "you don't trust anybody, you look out for yourself," and found that it was reinforced in her dealings with the power brokers of her institution.

After graduate school she secured her present position at a large corporation in another city. She carried her graduate school philosophy of life with her and looked out for herself. She did what was necessary to maintain her self-image as being exceptional, competent, and confident. Her graduate school connections have paved the way for her to enter the job market at the upper echelon of management. She tried to secure projects assigned by and for the people at the very top level of management and worked over 70 hours per week to maintain her position. She spent little time socializing with others, gained 30 pounds, and presented a physical appearance that did not match her sense of security or confidence.

Ebony sought psychotherapy because she felt she was having anxiety attacks and experiencing episodes of depression. At times she felt overwhelmed by her job and responsibilities. She complained of sleeplessness, of feeling sad, of being tearful, of not wanting to go to work, and of not wanting to socialize with friends.

Therapist Background

Leah is a 34-year-old black female who has been in therapy practice for 5 years. She is an attractive, dark-skinned single woman of medium height and build. She was reared and educated in the South, where her parents own a great deal of land, which they farm. Although her parents are from several generations of farmers and sharecroppers and have experienced financial hardships with farming, she considers herself to have been reared in rural, middle-class black America.

Leah has seven siblings. Two of them are high school educated and have continued the family tradition of farming. Five are college educated, but Leah is the only child with a doctorate and the only one living in the Northeast. She came to the Northeast for her graduate education and has made her home there. She visits her family at least twice a year and keeps in close contact with her siblings.

Forming a Relationship

Ebony had been referred to Leah by a well-established black psychologist in the city who was not accepting referrals at that time. Ebony, who had spoken briefly to Leah on the telephone prior to their initial meeting, indicated that she had been experiencing recurring episodes of tearfulness and had been having difficulty sleeping. Ebony also volunteered that she had deliberately sought a therapist of the same race and gender because she wanted to have a therapist who would be familiar with and sensitive to her experiences as a black woman. Upon further inquiry, she also noted that it was important for this person to understand how the "system" works and the dilemmas posed for black women interacting in these systems. Leah responded that she was a black psychologist and that one area of expertise for her was the psychological effects of racism. Ebony appeared to be reassured by that remark.

For their initial session, the therapist greeted Ebony in the waiting room and escorted her to her office. Ebony wore little makeup and her hair was not fashionably styled. She was businesslike when greeted, giving a firm handshake and a slight smile. Leah asked Ebony to share with her once more why Ebony sought therapy at that time. Ebony responded by reviewing her background and accomplishments, highlighting that she was from a middle-income background, that she had excelled academically, and that she had a senior position in her company. She concluded by indicating that, because of her position, she had to cope with tremendous pressure and stress, which she felt were causing her depression and periodic bouts with anxiety. For the remainder of the session, Leah sought more information about Ebony's depression and anxiety attacks, about any recent significant life events, and about her social supports. Ebony shared that she had been dating a white male but they had broken off the relationship several months ago and that she had few friends and socialized mainly with whites from her job. She also expressed strong feelings about maintaining a self-image as a competent and exceptional black person.

By the end of the session, Leah had formed the following hypotheses about Ebony: (1) Ebony was experiencing a racial identity conflict—she had requested a black therapist, yet has mostly white friends and has dated white males; (2) below the surface, Ebony was not as "together" and as powerful as she tried to project—Ebony's description of her job and her aspirations did not fit with her appearance.

Leah felt some connection with most of her clients during their first meeting; there was none with Ebony. In thinking about why, Leah realized that the session felt more like an interview to determine credentials and worth rather than an initial therapy session. Leah concluded that either Ebony did not feel comfortable enough to be vulnerable during that first session or Ebony felt that she had to establish her value and worth to Leah prior to sharing her vulnerabilities. What Leah did not consider at this point was that part of her assessment of Ebony was based on Leah's assumptions about Ebony's racial identity development. From Ebony's request for a black therapist, Leah had assumed a level of sophistication that did not fit with her experience of Ebony.

Over the next several sessions, Ebony reported feeling particularly depressed and tired. She focused on her pressures at work. Her routine consisted of arriving at work at 7 A.M. and leaving work between 8:30 and 9 P.M., eating fast food that she had picked up along the way, and going to bed. She went into the office on most Saturdays and slept all day Sunday, even though she had grown up in the church. Her contacts with others outside of work consisted mainly of telephone calls to family and a couple of old college and graduate school friends. Her parents were concerned about how hard she worked. Her sister, who had risen to success on the corporate ladder, was sympathetic. Her older brother was less sympathetic. He felt that she was doing five times as much as the whites in her organization and was reaping little from it. He also felt that she was not living, but avoiding her life by hiding behind her work. Ebony felt that he didn't understand her particular situation because he was a man and that the "game" was different for black women.

The recurring themes of these sessions were work, stress, and systems racism. Ebony struggled to justify her work stress and discount the possibilities of racism. Attempts by Leah to identify discrepancies in organizational power and racism were met with resistance by Ebony, who would reinterpret any racist situation (e.g., an inappropriate racial joke) as part of the job culture and the game.

Leah found that she was spending excessive time processing Ebony's case and realized that she was frustrated by Ebony's unwillingness or inability to face individual racism on the job. Ebony recognized individuals' particular personality quirks and their sometimes racist remarks, but she accepted those aberrations as part of the system and expected Leah to assist her in dealing with them without confrontation. Leah's style was confrontational; she felt that there were times when systems and individuals should be confronted. Listening to Ebony's work scenarios became increasingly more difficult for Leah.

By this point their relationship was characterized by conflict. Their philosophies on how to define the nature of and cope with racism differed and was causing each to feel frustrated. Ebony, an assimilationist and integrationist, believed that to succeed in life black people must discard their world view and replace it with the world view of whites. Leah, a separatist, believed that blacks are as likely to succeed as a people by establishing all black institutions as they are by integrating white institutions.

In the fifth session, Ebony described a work situation in which her white female coworker and friend had forgotten to mention to their boss that Ebony developed the majority of the ideas for a major presentation. Ebony did not confront her coworker because Ebony knew that her boss had seen her working on the project late the previous night and was aware that Ebony had done the bulk of the work. Also, Ebony indicated that this kind of thing happens all the time as part of the business culture in which "if you don't constantly watch your back you will be doomed." Ebony described this incident with a great sense of accomplishment and boasted that her coworker took her out to dinner that night, presumably because she felt guilty. Ebony had accepted the dinner invitation, as she felt that she had nothing to lose and would get a free, gourmet meal.

Leah responded from her own perspective with "how absolutely awful. Isn't it awful what people do to each other for the name of recognition? How did you make it through dinner knowing that she has no respect for you?" Leah knew that her perspective was different from Ebony's, but she felt that not commenting would have been dishonest on her part. She did not acknowledge their differences, but made her assessment as an unbiased statement of reality.

Ebony began to cry and eventually began sobbing. Leah was taken aback. She neither realized the power of her statement nor knew what part or parts of her statement had triggered such a painful response. At first Leah sat and observed Ebony, in the manner in which she had been taught in her training, but she noted that she felt cold and distant in doing so. Leah decided to reach over and touch Ebony's arm to comfort her. Ebony held her hand, but took about 10 minutes to feel composed and to stop crying.

As they discussed what was so painful about Leah's comment, it became clear that the key phrase was "how did you make it through" and that the key word was respect. Ebony had had the respect of others through graduate school, but since then there appeared to be no consistent way to gain "respect" or to be valued or to be a superstar. She sobbed, "Day after day you struggle and I don't know how I keep making it. I'm just so tired of it all." With that statement Leah connected with Ebony. She converged with Ebony's sense of periodic weariness of struggling against forces, like racism, that one cannot always readily see. Leah also understood that Ebony did not recognize the fatigue factor as a response to racism. That is where the two differed. But they had converged on the universal feeling of what it is like to struggle and not to have the respect of others.

Leah felt that Ebony needed to be given to. She told Ebony that the strategies that she had been using to cope apparently were not as effective as they once had been and suggested that they start looking at strategies for self-protection. Ebony agreed, but at the next session she reported that she had had a good week and that her tearfulness the previous week was probably due to premenstrual syndrome. Nevertheless, Ebony did pick up on the concept of self-protection, so they began to discuss strategies of how Ebony could protect herself at the work place. The focus on self-protection proved fruitful, and Ebony continued to report feeling less depressed and sleeping more soundly. She also used the new framework to reinterpret the job situation in a manner that did not allow for her exploitation and enabled her to feel respected.

Had Leah and Ebony formed a relationship? Leah felt that she and Ebony had converged on a theme around which to work but had not formed a therapeutic relationship. From Ebony's perspective, she had found someone with whom to strategize, and that task, in and of itself, defined and formed the relationship. From an EVM framework, the relationship had converged on a common goal or activity to create and refine strategies of self-protection. This task was one that both Leah and Ebony had agreed upon. They approached that task, however, from two different vantage points. Leah felt that through their therapeutic relationship she should provide Ebony with linkages to the black community, affirmation as a black person, and ways to guard against feelings of alienation. Ebony felt that she needed help understanding the rules of the white business establishment and the guidelines for surviving its competitive cultures and environments. This discrepancy represented a significant difference in world view, but this divergence does not negate the fact that they had begun to form a relationship. From an EVM perspective, the potential for a therapeutic relationship had been formed, even though Leah continued to struggle with the divergence of their world views. If Leah could have discussed with Ebony the areas around which their world views diverged as well as converged, both of them could have gained a broader perspective.

Sustaining the Relationship

Despite their differences in world view, their therapeutic relationship was beneficial for Ebony and was rewarding and challenging for Leah. The issue that continued to resurface as they worked to utilize their therapeutic relationship was how they connected as black women. On the surface this issue was more problematic for Leah than it was for Ebony. Leah found it difficult to understand how Ebony saw herself in relationship to her ecology. More importantly, Leah continued to struggle around why Ebony wanted a black female therapist and what Ebony valued about this particular relationship.

Leah struggled with two hypotheses. The first was that Ebony had not consolidated her racial identity. While growing up, Ebony had received clear messages that she was to be proud of being black and of being smart. It seemed to Leah that Ebony may have learned to value the competitive smart part of herself more than the black part. Consequently, when she entered competitive environments, she worked to maintain this part of her identity. In contrast, others in her new ecologies had responded to her black self more than to her smart self. In coping in these new environments she had been ineffective in incorporating this information into her ecological schemata. The second hypothesis was that perhaps race was not an issue for Ebony; it was an issue for Leah. Perhaps Ebony had successfully assimilated the values of the white American culture. At the very least, Leah needed to view Ebony's ecology from Ebony's perspective and not focus exclusively on the possible racial dynamics.

During this phase of their therapy relationship, Ebony reported that another black female had been hired at her company. This woman was at a level comparable to Ebony's level, although she worked in another division. Ebony reported that she had heard from the grapevine that this new person was not very bright and, if the woman was not bright, she did not plan to get to know her. Ebony also noted that she was annoyed because everyone thought that Ebony had met the new employee because they were both black. Leah was annoyed by Ebony's comment, felt that it demonstrated Ebony's colonialized mentality, and asked Ebony on what basis she would get to know the new employee. Ebony essentially said that she would get to know her if she had something to offer either through business or social connections.

Leah suggested that Ebony had similar attitudes about a fellow black employee and was using the same criteria for judging that white workers had applied to Ebony. She also added that it appeared that Ebony's criteria for valuing human relationships was materialistic in nature. Ebony strongly disagreed with Leah's interpretation. She defended herself by stating that she had many friends whose relationships she valued because of their personalities, not what she could get from them. Ebony also noted that she resented the implication that she was racist or an "Uncle Tom," and that she was aligned with the more negative and oppressive elements of her work environment.

Leah apologized to Ebony for offending her, then added that she and Ebony differed greatly on their views about what it means to have a relationship with another person and what it means to have a relationship with another black person. Leah went on to say that in her world view the only consistent and reliable system of support blacks have had has come from other blacks. She noted that all blacks are not good and all are not bad, but that when individuals are feeling isolated and abused they tend to look to and look for the black community's support. She added that from her perspective she would have viewed this new employee as a potential ally; the whites in the dog-eat-dog world of business have allies. She argued that "everyone deserves an ally. Everyone needs support. You have been there for over 2 years and you have no consistent ally. And yes, because she is black and female, I think that she has the potential of being an important ally and friend." Finally, Leah added that she was concerned that Ebony only talked about relationships in terms of what was given and received. Relationships are give and take, but they are typically not balanced.

With this sharing of her world view by Leah, Ebony began to share her own world view. She viewed the world as a competitive place. In her opinion race has been used as a psychological handicap and had kept too many blacks out of the race for success. She felt that racism was a reality and that if she constantly recognized it she would become paralyzed by it since she could not eradicate it. She felt that to survive she could not afford to be friends with blacks who feel burdened by racism.

Out of this exchange they did finally recognize that both agreed that the environment responds to one's race and that coping mechanisms are needed to respond to that reality. However, the divergence of their views about being black in America was becoming clearer to both of them. The divergence pertained to how to cope with racism and how to relate to one's own blackness and to other blacks in shielding oneself from racism. Leah expressed her opinion that Ebony could not cope effectively with her environment unless she was willing also to deal with racism, to risk feeling the pain of racism, and to explore how it makes her vulnerable. This particular session ended with both client and therapist having a better understanding of their similarities and differences around racial issues.

In the next session, Ebony indicated to Leah that she had thought about their differences in seeing the world and that she recognized the value of Leah's perspective, but that she was unable emotionally to cope with racism and her black identity at that time. She felt that to confront these issues was the next step for her but that she needed some time to cope with them.

Leah agreed to approach these issues with Ebony in a less intense manner and to work to use their therapeutic relationship as a supportive one for Ebony. In essence, Leah switched to investing more in sustaining their relationship and pushed less strongly on using it to work out Ebony's problems. She suggested that they use this support to build the trust and courage needed to explore difficult issues. Ebony agreed to this new focus and, during the course of sustaining the relationship, Ebony confronted the ugliness of racism and developed a framework for coping with racism on the job.

Over a period of several months Ebony continued to feel good about the way she had been managing her life. She had become friends with the black employee at work and, through this friendship, had extended her social network to include blacks and whites. She began to refer to building relationships that felt like home in which she was not accepted because of star status. She was accepted because of her qualities as a person. Within Ebony's network of white friends, she became more selective. She nurtured only those relationships in which there was mutual support and respect.

Terminating the Relationship

By the time Leah and Ebony discussed termination, most of Ebony's friendships were based on a noncompetitive, nonmaterialistic framework. During the termination period, Ebony met two men, both of whom were interested in her. One, a black man, went to her church. The other, a white man, was a friend from work. Ebony realized that she had romantic feelings for the white man rather than the black man.

When Ebony discussed her choice of the white man over the black man, Leah was disappointed. Later when Leah discussed this issue in peer supervision, she realized that her disappointment was twofold. First, Leah felt proud of her work with Ebony. She felt that she had assisted Ebony in integrating her ecologies and thereby consolidating her identity. Leah felt disappointed because Ebony's choice of a white male for her partner negated Leah's feelings of accomplishment in helping Ebony to come to terms with her identity. Second, she believed that if a black person has a consolidated identity and is proud of his or her heritage, that perspective is demonstrated not only by how one treats blacks and whites but more importantly by whom one chooses to love.

Thus, Ebony's love for a white man over a black man was a contradiction for Leah. Leah's disappointment then was also a reaction to being challenged about her conceptions of racial identity and her knowledge of the literature on black personality development. She could not consolidate her book knowledge and her experiential knowledge to come to some understanding about Ebony's choice. Leah did not share her disappointment with Ebony, since she knew that it was her internal conflict and not Ebony's.

Commentary

Both Ebony and Leah grew from this therapy relationship. Ebony broadened her perspective of herself and of how she responded to her ecology and of how her ecology responded to her. In graduate school and in her work environment, she had begun to think of herself and relate to others as objects. In therapy she reexperienced a model of human relationships with which she grew up, one which valued human beings regardless of what they can give you. When she entered therapy, she could no longer recognize or rebuild such relationships in her new context. In her therapy Ebony allowed herself to be given to, to be vulnerable, and to trust. She also developed ways of coping that recognized her environment instead of ignoring it.

Leah also grew from her relationship with Ebony. Leah had defined for herself what it meant to be black and had developed this understanding in conjunction with the literature on black personality development. However, Ebony challenged her definition of blackness and of the ways in which one could function competently as a black person in America. Leah's relationship with Ebony forced her to deal with how she defined herself and rethink her understanding of viable ways in which blacks could experience self–world relationships. In her work with Ebony, Leah experienced a divergence in the ways in which blacks could experience themselves in the world and function competently. It was Leah's learning to accept that divergence that served to maintain the therapy relationship.

There were several issues not discussed that would have enhanced their personal growth. One issue pertained to the issue of their gender. Leah never asked Ebony why she preferred a female therapist. To have explored the reasons why Ebony wanted a female therapist may have given Leah more information about how Ebony saw herself and constructed her reality and self–world relationships. Also, as in the case of Mary and Sarah, the gender issue would have informed the therapist further as to the dynamics of their therapeutic relationship.

Black Therapist–White Client Dyad

Background Factors

Client Background

John is a 26-year-old white male who is married and has three young children. He is a high school graduate who works on the assembly line in a local factory, while his wife, Susan, works part time in the public school cafeteria. Their children are 6, 4, and 3 years of age and are cared for by Susan's mother when Susan is at work.

John has never lived outside of the city where he was born except for 3 years of military service. The third of five children, he has two older sisters and two younger brothers. His father worked as a laborer during the week and, as John puts it, "raised hell" all weekend. John's father had a heart attack 4 years ago and was so frightened by his illness that he sought help for his alcoholism. He has been alcohol-free since then, but his moodiness has increased and his temperament has oscillated between being reserved and having angry emotional outbursts. John's mother and siblings consider father's angry outbursts as part of his father's behavior pattern that existed prior to his heart attack.

Throughout his school career, John was an average to below average student who was well liked by his teachers and peers. Nevertheless, there were several instances in elementary school in which John had become angry with a classmate and had a tantrum. These outbursts were of concern to school officials and he had been referred to counseling.

John and Susan met in high school, started dating, and married when they were both 19. For the most part John feels that he and Susan have a good marriage and that they get along most of the time. He did complain that she had too many women friends to whom she talked. John did not have any friends in whom he confided since he preferred to keep his problems to himself and work them out alone.

John entered therapy because his wife left him. Recently, he had experienced periodic outbursts, some of which he related to alcohol overuse and some of which he related to having a bad day. After his last outburst in which he broke a door and damaged a wall, his wife told him that she would not come home unless he got help.

Therapist Background

Henderson is a 45-year-old, medium-brown complexioned, married black male. His children range in age from 10 to 20 years. He has lived in the same city all of his life, feels very well connected in the city, and is familiar with the city's ethnic boundaries and neighborhoods. He has two siblings, one of whom lives in the same city. The other moved to another city over 20 years ago. Henderson grew up in a predominantly black but interracial neighborhood. He now lives in a predominantly white neighborhood in a suburb of the city. He is active in community politics. His wife is a teacher in the school system and is from the Midwest.

Forming a Relationship

Henderson greeted John in the waiting room, escorted him to his office, and asked about his reasons for entering therapy at that time. John explained that he was having a great deal of stress on his job and at home and recounted the incident that had led to his wife's leaving. He explained that his behavior really frightened him and his family. When he calmed down, he tried to apologize but his wife was afraid. So she and his three children left to stay with John's in-laws. Susan said that she would return home only if John went into therapy. John had had previous outbursts of screaming and yelling but had never become violent. Because he loved his wife and wanted his family back home, he decided to come to therapy.

During this first session, Henderson explored John's home and work situation. He also took some history and background information and asked John if he had ever been in therapy before. John reported having been sent to counseling once after having trouble in school as a boy. He remembered it as an okay experience. "We just talked a lot. I don't know what I got out of it. Things did get better over the course of the school year."

Henderson ended the first session by asking John if he had any questions about therapy and by sharing with John the center's therapy policy. The center allowed for 12 therapy visits, after which a client was either referred to group therapy or, under special circumstances, could continue for a maximum of 12 additional therapy visits. He told John that the first few visits would be used to get to know each other better and for Henderson to get more information about John's particular life situation.

Henderson did not raise with John the issue of their race difference, although he knew that this could be a potential issue since John had grown up and lived in a section of the city known for its prejudice. Henderson decided to discuss the issue of their race difference only if it arose as an issue in therapy. Henderson felt that in conducting short-term psychotherapy it was not advantageous to raise more issues than could be adequately addressed in such a short time period. Moreover, he felt that racial issues are complex and often require more time than that allowed in short-term psychotherapy.

Over the next two sessions, John gave Henderson more information about his life circumstances. Henderson learned that John grew up in a home with alcohol abuse and violence and heard from John the various strategies that he used to cope with this environment. He also learned of John's tendency to abuse alcohol when under pressure. Henderson concluded that John fit the category of an adult child of an alcoholic and was at risk of repeating his father's pattern. John seemed to be a basically good man who was struggling to learn other ways to cope. His wife was a symbol of his ability to align himself with positive people as well as a reminder to him of his insecurities and his low self-esteem.

After the third session, Henderson shared his view with John and focused on John's struggle to be different from his father. He also shared with him the current thinking on the problems facing adult children of alcoholics. John replied that Susan had mentioned this pattern to him. She had seen two television talk shows on children who grew up in homes with an alcoholic parent. He had told her it was "baloney" but now thought maybe he should have paid closer attention to what she had to say. They agreed to focus on John's life growing up and on how, in camouflaged ways, he had translated his old coping skills to new situations.

Sustaining the Relationship

Over the next several weeks, Henderson and John focused their sessions on examining John's coping strategies at home and at his place of employment. Henderson provided John with some mini-lessons on stress and on the psychological and physiological ramifications of prolonged and intensive stress. They also discussed situations that had come up at home and at work and reviewed various ways to handle the stress.

John was assigned tasks and homework around his stress management. Most of these tasks involved finding periods of relaxing and finding ways in which he could enjoy his family without increasing their financial burden. John was compliant with most of his tasks. He appeared to be handling his life circumstances better and told Henderson that he felt that being able to talk about his problems really helped. He confessed that he was not sure that therapy or just talking would do any good, but that it had helped him.

Terminating the Relationship

The termination phase of the relationship took several weeks. Over this period Henderson and John focused on setting up continued supports for John. John had come to realize that he was fairly isolated and that he tended to have superficial relationships with his friends. He also tended to hold his problems within because he did not think anyone would care enough to help, and he did not think anyone could help. Henderson felt that a group for adult children of alcoholics could provide John with the continued support that he needed. He encouraged John to attend such a group and to take his wife with him to some of the meetings. By the time they terminated, John had attended one group meeting and Henderson had arranged to see John in 2 months for follow-up.

Commentary

In the above case, there was no reported instance of conflict during the therapy process and no instance in which the therapist or the client appeared to experience difficulty due to their race difference. Despite their very different backgrounds, convergence appeared to be the norm throughout the interchange between the client and therapist. As this case reflects, many therapists participate in cross racial/ethnic psychotherapy dyads and report conflict-free, effective, and satisfactory relationships with their clients without ever discussing their ethnic/racial difference.

The reasons therapists give for not mentioning race include: (1) The client's issues are universal and are not wed to any particular culture or groups; (2) Race is not the salient variable in therapy. Instead the central issue is the quality of the relationship that the therapist is able to establish. Warmth and empathy are two variables that have been identified as central therapist attributes in this regard; (3) The structure of the therapy does not allow for a discussion of race unless it is an issue (e.g., short-term psychotherapy); (4) The therapist is not comfortable with discussing race and does not know how to approach the issue.

Our position is that the choice not to discuss ethnic or racial differences has a cost associated with it. That cost is the degree to which the therapist and client both grow to recognize and understand the multiple influences and variables that shape each person's humanity, uniqueness, and world view. We do not view race issues as excess therapeutic baggage or as a complication. Race informs us about individuals' understandings of themselves and about the base from which they construct their reality. If we do not recognize that part of who we are or that part of others, we have limited the breadth and depth of the relationship.

The short-term structure of therapy significantly contributed to shaping Henderson's and John's therapeutic ecosystem. The health center had clear guidelines about individual therapy. Both the client and the therapist understood that they had limited time to work through problems in their relationship and in the client's home and work life. Consequently, they converged around the structure imposed on them. They had 12 sessions in which to address John's issues. It is important to note that it was Henderson's processing the meaning of the 12 sessions on their therapy relationship that made the 12-session limit such a powerful ecological structure. Short-term therapy does not negate EVM strategies. In fact, one of us teaches EVM psychotherapy within a short-term psychotherapy model.

The other factor that shaped Henderson's and John's experience was that both client and therapist were males. There was a shared implicit understanding about what it meant to be in control and to maintain one's esteem as a man. That is, their gender identity as males provided a basis for convergence. They also implicitly understood the rules of negotiating power from a male perspective and they both understood the aggressive ways in which men assert themselves at work. Being a male in America provided a framework for convergence.

Another factor that contributed to their achieving convergence was the distress that John was experiencing. Henderson could respond to John's distress and did so in a way that made sense to John. The profile for adult children of alcoholics fit closely with John's understanding of his reality.

In spite of these areas of convergence, the choice not to recognize openly the ethnic and/or racial differences between therapist and client limited the therapist's understanding of the client's ecology and culture. Both client and therapist missed the opportunity to move beyond their particular perspective and to bond on other levels. For example, it is possible that by acknowledging their racial differences Henderson would have learned about racial issues at John's job and about whether these issues contributed to John's stress. Also, in one of his sessions, John mentioned that the black employees at the factory seemed to handle their stress differently. Henderson responded by asking him how it was different and whether there were other individuals who seemed to handle their stress differently. Henderson could have used this statement by John to address more directly coping styles that are the same and different for different cultures, races, and genders. Moreover, such a discussion could have assisted John in isolating the nuances of his particular ecological set and in formulating strategies that might be adapted from other groups but were particular to his circumstances.

Essentially, the racial-avoidant pattern of their therapy relationship placed a ceiling on and boundary around the ways in which both individuals could grow. They did gain, however, in that each had a gratifying experience with someone of a different race. And it is possible that this experience may generalize to other areas of their lives. However, their loss was the experience of furthering their understanding of their racial ecosystem and how it influences their ways of relating and coping.

White Therapist–Black Client Dyad

Background Factors

Client Background

David is a 37-year-old black male who is married and has four biological children. Two of his children, ages 20 and 17, are from a previous relationship. His wife, Dora, age 35, has a 10-year-old child from a previous marriage. David and Dora also have two children, ages 6 and 3. The three youngest children reside with David and Dora.

David grew up in the projects of a major metropolitan area as the youngest and only male of five children. His father died from a heart attack when David was 20 years old, but his mother is still living and working part time. David's siblings felt that he reaped the most financial benefits from his parents' hard work. As the youngest he received more material goods and attention. His older siblings called him spoiled and attribute his pampering to his male status. David felt that he had an easy life. He described himself as a below average student who was a "good enough" kid that he managed to get by in classes because he was relatively well behaved.

His family was extremely disappointed in him when David became a father while he was in the twelfth grade. Neither parent insisted that he marry his girlfriend, Dionne; they did insist that he parent and support his child. Dionne and David had a stormy on-and-off relationship, which ended several years later, after the birth of their second child. David has maintained his parenting commitment to his children over the years, and he and Dionne have a "friendly enough" relationship.

David has worked since the birth of his first child. He does not consider himself to be smart, but he does feel that he is a good worker and gets the job done. He also feels that "a man is not a man" unless he works and puts food on the table. David met his wife Dora 8 years ago and, after dating for about a year, they married. David feels that they have a good marriage and that Dora has put up with a lot from him recently in terms of his drinking and going out with his friends.

Therapist Background

Harry is a white male, age 40, who grew up in the Midwest as the second of three children. He has fond memories of childhood until the age of 10, when his father's small business nearly went bankrupt. During that time the family underwent an economically difficult period, his father began to drink heavily, and his parents' marriage began to disintegrate. By the time he was 15, business had begun to improve, his father's drinking became more tolerable, and at least at this point his father and mother were not arguing.

Harry was a very good student who was considered by his teachers and peers to be "an all round good guy." Harry feels that his intellectual abilities and willingness to work hard enabled him to obtain competitive academic scholarships so that he could complete college and graduate school. While in college, Harry met and married his wife. They have three children and live a comfortable life in the suburbs.

Forming a Relationship

Harry met David in the waiting room of the mental health clinic of the health maintenance organization (HMO) and escorted David to the office. Once settled in the office, Harry asked David why he sought therapy. David told him that he was referred to counseling by his job supervisor and manager because he had been having difficulty at work. He had also been experiencing a great deal of stress because of financial pressures and marital problems. David said that his manager felt that his personal problems were interfering with his job performance and with his ability to be a team player. David had been employed by the company for 10 years and had a reputation as a good worker, but recently David had been tardy from lunch on several occasions and his supervisors had smelled liquor on his breath when he returned from lunch. The supervisor, who wanted to give him a chance to get help for his problems, contacted the company's employee assistance program, and they referred David to the HMO.

When Harry asked about his job and his home life, David shared that on the job many of the men whom he had started working with had been promoted or had moved on to other areas of the company. Over the years, he had received pay increases but he and another, much older man had not been selected for job promotions. They were the most senior members of the loading dock crew. The newer employees on the dock were young black and white men in their early twenties who did not appear to care about getting ahead. What angered David was that the white employees seemed to get promoted, regardless of their efforts. David would train the younger employees only to have them promoted to supervisory positions. David often got into arguments with fellow black employees, did not receive promotions, and did not seem to care. He felt angry at most of the black employees because of their attitude and felt angry with the white employees because of their privileged status.

At home, David was experiencing financial pressures. He paid child support for his 17-year-old and had three children at home to support. His wife had been laid off from her job and had been looking for employment for 3 months, although David wondered at times how hard she was looking. He noted that he and his wife had numerous arguments about finances, which had significantly interfered with their relationship. Finally, David was worried about his 17-year-old son, who was starting to become friendly with teenagers who, according to David, were going "nowhere in life." David had begun to drink more than usual and to stay out late as a means of coping.

Harry could hear in his voice and see in his face how overwhelmed David was. He considered the possibility that David might be experiencing prejudice and discrimination around being promoted at work. However, it was hard for Harry to believe that David could be passed over for 10 years for no other reason than his race. Harry wondered if more was going on at David's job than what he was reporting. Also, Harry noticed that David spoke in black dialect and that his grammar and diction were poor. Harry wondered if these factors could have contributed to David's being overlooked for promotion.

The session ended with Harry explaining the HMO's therapy policy. David would see Harry every 2 weeks. Their sessions would be confidential and not part of his employment record. Any information requested by David's employer would be released only with David's approval.

In the following weeks Harry became more familiar with David's background and routine at home. He listened to David's life and thought about how cumbersome and disorganized it all seemed—trying to manage two families, plus an extended family and his job. He also felt that this pattern was to some extent typical of black families.

Harry and David agreed upon treatment objectives. They decided to deal with David's job first rather than address his home life. Dora had recently gotten a job, and things were better at home with the knowledge that another paycheck woiuld be contributing to managing the household.

Harry had David describe the nature of his work, tell him about all of the employees with whom he had the most contact, and describe the qualifications and previous job experience of the employees who had been promoted over David. He also asked David about his style of interacting with people, how people reacted to him, and how David handled problem situations or his anger on the job. Harry felt that once he had identified every possible explanation for David's not being promoted, he could then deal more directly with the discrimination hypothesis.

As Harry questioned David, David became more annoyed and agitated. Finally, David looked at him and said "Man, you are a white boy for sure." Harry was taken aback by David's comment and intimidated by his angry face and large bulk. Finally he asked David what he meant by his statement. David responded, "You know what I mean. You tryin' to say that they justified in not promoting me. You tryin' to find every reason in the book to get them off the hook! I thought you suppose to be on my side. I was stupid to think you anything else but white!" With that statement David got up to leave. Harry asked him to stay but David just looked at him and walked out.

From an EVM perspective, David and Harry had generated a crisis and conflict in their therapy because of cultural differences in problem-solving style and because of the legacy of their particular ecosystems. David interpreted Harry's questions as a betrayal, which was very much a part of David's expectation of black–white relationships. David had concluded that Harry's race—his whiteness—had proven to be the most important variable in how Harry was defining their therapeutic relationship. David had entered the therapy with a relationship history with whites that needed to be explored during the first session. If it had been, it might have provided a forum for addressing David's expectations about their cross-race relationship. Although Harry had been socialized to treat all people in a nondiscriminating fashion, his assumptions and stereotypes of black culture implied that he did hold some inferiority assumptions about blacks.

Within an EVM framework, a discussion of their racial ecology would also have involved a discussion of their knowledge limitations and assumptions about the other's culture. David made assumptions about Harry and Harry made assumptions about David. If there had been a sharing of the general frame of reference from which each person was communicating, then they could have succeeded in shaping a context for attributing meaning to questionable statements and inquiries, and they could have formed a context for convergence.

The next evening Harry called David, explained his intent in asking the questions and apologized for offending David. He also said that he wanted to maintain the therapy relationship with David, if David felt that they could work together. David accepted his apology, said that he would give it another try, and apologized for walking out of the session.

From Harry and David's perspective, the next session went well. They reiterated that they did not intend to offend and/or disrespect each other and agreed to discuss their differences openly but did not review their angry interchange. They began to reexamine David's situation at work and experienced a sense of convergence because they had established a context for understanding their exchange.

Sustaining the Relationship

The middle phase of the therapy relationship was marked by the two men dealing with a number of areas. The first was David's self-esteem and how his esteem influenced his relationship with his fellow employees and his family. The second was David's use of alcohol and marijuana as a coping mechanism for his depression. And the third was David's management of his anger.

During this phase of therapy David and Harry continued to work through issues of divergence, but they did not experience additional conflict. Their established convergence around their acceptance that each other's intent was honorable and without malice, so they had a basis for coping with their differences.

For instance, Harry felt that role definitions in David's family, especially his extended family, were not clear and caused stress for David and his immediate family. David was involved in disciplining his sister's children, and that seemed to Harry to be unnecessary. When David's 10-year-old nephew had gotten into a fight at school, his mother asked David to come over to her house, talk to her son, and set up a punishment for him. David complied with the request, as the boy's father lived out of state. Harry felt that David's sister was abdicating her parenting responsibilities. David told Harry that he could hear what he was saying but that was not how he and his family operated. Moreover, what Harry was suggesting did not feel right to him. After much discussion, they were able to agree to disagree.

In future sessions, David continued to mention his nephew and his involvement in his sister's family. Harry continued to point out concerns from his perspective. Some of Harry's suggestions felt right to David and he acted upon them, and some of them did not and he did not act upon those. This pattern proved to characterize all areas of divergence experienced in their therapy and to be of value to both of them.

Terminating the Relationship

After a year of therapy David began to feel more in control of his life and his work situation, so he discussed with Harry the notion of ending therapy. By this time David was managing his stress level, had ceased drinking on the job, had decreased his social drinking, and had a clear sense of the requirements for promotion. He also enrolled with his wife at the community college in a night course on parenting. David felt that therapy had helped him to increase his confidence and to confront his problems without internalizing them. He also stated that he felt better about himself and that he was able to interact with his wife and children with greater ease and patience.

As David introduced termination, he also introduced the idea of keeping in contact with Harry on an informal basis—"Maybe we could have lunch or something." Harry told David that he liked him a lot and had grown to have tremendous respect for him, but that he had established a policy not to socialize with his clients in order to protect the possibility of a future client relationship. David did not understand what the problem was in talking over lunch, stating that it would not be often, maybe only once a year. Then David told Harry about a cousin of his that he only sees once a year—but when they got together they "could really talk." As David explained this relationship to Harry, Harry interpreted David's feelings concerning his bond with his cousin as a statement of David's bond with him. Harry hypothesized that David experienced him as a family member and wanted to know how that bond could be preserved.

Harry told David that they had a relationship that was unique because of the personal nature of things they discussed and the level of sharing that took place. He went on to say that therapy relationships feel like family relationships and that it is often inconceivable to say good-bye to family. He then suggested that maybe the issue was not whether they must say good-bye, but how they could maintain contact. With this reframing, he and David worked out a way to maintain contact with each other that was comfortable for both of them. They decided that

Harry would call David in 2 months to see how he was managing and that David would write him a note or give him a call as a means of keeping in touch after that.

Commentary

What seems most striking about this dyad is that David and Harry gained a great deal from each other and also missed repeated opportunities for growth. They learned that they could achieve a relatively harmonious relationship with someone of the opposite race. They also learned that they could experience racial conflict with a person and then resolve that conflict.

Nevertheless, they never dealt directly with the issue of race and culture and therefore lost the opportunity to grow beyond their respective world views and beyond their ethnocentrism. This limitation placed boundaries on the extent to which they could develop trust in their relationship and communicate effectively. For instance, Harry never confronted his personal prejudices and stereotypes about black culture. Nor did he confront David's perceptions of his whiteness and what that meant to David. Because Harry proceeded with therapy without exploring the issue of race for himself or for David, he missed the multiple meanings of some of David's statements. For example, David discussed his relationship to his nephew and to his sister. Harry missed that part of the communication that emphasized David's sense of family responsibility and commitment. More importantly, he missed the connection between the role that David had in the family and role definitions within many black families. When David raised the issue of his nephew, he was not complaining about his family role as uncle, he was communicating to Harry his concern about his nephew.

David also had strong beliefs about whites, which were not explored and which continued to limit his level of growth in therapy. At some level, David expected Harry to misunderstand his particular job-related concerns and to think about his concerns from the perspective of white authority, and he never looked at those expectations. David also missed the opportunity to sort out his thinking about his relationships with his fellow black employees whose attitudes about work and advancement had disappointed him. In hindsight, Harry realized that he held similar images of the "typical" black worker. Consequently, Harry did not identify this intragroup conflict as a problem area for David. However, it was an area of difficulty because David's understanding of what it meant to be a black man was being challenged by members of his racial group and support network.

None of these issues were addressed because Harry and David were unable to discuss race, though they both were responsible for bringing it up. Harry, of course, bore the greater responsibility because of his position of power and authority in the dyad. Nevertheless, both Harry and David reported a gratifying and satisfactory experience in working together.

Summary

For each of these dyads the therapist and client were presented with opportunities to grow beyond their current understanding of themselves as ethnic and racial beings. Moreover, the therapeutic ecosystem provided an opportunity to explore their self–world relationships given their ascribed status in society, their gender, their socioeconomic status, and how they defined themselves. The client's growth is the focus of therapy; however, the EVM framework emphasizes that within any human exchange where individuals contribute their multiple realities and experiences to form an effective relationship, the therapist learns and grows as well. In these instances that was the case, and it seems to us to have enhanced the client's gains, not diminished them.

10

Teaching, Learning, and Applying an EVM Approach

Individual Psychotherapy and Related Activities

Throughout this book we have been writing about ethnic validity issues that arise in counseling and psychotherapy. In doing so we have paid particular attention to therapist–client relationship patterns. We have also addressed their role in teaching contexts and in supervisor–supervisee relationships. We have noted that teachers as well as students must learn to attend to ethnic validity perspectives to become an accepted part of the psychotherapy world. In this chapter, our goal is twofold. We want to attend specifically to the teaching–learning process. We also want to outline how the ethnic validity approach can serve as a model for teaching and practice in a range of intervention contexts and with diverse groups of people engaged in human helping activities. Calling attention to these few topics provides a bridge to a wider range of applications for the ethnic validity approach.

Teaching Themes

One of our objectives in this book has been to demythologize and rehumanize psychotherapy and our understanding of it. We have stressed that the therapist and the client are both somewhat autonomous individuals, but they are also embedded in their particular cultural and ethnic/racial framework. As we turn from describing an ethnic validity approach to psychotherapy to applying it to training therapists and to related activities, we want to focus on three themes that are basic to our approach.

Theme 1: We Are All Part of the Ecology

In teaching others to conduct therapy we have to teach them to become aware of their own ecology as well as that of their clients. At the most general level, we provide people a means of learning about their ecologies by exposing them directly or vicariously to human diversity. One direct approach to exposure is to teach psychotherapy in a context that includes a diverse group of students and a diverse group of clients. Indirect approaches include assigning readings about different cultures and the experiences of people from both culture-defining and non-culture-defining groups in those cultures. Anthropology, sociology, history, and literature are valuable sources. Other sources are the dramatic arts, including the theatre and movies. An even richer indirect source is diverse life experiences, but those cannot usually be prescribed as part of a curriculum.

Teaching and learning also take place in the context of doing psychotherapy. One of the authors tells his graduate psychotherapy students that it is important and essential that they (1) acknowledge their awareness of their ecological identity, and (2) be quite willing to explore the relevance of their identity to the therapeutic relationship that they are establishing and to the therapeutic interactions that will stem from that relationship.

Each of us has racial, ethnic, gender, age, class, and other status characteristics. It is important that we learn to acknowledge their existence and discuss their relevance to the therapeutic relationship and process for at least four reasons. First, they may have special relevance. Second, it is easier for our clients to discuss ethnic/racial topics if they know that we are aware of their potential relevance. Third, it is easier for our clients to discuss them if they know that we are open to discussing them. Fourth, it is easier for us and our clients to discuss them if we have learned how to do so comfortably and skillfully. We learn to be comfortable with and skillful about dealing with ethnic/racial and other ecological factors through working at it. Our effectiveness rests in part on the normative accuracy of the ways we interact with others. That normative accuracy includes an understanding of other people's perspectives and consequently of what kinds of behaviors are appropriate in interacting with them and what kinds of responses it is realistic to expect from them.

An example may be useful in clarifying our point. Most therapists are white males. Therapy operates on the basis of interpersonal trust, and therapists encourage clients to develop trust in them. A legitimate question arises as to how much a female client, particularly one from a minority status group, should trust a white male therapist. After all, minority group members have more than enough reasons to be skeptical of the trustworthiness and benign intentions of white people. To the extent that her therapist is more trustworthy than other white males, he may lead her to be more trusting of other men, white men in particular, than is in her interest or is appropriate in her world.

Therapists also judge a situation from their ecological status. White males may be inclined to expect that their perspective is valid and unbiased. Their life circumstances have generally supported that view. As therapists, and therapists in training, they are generally taught to believe in their own objectivity and benign intent. They are taught to view client distrust as a manifestation of paranoia. Ridley (1984) has pointed out that in the psychotherapy literature minority clients are viewed as somewhat paranoid. He then suggests that that paranoia may be healthy. The white male student (or any student) therapist can acquire an experientially as well as intellectually accurate sense of how clients react to his race/ethnicity, how he reacts to it, and how he reacts to various clients only through actual experience, preferably in a context in which supervision and feedback can be provided.

Our point is that part of teaching someone to be a therapist is engaging that person in exploring life directly, in reading widely, in observing and listening carefully, and in trying out a variety of formulations of who he or she is and how he or she is perceived by others. Approaches available for teaching students how to identify, understand, and figure out how to know and utilize their ecological rootedness include workshops, role playing, and conducting therapy under supervision. Those same approaches can at the same time teach students how to be sensitive to the ecological rootedness of their clients.

Theme 2: In the Words of a Student, "I Have to Fix My Own Puzzle First, Then I Can Fix Theirs"

At a more general level, the student's point is that we each have to work out for ourselves ways to deal with an issue before we can be of help to someone else. We do have to *fix* our own problems. We do not have to, and cannot, *fix* theirs. We can, however, help or facilitate their efforts. The issue is that to become, or be, useful therapists we need to be prepared to learn and to change, and we need to expect to change. We need to commit ourselves to an ongoing process of assimilating new experiences and perspectives. From an EVM perspective, that learning and teaching must incorporate learning about our ethnic/racial nature as well as our individual nature. Further, even when we do focus on the importance of students learning about themselves as preparation for becoming a therapist, we usually think of recommending therapy for therapist trainees. There are, of course, instances in which therapy can be of value in facilitating the student's development as a therapist, and it can be appropriate. Yet even in those instances, conventional individual therapy approaches tend to be limited in two ways. They are usually focused on the intrapsychic and interpersonal aspects of an individual's life and slight its psychosocial or sociocultural aspects. Further, the recommendation to seek therapy usually implies a need to look at deficits that, by definition, are to be labeled and considered in some sense pathological. We are suggesting that students need to be provided an ethnic validity perspective, a means of attending to racial/ethnic identity, ecological identity, psychosocial competencies as well as limitations, and resources to use as well as deficits to overcome.

If the student is to fix his or her own psychosocial or sociocultural limitations, biases, or distortions, he or she needs to have that task introduced as part of the general task of becoming a therapist. Further, that point needs to be particularly stressed as we try to provide effective psychotherapy for ethnic minorities and as we try to provide effective psychotherapy training for ethnic minority students. We are all going to be changed by that effort, or we are not going to accomplish that goal. As individuals, we will need to change in quite different ways. For example, it is easy and obvious to see that a white male therapy trainee must change in so far as he is a member of the majority with its insensitivity to its own biases. In that sense, he does not even qualify as ethnic, let alone as minority. He is the oppressor in an ecological sense, even if not in a personal sense. Obviously, he must become aware of that aspect of his identity to help a member of an ethnic minority group or of another culture grow in humanity and well-being. The part that is more difficult for all of us to accept is that he has an ethnic identity too. Yes, if all that we do is make him aware of everyone else's ethnicity, we may simply make him so hypersensitive that we immobilize him so that he can neither help himself nor anyone else. Further, unless others can be helped to see him as also having an ethnic identity, they are limited in their capacity to relate to him or others like him. They are also limited in their capacity to define their individual and ecological statuses as part of a broad social ecological context that includes everyone in a nested way. It is, needless to say, frequently difficult to work out an approach to our individual and collective conditions and interactions that is more humane for all of us. Nevertheless, as we strive to learn to become therapists or to teach others to become therapists, we need to undertake this balancing act in a fairly direct and explicit way.

Theme 3: There are Trade-offs, Triangulations, and Multiple Truths

Our task as teachers is to work out and implement an approach to training others to become more self-aware individuals. That self-awareness is needed so that they can integrate these individual and broader ecological factors that influence the ways they live and can then use that broader perspective in understanding clients and helping them accomplish a similar task in their own lives. To guide that teaching and learning process, we as teachers need to formulate a conceptual framework that is consistent with our experiences as persons, therapists, and teachers of therapy. The ethnic validity framework and the psychosocial competence configuration perspective on which we have based this book have served as that basis and are what we use in teaching others to be therapists. Nevertheless, that framework is just that—a framework. It does not provide an answer to all of our questions. It does provide a way of thinking about them, of keeping in mind the considerations involved in seeking answers to those questions, and of going about evolving at least tentative working answers to some of those questions.

In applying the idea of ethnic validity to therapy we have tried to speak of the trade-offs—the gains and limitations—of any therapist–client pairing. We have also spoken of conceptualizing therapist–client interactions in terms of convergence, divergence, and conflict. That is, no matter how different we are ethnically we can potentially find areas of convergence—areas of agreement, of commonality. If we can transcend our ethnocentrism we can also grasp that individuals will diverge in ways to live—they will be different. Finally, we arrive at a position in which we can acknowledge that our perspectives conflict in some ways, but that there are many potentially constructive ways to contain those conflicts. We need not subjugate or destroy one another to survive. In teaching we focus on sensitizing students to this way of formulating their relationships to their teachers, their fellow students, their clients, and the issues that arise in the course of conducting therapy.

In a similar way we have come to emphasize the importance of trade-offs, triangulations, and multiple truths. As we have been stressing throughout our writing, any position we may take has both advantages and limitations; it embodies trade-offs. Further, we often cannot directly challenge or verify an observation or interpretation of events.

That may be because we did not observe it as we weren't present at the appropriate time and place. On the other hand, it may be because it simply does not permit direct observation, as is often the case with anyone's sense of her or his own or someone else's inner reality. In those types of instances our only recourse is to use a process similar to that which surveyor's use—we triangulate. We get a fix on something by making a set of at least three indirect measurements or observations.

Nevertheless, even using this type of approach does not enable us to transcend the possibility of multiple truths, each of which has at least some validity. In teaching we focus on the importance of learning to accept, live with, and build constructively on those multiple truths. In teaching a semester-long course on individual adult psychotherapy one of the authors includes several workshops. The following is an account from one of those workshops that illustrates the importance of attention to these factors:

> One such workshop involved me and four student therapists of whom one was a white female, one a black female, and two were black males. We were focused on the general question of what we are trying to do with therapeutic relationships after we have established them. In doing so we were referring to the clients we are seeing. The black female student was discussing her dilemmas in working with a black female client who has had her feelings betrayed many times so sees no point in talking about them. To her the only solution is to describe events and go on with life without feeling. The white female student stated emphatically that, when a person is dealing with feelings such as those of loss or betrayal, the feelings must first be expressed and dealt with totally as feelings before any attempt to deal with them cognitively can be helpful. After some discussion I indicated that the white student's perspective is consistent with traditional therapeutic views and with a middle-class Anglo world view and may indeed be appropriate for people with such a background. I then added that this view is culture based and there may be other approaches. She responded strongly that I am authoritarian, racist (biased against whites), not open to change, and unwilling to teach real (traditional) therapy. She went on to point out that I was always putting down white people and related that to my origins at a particular time in the history of psychology and to my own inner dynamics.
>
> In all fairness to her I do believe that the dominant Anglo ethos in American society is often ethnocentric and Anglos are often unaware that they are members of a culture based group just like everyone else. I also think that American psychology and Western (European & American) therapies have grown out of that ethos and have viewed it as the universal nature of people. I have even said as

much in person and in print. I have also said that I believe we Anglos bear a special responsibility because of our dominant position to correct our biased theories and practices. The question is whether I have a broader view of Anglo and other cultures or whether I do hate myself and other Anglos and need to engage in flagellation of myself and others like me.

It might be easy to dismiss her charges by responding that she is the one who has internal conflicts, not I. That seems to me to be unfair to both of us. She does have internal conflicts but so do I. We do belong to different cohorts so have been socialized in different periods of historical time. We have struggled with different social issues. We are also both products of that very Anglo heritage to which I referred. So how are we to resolve our differences.

I would argue that we need to triangulate. We need the input of others, some with a similar perspective and some with a different ethnic perspective. In this instance the views of the black students provided the only other perspective we had available so I suggested that we check with them. The two males said that this course had provided for them the *only* occasion they had experienced in their psychology training in which the professor had *not* presented and defended the Anglo perspective as the "true" or valid one. They said that what they valued was being in a context in which the Anglo perspective was represented as one of a number of yardsticks against which a person could measure behavior but not the only one nor necessarily the best one. The black female seemed to agree that I was biased. That is, she said that the white student could consider this a good experience. Now the white student could know what it is like to be a minority and have her perspective put down.

Am I biased? The question seems unresolved in an ultimate sense and probably always will be. In a more immediate and specific sense, there are differences of opinion. Two women think I am and two men think I'm not. I believe the more general points are these: (1) As two Anglos arguing about our views we were both trapped in our Anglo perspective (2) As a man and a woman arguing we were speaking from different sexual/social perspectives. (3) The black students have their own biases but they also have a different (non-Anglo) perspective on the behavior of the two of us. (4) There is no position that any of us could have taken that would be considered to be unbiased by all observers. (5) Since we were able to discuss our perspectives we all could learn something about our ethnicity and each other's. We could also learn about how our ethnicity influences how we think about, feel about, and conduct therapy. (6) It is very doubtful to me that any of us could have worked through these possibilities with clients of our own ethnic identity or of a different one. In short, to transcend our ethnic perspectives we need to interact with *therapists* who are from similar and from different ethnic

> perspectives than our own, not just with clients. (7) Unfortunately, this particular interaction was confounded by my faculty status in relation to their student status. In fact the white student argued that the black students would not be willing to challenge me as they knew I was going to give them a grade. They accused her of being unfair to them and not respecting their integrity. Perhaps they did challenge her position because they respect mine. Perhaps they were stung by her insult and struck back. (8) To sort out those possibilities I need peer challenges and feedback, not just feedback from students. I also need hierarchical feedback from supervisors and others more experienced and knowledgeable than I. (Tyler, 1986, pp. 9–12)

There are undoubtedly many more examples that could be used to illustrate the points made here. In fact, it is our hope that the one described above will serve to stimulate the thinking of teachers and students about disagreements and interchanges in which they have participated. A very powerful, if not essential, component of teaching and learning is our involvement in the learning process with our students.

We are also convinced that there is merit in viewing therapy as having ecological, ethnic/racial, and individual components and incorporating that perspective in our teaching. That does not mean that there are no important therapeutic gains that can be achieved by identifying and examining convergences in human experience that transcend ecological and ethnic/racial barriers. Of course there are. There are also important therapeutic gains that can be achieved only by identifying and examining divergences in human experience that are specific to ecological and ethnic/racial barriers. Finally, there are other important therapeutic gains that can be achieved only by identifying and examining conflicts in human experience that are a function of ecological and ethnic/racial barriers. Our point is that a significant aspect of our teaching is to alert our students to these distinctions and to explore them in the teaching context.

Unfortunately, at present we have only a limited awareness of the import of these positions because we have only begun to explore them. We have had to do a lot of exploring and sorting to identify cross-ethnic/racial convergences. And we have found them by struggling with our divergences and our conflicts, not by ignoring them. It is that kind of approach that we want to introduce as we look at the actual process of trying to help someone learn to become a therapist. That is, we approach the teaching of therapy by looking for convergences, divergences, and conflicts. We look for competencies as well as limitations. We look for cultural, racial, ethnic, gender, and other social factors as well as individual ones. Above all, we approach it by saying that we are all humans struggling to make sense out of our lives and learning to become a therapist is best achieved with that point central in our awareness.

Summary

What we are trying to emphasize for the therapist in training and the therapist trainer is that when two people interact, they do so at many levels. The teaching–learning involved in the process of assisting someone to become a therapist needs to attend in some way to those realities. In actual situations, all of these explorations, consolidations, and adaptations are occurring more or less simultaneously and often in contradictory ways. The client and the therapist are utilizing interpersonal influence and problem-solving skills to shape their interactions in directions that will accomplish their respective goals. In doing so they also exhibit to themselves and to each other contradictory and dysfunction behaviors, feelings, and reactions, as well as constructive ones. It seems likely that anyone, inexperienced or not, would be overwhelmed if he or she tried to attend to all of it at once. And we are not proposing that anyone should. We are saying, however, that therapists (trainees or experts or trainers) need to be sensitive to cues that any of these factors are operating in any therapeutic interaction. Consequently, one of our goals in teaching therapy is to assist trainees in their efforts to acquire those sensitivities.

That task is a complex one that continues as long as any of us works in a helping or teaching capacity. Being an effective teacher requires that to some degree we extend our own world views at a cultural or ethnic/racial ecosystem level, at an interpersonal or personal level, and at a level of interacting with the world of work and society at large. In other words, we as teachers, our students, and our clients are involved in extending our personal competencies as well as our self- and world views. Those tasks are demanding and difficult at best. Facing them leads us back to where we started. We (teacher, student therapist, client) have to learn to triangulate to get a fix on who and where we are, what we are involved in, and what we are doing. We have to learn to assess and work with the trade-offs involved in understanding and changing ourselves and others, and we have to learn to relate differently to the multiple truths that characterize the human condition and human internal and external relationships. Much of the process of teaching–learning in relation to the task of becoming a therapist is focused in one way or another on that agenda, which is central to our approach to helping anyone learn to be a better therapist.

We cannot attend simultaneously to all of the aspects of such a complex set of processes. Consequently, we will look first at understanding therapy as a human interaction process, then at the sequence inherent in a therapeutic session or course, and then at supervisor–supervisee interactions as a special vehicle for that learning. There is inherent overlap in this ordering, but we have tried to keep it at a minimum without losing sight of our goal to provide an integrated picture of these interrelated facets.

TRAINING GOALS: UNDERSTANDING THERAPY AS A HUMAN INTERACTION-BASED CHANGE PROCESS

Throughout this book we have stressed our view that psychotherapy is a change process that occurs through the medium of human interaction. Also, it is a process in which the most basic goal is that of improving the soundness and well-being of the client's humanity as a person. Those ideas are compelling to us, but just stating them does not answer the question of how we teach them to students. In the final analysis, each teacher and each student must work out a solution for themselves. What we want to provide is encouragement and guidelines for paying more attention to humanness and human interaction in therapy and in the process of learning to do therapy.

The Human Factor

Traditionally, a fixed role has been advocated as most appropriate for therapists. Emphasis has been placed on the therapist interacting with the client in a unilaterally controlled way that precludes their knowing each other as persons in the more usual sense. We are going to outline a contrasting approach in which the reality of the therapist's humanness is acknowledged and accepted as part of the therapeutic reality.

We have created ourselves as psychosocial beings, we express that part of ourselves in all of our interactions, and we also differentiate our roles and define boundaries in our interactions. The student's task is to learn to establish and maintain a pattern of personal and role integrity as a therapist. The teacher's task is to facilitate that process. We are going to suggest one way of structuring that task. This approach can be used as part of a course requirement or as a set of questions for a student, a supervisor, or a practicing therapist to address with some regularity. For purposes of presentation, we outline our approach as a term paper requirement in a formal psychotherapy course that combines didactic and practicum components. It can also be a task to undertake in a workshop, or as a regular review exercise throughout a course, an internship, or as a guide to self-directed learning.

The student must answer the following five questions. The answers may be based on theory, technique, or personal experience and preference and to some extent will involve all three. Except in rare instances in which the student's view is quite idiosyncratic and potentially destructive, what matters is for the student to identify his or her general view of therapy and formulate a sense of comfort with that view as an organizing framework.

1. *Why am I becoming a therapist?* In this section, it is important to articulate what kinds of ecological, ethnic/racial, community, interpersonal, and intrapersonal factors converged to lead the student to direct his or her energies toward becoming a therapist. The point of this question is that unless each of us confronts it, we and our clients are unwitting victims of our unawareness.

Also, it is of value for the student to learn that there is no necessary benefit nor harm in wanting to become a therapist because of having been helped by a therapist, of seeing therapy as a vehicle for helping others or changing society, or as a way of earning a living. There potentially is harm in not being aware of these motivations and of implicitly or, for that matter, explicitly expecting clients to respond in ways that validate our commitments. For instance, if it is important to us as therapists that our clients get married because getting married improved our lives, then we have imposed our values, not helped our clients to identify their own.

2. *What do I think therapy is about?* Anyone who tries to become a therapist brings to that undertaking a background of personal experiences plus formal instruction and exploration of the literature about therapy. Students need to formulate a specific sense of what they think they are doing. Many aspects of what a student is about will only become apparent as the teacher, the student, and the client observe what the student is doing. Nevertheless, it is only by answering that question explicitly that any of us articulates a coherent reference point from which to guide, assess, and modify our approach to therapy. We need to state for ourselves the who, what, how, and why of taking initiatives; of forming and using relationships; of seeking patterns of interaction; of introducing, excluding, or responding to racial, ethnic, social, gender, or other concerns.

3. *What is my role as therapist?* A therapist should have a coherent sense of his or her role as a therapist. The student begins to define that

role by trying to express it, by asking, "What do I think that I want to do or am supposed to be doing? Is my role reactive and fixed? Is my role a flexible one that is outcome as well as process related? Am I to try to meet the client's expectations of my role?" Learning can proceed more quickly and more effectively as we define our starting points.

4. *What is the client's role?* The student needs to formulate his or her views about the client's rights and responsibilities to define the relationship and the meaning of events in therapy and in his or her life. Other questions to answer include our expectations as therapists about what the client is expected to do or permitted to do outside of the therapy situation as well as inside it. What are the client's rights and responsibilities to establish and monitor behavioral guidelines?

5. *How do we conceptualize the nature of a total therapeutic interaction process? What are its phases?* Therapy is not ordinarily thought of as a process without end. Rather, it has a clear beginning; at some point it becomes a working relationship; at some more distant point it ends. If we are to teach someone else about being a therapist, or learn about it ourselves, then we need at the very least to outline for ourselves what we understand to be the *natural* course of therapy. As an aid to accomplishing that task, we will outline some of the issues to which a student needs to attend in each of those three phases.

Phase 1: Forming a Relationship

The questions that a therapist must consider include whether he or she is going to view the client's dysfunction as a disease (neurosis, etc.) or as a problem in living. In either case students need to ask what kind of relationship they believe needs to be formed and how they are going to account to themselves and others, including their clients, for forming a relationship of that particular type. They also need to ask and answer how that relationship will get formed, what they need to do to enable it, and how they will know when it has been established.

Phase 2: Sustaining and Utilizing the Relationship

The first question that confronts the student therapist once a relationship has been established is "What do we do now?" We live in a society that believes in "They lived happily ever after." The student therapist must ask what he or she and the client need to do to accomplish their therapeutic goals. A related question is "What are the similarities to and differences from a therapeutic relationship of any newly formed relationship?" Other questions include whether therapy may have a variety of goals and outcomes and proceed in a variety of ways. Or, does the student believe that there is a *natural* or *ideal* process or outcome that will evolve or should evolve in the course of therapy. The student needs to consider whether he or she is going to focus on the client's past, present, or future; and whether priority will be given to lack of opportunity, inaccurate or conflicted learning, inadequate psychological resources, or destructive impulses as organizing themes in defining and working toward therapeutic goals. In other words, the student needs to identify and spell out a theoretical framework and justification for his or her view of what the work of therapy entails and of how to guide it as therapist. The student also needs to answer on what grounds he or she can use the relationship established to derive and proceed toward therapeutic goals that make sense both to the client and to the therapist.

Phase 3: Terminating the Relationship

The decision to terminate a therapeutic relationship and the process of doing so raise a number of questions that all too often are not scrutinized particularly well but that also need to be spelled out. "How do we (the client and I) define what we have accomplished and whether we have accomplished what we set out to accomplish? How do we define the completing of a process and relationship? How do we go about terminating, and what are we terminating? What have we gained/lost in the termination? What has the client gained/lost in the termination? What have I (the therapist) gained/lost in the termination?"

Again, we are faced with the question of whether there is some process that will automatically lead to a psychologically mature natural outcome at which point the client and (the student) therapist will know that therapy is complete.

What the students need to do with these questions is to formulate their chosen theoretical, societal, and personal views on which they base their answers to these questions. They then need to formulate their answers and decide whether and how to include their clients in that understanding and the process itself.

Our point is that student therapists need to formulate some basis for guiding themselves through the process of arriving at the decision of whether termination is indicated and of communicating with a client about that judgment. If the therapist and the client don't agree, they need to devise guidelines for working through that conflict, including their different perspectives. The student also needs to understand how focusing on termination involves their relationship and involves redefining it.

If students can put together a somewhat articulated answer to these questions, then they have a framework for guiding themselves and their clients through those activities and tasks. They also have a framework for responding to and guiding their clients. Termination does involve both a process and a task that is to be completed. The therapist has been acting as model, mentor, sage, listener, educator, and recourse of last resort (or at least an important recourse). Whatever these combinations may be, it is important for the would-be therapist to think about them as he or she begins to learn about or enhance previous learnings and experiences about the reality that therapeutic relationships do terminate, and should. Students need to formulate an understanding of termination that enables them to manage it constructively without burdening their clients or themselves in ways that diminish either party or what they have accomplished together. That very process can be a positive and productive one for both the therapist and the client.

The Structure of Therapy Sessions

We have already talked about therapy as a sequence. We have talked about the beginning, the middle, and the termination. Now we are going to focus on the idea that each session is a sequence that can also serve as a model for the overall therapy process. Each session has some special characteristics, but it also has the general characteristics of a beginning, a middle, and an end. What follows is a sketch of how to think about and organize a therapy session. A teacher can use it as a guide for a lecture, workshop, or role-playing session. Students can use it as a model or a stimulus for developing their own approaches. For purposes of illustration, we are going to use the first interview as a model. It contains all of the elements, is particularly important for newly aspiring therapists, and is the point at which we begin learning as well as doing therapy.

A First Interview

Objectives. Our first objective is to greet and introduce ourself to our client. After all, we are strangers. As we have said earlier, that first greeting conveys an entire ethnic/racial and social message. We convey our presence and acknowledge the presence of our client. Clients convey their presence and acknowledge our presence. To the extent that we can make that greeting a humane, nonthreatening event, we can make the beginning a humane nonthreatening enterprise. That is all the more reason for us as teachers to help our students approach that first meeting in a relaxed and comfortable way. After all, it is our presence that enables them to have a model and a sense of support. It is our manner that conveys that therapy can be a humane nonthreatening enterprise.

After we greet a client we take on a special responsibility. It is our task to explain to the client the nature of the setting, the nature of what we will undertake as we begin to work together in a therapeutic relationship, and the general way in which we will go about it. We then need to get the client's specific agreement to proceed in that fashion.

Our next task is one of inquiry and assessment. In developing the psychosocial competence perspective, we have written of *search and organize* as an initial stage in most phases of the activities that characterize living. The search is our task in the beginning of any therapy session. One area in which we need a fuller understanding is that of the client's complaints. Usually the presenting complaints are an initial focus and, although they are usually recorded in an intake report, it is important to check on the client's views of them at this moment. Aspects of those complaints to be explored are their nature, what precipitated them, what have been their consequences, how have they been handled, and what are the client's concerns about them at this time.

It can also be useful to explore whether these complaints have occurred before. If so, then the same questions apply to learning about those earlier occurrences. A question to be added is that of what the residues from those earlier occurrences are and how they bear on the present situation? Then it can be appropriate to explore whether there are other problems the client is thinking of. If so, then they too can be explored or a decision can be made to defer considering them until some more appropriate time.

A next, and important, focus is that of exploring what led to the client deciding to seek therapy at this time for these problems. What does the client hope to gain from seeking therapeutic help? Asking these questions does not imply that we expect the client will necessarily have clear and coherent answers to them. Nevertheless, we need to know what the client's answers are. Further, asking the questions turns the client's attention to the relevance of those questions and their answers.

Particularly in the first or other early sessions of therapy, it can be of value to ask for a general informational background from the client. It is unrealistic to expect that all of the information that will eventually appear to be relevant will spring spontaneously from a client's lips in the first session. Actually, it is more likely that a client will want more structure than a simple "tell me about your life up to this point." Even so, it is worth trying. Other useful avenues of inquiry include asking the person to describe a typical day; to describe his or her present life situations; to outline his or her strengths and limitations; to summarize his or her goals, hopes, and fears; to describe how he or she typically negotiates the events in his or her life; to identify the best and worst events in his or her life; or to identify his or her first memory. Any of those areas can be explored as a means of learning about the client's life and approach to it. They also serve to orient the client to the view that life has continuity in it. Today's events do not spring into existence separately and apart from our past.

Structuring Therapy. Our next step after searching is to organize what we have discovered and relate it to the possibility of undertaking therapy with this particular client. That task involves structuring with the client what we have to offer in the way of therapy, how what we have to offer may be of value in helping the client to improve the quality of his or her life, and what kind of relationship we see as crucial to accomplishing some therapeutic gains. That structuring includes outlining what we see as our role and what we see as the client's role. What we as therapists have to say depends on how we view those roles. For example, as was mentioned earlier, one of the authors usually points out that he cannot tell the client (or anyone else) how that person feels. He can suggest that other people in such a situation have certain kinds of feelings, and even that they have found certain ways of dealing with those feelings to be effective. However, it is up to the individual to explore and decide just how he or she feels and what it makes sense to do with and about those feelings.

Some therapists do not say anything about their role or the client's. It is our view that such an approach leads to developing a covert set of definitions and rules about therapy. We think it is more efficacious to outline those issues overtly. We also think that addressing the nature of these roles provides a particularly valuable opportunity to address ethnic, racial, gender, and even personal factors that may influence the therapeutic interactions. Whichever approach one takes, in one way or another a pattern will begin to be developed. Further, we think it is of value to check explicitly with the client as to whether our perspectives seem acceptable, what problems they present, and what the client likes about them. Finally, we need to work out some shared sense of how we are going to proceed.

Tasks to Address in the Session. The above issues are important for searching and organizing. We think they are part of the beginning of every session. But, something needs to be accomplished during a session too. In fact, a sense of accomplishment is particularly important early in therapy. So, at least one goal in our first session, possibly in most sessions, is to accomplish something concrete and immediate for the client and for ourselves. Let us start with the client.

Often for a client, there is a crisis. Explaining what a crisis is and conveying a perspective on how to manage that particular crisis can be of short- and long-term value to a client. It may even make a difference in whether that client returns for further sessions.

Other possibilities include listening to the client's doubts about therapy or about the possibility of working out his or her problems successfully. Accept the legitimacy of those feelings. It can be of value to indicate that therapy can be helpful, but it is usually counterproductive to be excessively reassuring. It can also be helpful to elicit questions from the client about therapy or about one's approach to therapy and to answer them as openly and fully as possible.

It is also important to accomplish some goals for yourself as therapist. It can be of value toward the end of the first session to sum up how you see the session and what you feel has been accomplished. Such a summary need not be lengthy and should not be technical. It can simply involve noting that you have been able to learn some things about the client and that that knowledge provides a basis for a better understanding of the client and the client's issues. It can focus on the client's openness or thoughtfulness or any other constructive contribution or attribute.

A summing up of this kind also serves to establish a pattern of thinking of therapy sessions, and of life, as having definable phases and events that have identifiable characteristics that can be attended to as markers. It can begin to establish the value of summing up the import of events as a way of understanding them and building on them.

In conjunction with summing up, it also makes sense to seek a commitment on the part of the client to returning for further sessions. There is value in exploring feelings about that possibility and in expressing one's judgment about the potential value of it. It is important to emphasize that continuation is an open issue that involves both the therapist and the client. To assign the sole responsibility for that judgment to either the therapist or the client is to reject the assertion that therapy is an interaction.

In working out an agreement to continue, it makes sense to be somewhat explicit about the terms of that continuance. We may want to agree to continue for one more session, for a fixed number of sessions, or for an indefinite period until we have accomplished some more or less explicitly defined objectives. Again, it is important to be consistent with our assumption of an interaction and involve both therapist and client in establishing the nature of the agreement. We may work in a context in which limits are defined. For example, there may be an agency policy about the maximum number of sessions allowed. If so, we should make those limits explicit.

Another goal that can be aspired to is that of setting some interim goals, something concrete to orient toward. It may be that therapist and client agree that the client will decide which of several problems mentioned he or she wishes to begin working on in the second session. Or perhaps we have agreed on what topic will constitute our initial focus. We may then want to establish something the client can do to work on that topic before the next session. For example, we might arrange with a client to observe his or her reactions to that issue (e.g., being ignored) over the ensuing time and remember particular feelings about it or patterns of interaction in it. It might involve trying to react to the situation or event in a new or different way.

Possibly nothing as specific as the suggestions in the above paragraph seems appropriate. In such a case it can be meaningful to focus on getting better acquainted or learning more about each other and how we interact. It can be of value to point out to the client the importance of learning about him or her in order to be of help. It can be noted that it may simply require more general talking and exploring before the client will be comfortable focusing on some particular aspect of his or her life to begin to work on changing. The issue is not that some specific goal needs to be set. The point is that it is of value to the therapist and, for that matter, to the client to begin to formulate a sense of organization and direction in their interaction. Establishing that sense of direction can be more useful if it is done explicitly. Otherwise it will be done covertly. If it is done explicitly, there is less chance of misunderstandings and of a sense of hidden agendas.

Finally, a task that may be of value to both therapist and client is that of assigning activities to be undertaken between the sessions. Working out with the client something that he or she can think about or do between sessions serves several purposes. It helps provide continuity between the sessions. It also helps relate real life and therapy to each other. It helps establish an active role responsibility for the client and also for the therapist. If we focus together on establishing such interim active links, we both stay actively involved in the direction of the therapy. Neither can assume a passive stance and assume that the other is directing it all or that therapy will just naturally happen.

Subsequent Interviews

All sessions will have a beginning, a middle, and an end. The elements and emphases will differ, but this framework is a useful one for directing our thinking about such sessions. Each session begins with greetings and mutual assessments of each other. We then turn our attention to what has brought us together and what we hope to accomplish during this session. That search and organize process may include a review of the past week(s) but is focused on bringing us up to date. We then turn to our day's agenda, though we do not call it that. That agenda may involve a deeper exploration of past events and experiences, it may involve an effort to work out more fully future hopes, fears, directions, or courses of action. As we approach the end of a session we shift our focus to culminating, concluding, and redefining. Those activities may not be monumental toward the end of each session, but they do involve at the very least pulling the session together and looking ahead to the interim period and to the next session. In a final termination session, those issues become our central concern, and the period of looking ahead takes on a much more indefinite character. We are going to get on with our lives and our work, and so are our clients. We do that after every session, but in this final one that issue looms much larger. Nevertheless, regardless of the emphasis in any session, there is (or should be) a phasic pattern to it. Keeping that in mind can be of very substantial value to any therapist in training. It helps him or her to have a sense of the session and to guide the flow of the session. It also provides a very realistically and therapeutically valuable model for our clients.

Supervisor–Supervisee Relationships

We have written at some length about the ethnic validity issues that arise in counseling and psychotherapy. In doing so we have paid particular attention to them as they bear on therapist–client relationship patterns. We have also touched on issues of supervisor–supervisee and supervisee–supervisee relationship patterns. At this juncture, we want to give them more systematic attention. A core aspect of learning to become a therapist is the very specific learning that comes from direct feedback. Supervisors are the more experienced individuals who provide that essential detailed observation, feedback, and instruction about the student therapist's understanding of and conduct of his or her therapeutic activities.

In our traditional approach to teaching, it is the supervisee who is subject to scrutiny and the supervisor who is protected from it. That pattern has also held in the therapist (student or otherwise)–client relationship. We have proposed instead that we conceive of the therapist–client relationship as a collaborative resource exchange process. We want to reconceptualize supervisor–supervisee and student–student relationships in a similar fashion. And we want to do so within an ethnic validity framework.

Helms (1985), in her writings about racial identity issues, has pointed out that therapy is likely to be counterproductive if the client's racial identity awareness is more advanced than that of the therapist. The same logic may be extended to the supervisor–supervisee relationship. A supervisee who is more concerned with and sensitive to ethnic validity issues than his or her supervisor is placed in a difficult position that may seriously limit the student's possibilities for learning. It may also reduce the supervisor's effectiveness as a teacher and growth as a professional. Such situations become increasingly difficult to the extent that the domain of learning involves matters that relate to our humanity and to our related beliefs about the human condition. Particularly difficult are issues about our senses of personal dignity, our moral views, and our senses of social equity and fairness. That difficulty is compounded when the supervisor is resistant to acknowledging its relevance or to dealing with it. We do not want to minimize the difficulties the student faces nor deny that the student may justifiably feel that the situation is unfair. On the other hand, we do not want to portray all supervisors as white racists and all students as paragons of transcendism. It seems more likely that both have strengths and limitations, insights and blind spots, areas of understanding and of prejudice. What can we do?

Convergence, Divergence, Conflict

Our answer is that any of us, supervisors or supervisees, can take an ethnic validity view and work to transcend our ethnic/racial/cultural limitations. It is easier, but not essential, if this process is shared. Our efforts to transcend our own ethnic/racial limitations are likely to be more limiting and more scarring if we have to make that effort solely on our own or in the face of opposition. Consequently, our goal may become one of surviving difficult cross-ethnic learning (and life) situations with a minimum of harm. Even that is a worthy goal.

We begin with the assumption that as supervisors and as supervisees we will find areas of convergence as well as areas of divergence and conflict. We seek out the areas of convergence and try to build on them. In reality we often have difficulty in doing so.

For example, a white male supervisor who was not religious was supervising a young black male therapist trainee. The trainee was seeing a black male college student client who was having a harrowing inner and outer struggle among his fundamentalist religious beliefs, his self-doubts, and his desires for heterosexual contacts. The client had largely immobilized himself as he feared doing anything sinful, yet he could not decide whether he really believed the fundamentalist creeds he had been taught. He was struggling vainly to get some indication, including a sign from God, as to what to believe and how to proceed. He also knew that the trainee therapist was a singer in a gospel choir and told his therapist that he felt inhibited from expressing some of his thoughts. The trainee was having tremendous difficulty responding to the client's distress, defining his own position, or engaging the client in exploring how to develop a course of action. The supervisor knew that the trainee was sensitive to being pushed by white faculty and supervisors and also believed that the trainee needed to take some initiatives on his own. The supervisor also felt uncertain about questioning the role of religion in the trainee's and client's lives. It was only after much tentative exploration that it became possible to discuss the issue. In a group supervision session, another black male therapist trainee took the initiative to ask about how to differentiate the roles of spiritual advisor and therapist. The supervisor, the other trainees, and the trainee therapist then discussed the differences between those roles. That discussion enabled the trainee therapist to sort out his own conflicts and to proceed in working with the client.

It was months later (after the client had been terminated) that the trainee volunteered the information to the supervisor that he had been immobilized because he did not want to say anything that would lead the client to abandon his faith. Yet he did not feel that as a therapist he could encourage the client in that faith. In retrospect, the supervisor came to realize that his own tentativeness about exploring the issue of the trainee's seeming difficulty came from his own uncertainty. The supervisor realized that he had not figured out how to explore the basic role that religious faith seems to play for many black people in the USA without being accused of insensitivity to both ethnic/racial and religious issues.

The supervisor was faced with exploring the parameters of his own value system as he confronted the challenge of his supervisee's uncertainty. Both were struggling with common or convergent themes such as

What value does religion hold for me? What do I see as religion's strengths and limitations for others? Is it appropriate as a therapist (by whatever definition the client and therapist have reached) to provide religious guidance? What is the value of religion as seen by the black community? Does it re-create oppression or does it provide a medium for effective functioning? In this example the supervisor immobilized himself by denying his uncertainties and sensitivities about racial and religious matters and attributing the problem exclusively to the trainee therapist. The supervisee did need to explore his uncertainties about the relationship between his role as a religious counselor and his role as a therapist, but that task was made more difficult by the supervisor's stance. When the therapist–religious counselor issue did get identified, the supervisee and the supervisor did begin to converge on clarifying the supervisee's therapeutic relationship with his client. When the therapist later identified his own racial sensitivity about religious issues, he was able to participate more fully with the supervisee (who was the one who initiated it) in finding a convergent basis for exploring the supervisory relationship as well as the therapeutic relationship.

A different pattern of racial/ethnic sensitivity issues is reflected in the example of a black student in a practicum setting who was assigned a white client. In the first session, the white client stated that she did not want to work with a black therapist. The student indicated that she would check with her supervisor about the possibility of a referral. The supervisee informed the white supervisor and said that she would prefer that solution also. She did not want to work with someone with such an attitude. The supervisor rejected that option, stating that the client was to be told that she would work with this therapist or not receive therapy in this agency.

The student therapist informed the client who accepted that decision and continued in therapy. The student therapist was able to be therapeutically effective, the client worked at the issues that concerned her, and the client improved. The student felt that both she and the client grew from their interaction. To some extent they did find some areas of convergence, including a capacity to reach beyond their desires for racial particularism. Yet neither of them mentioned the issue again during the sessions, and the supervisor never dealt with it further. We can only commend the supervisor for confronting the issue and requiring the student and the client to confront it. We can only commend the student and the client for working beyond their differences, their particularism.

Whose Responsibility?

What we are left with at this point is questions about what remains in the unspoken and unprocessed domains of interchanges. Whose responsibility is it to go further? It is everyone's, and no one's, so it is easy to say that it is someone else's.

We want to argue that the supervisor had a responsibility, and an opportunity, to explore those issues with the student. We want to argue that the supervisor had a disproportionately larger responsibility than the student therapist or the client. After all, the supervisor's professional role is one of defining the domain of therapy, the major issues therein, and the ways to address those issues. From our perspective the supervisor needs to be asking to what extent his or her perspectives are generational and not directly relevant to the student therapist's generation and to the somewhat changed world. The student needs to be searching also for those distinctions. After all, neither generation possesses all of the world's wisdom, nor all of the world's bigotry. Further, the student and the supervisor need to be asking questions about the extent to which our conventional theories of culture, personality, psychopathology, and psychotherapy are biased and constrained by the biases and constraints of earlier generations. The supervisor–supervisee relationship and the supervisee–client relationship are reciprocal, but they also are asymmetrical. The supervisor bears a responsibility to provide leadership and support as these issues arise. Issues need to be explored, and answers to them that reflect our more recent history and understanding need to be articulated by supervisors for themselves as well as for their students. Even from a universalist perspective of seeking presumed universal psychological processes, life is not totally content free. The client raised the issue of race and the student wished also to avoid this cross-racial interaction. It behooves the supervisor to be sensitive to those racial issues as interfering with therapy, at least in the form of traditionally conceptualized transference and countertransference issues. That is, it would almost seem to go without saying that what it means to be a supervisor is that a person in that role takes on a special overarching responsibility to help those being supervised and the people under his or her care. Further, that special responsibility involves most importantly helping them to deal with issues such as, in this instance, their cross-racial conflictedness that is interfering with their life functioning. Specifically, the client has sought professional help and the student therapist has offered it. Their initial prejudged aversion interferes with their capabilities of achieving those goals. The student needs to learn to provide therapy to a broad range of individuals; the client needs to learn to use professional resources on the basis of their professional competence, not other factors.

We want to argue that the student has a responsibility, and an opportunity, to explore those issues with the supervisor. Certainly the issues she confronted in this context are complex. These are issues for many non-culture-defining group therapists, and she knew that she needed to learn to contend with them professionally, not just personally. It is important that she at least explore the possible ways that this therapist–client pairing could provide her an opportunity to learn about working with an apparently prejudiced client. She could explore whether and in what ways the client's reaction is race related and whether it is based on a generalized prejudice or on specific experiences that were bringing this client to therapy. It can hardly be an issue that she never thought about again. She may well have felt that the supervisor was being insensitive, possibly racist. Even so, she has a responsibility to explore whether and how her own feelings about this cross-racial match might be affecting therapeutic and supervisor interactions. She also has a responsibility to ask on behalf of the client. At the very minimum she needs to know whether her racial feelings and the client's seem to the supervisor to be interfering with the progress of the client's therapy.

She could more understandably have felt reluctant to ask about the supervisor's unspoken biases; she could have seen asking about them as potentially threatening to her own career development. It is this latter consideration that presents the most complex and difficult issues for the student therapist. First of all, a NCDG group student has been enculturated and socialized not to confront CDG authority figures about issues, particularly issues of prejudice or bias on the part of those figures. Second, the practical issue of how to raise such questions is problematic. The student needs the supervisor's guidance and support to raise questions about difficult issues, and in this most critical domain feels that absence most crucially. Unfortunately, that difficult burden falls inequitably on the NCDG student. We can only note that it is important for the student to balance the risks involved against the professional responsibilities to herself and her client and try to clarify the ethnic/racial issues raised in this situation or similar ones.

What we have just said may seem harsh, even unduly so. It seems to place a disproportionate burden on the student. That burden may already seem disproportionate to NCDG students contending with several basic questions about therapy, therapists, and therapeutic approaches. They are grappling with whether they are being given a fair opportunity to become participants in a therapeutic profession and about whether mainstream therapeutic approaches are valid for them and other NCDG individuals. Their points have validity. They are heightened and accentuated for them. Nevertheless, in some respects they have commonalities with issues that CDG students are also facing. And in some respects their supervisors are facing those same or related questions. The difference is, of course, the central one associated with society's entrenched ethnocentric views about NCDG groups. It is important that we sort out both the commonalities and the differences that NCDG students have with CDG students in their efforts to be true to their own experiences, identities, and goals and at the same time acquire the personal and professional maturity and skills that they need to become effective therapists.

Perhaps we need to reiterate that we are emphasizing the importance of socializing supervisors, therapists, trainees, and clients to a world view in which the possibility of choice and human agency and assumption of active responsibility for managing one's life are central. We are also emphasizing the perspective that people can interact with others (and for that matter with themselves) in ways that seek convergence, accept and respect divergence, and work to contain conflict in nondestructive ways. The trainee is in the process of maturing personally as well as professionally. That maturational process involves to some extent a conflict with earlier generations, including supervisors. As we noted in discussing the supervisor's responsibilities, we believe that both the student and the supervisor need to be asking to what extent their perspectives are generational and not directly relevant to the student therapist's generation and to the somewhat changing world. Since neither generation possesses all of the world's wisdom, nor all of the world's bigotry, it seems to us that the supervisor and the student have much to gain from trying to converge on the task of exploring these issues together. In particular, the student and the supervisor need to be asking questions about the extent to which our conventional theories of culture, personality, psychopathology, and psychotherapy are biased and constrained by the biases and constraints of earlier generations. Nevertheless, we come back to the point that the student needs to be searching for those distinctions even if the supervisor is not.

Part of the hallmark of maturity as a student therapist, as a supervisor, and as a client, is learning to accept and continue to build one's own capabilities and perspectives within the context of one's own and others' limitations. In this sense, the student is faced with confronting the fact that supervisors have limits (as well as strengths) from which to learn. Perhaps the learning will focus primarily on how to handle conflicts, including supervisors' potential insensitivities to racial/ethnic and gender issues. Perhaps the learning will focus primarily on how to explore with a supervisor the bases of the supervisor's perspectives. Perhaps the learning will focus primarily on learning how to persuade supervisors to become more sensitized to their racial/ethnic and gender biases. Perhaps the learning will focus primarily on learning how to contain one's own sense of violation and the sense of violation of what are presumed to be a client's concerns (after all, neither the supervisor nor the client may see the issues the way the student therapist does).

At this point in our discussion, we emphasize heightened awareness of the possibilities of these conflicting and divergent perspectives. That awareness is perhaps the best protection any of us can have against getting locked into self and other destructive patterns. It is also a significant resource as a basis for contending with our own internal conflicts and our external ones with others, whether we are supervisors, students, or clients. That awareness is also an important foundation as a basis for identifying and building on our areas of convergence. At some level, we are all committed to the potential value of therapeutic approaches as a means of helping people in their efforts to alleviate their problems and improve the quality of their lives. Part of the particular responsibility of the student is to contribute to that endeavor as a highly talented and promising representative of a new generation and new perspectives. That responsibility carries some risks. We do not have a formula for guaranteeing smooth passage to maturity as a therapist. We do want to be sensitive to those risks, while still encouraging students to explore and act on that responsibility. We want to encourage supervisors to be sensitive to them also, and to explore and act on their responsibility. As a final comment to students, we want to reiterate the importance of taking some risks, learning from them, learning to accept that sometimes important issues will be treated cavalierly or unjustly (by supervisors and by themselves), and learning how to contain those defeats and continue to build one's life, sensitivities, and professional capabilities (we never said it was easy).

What was the client's responsibility? We ordinarily encourage clients to think about their own issues, not about us and ours. The therapist's potential difficulties with cross-race issues are not ordinarily a client's concern. Yet this issue was one of the client's issues. In fact, the client had said so in the beginning in voicing a desire to avoid working with a black therapist. It would have been an important gain for the client at termination, if not before, to *culminate, conclude, and redefine* herself and her feelings about cross-racial interactions. That client may very well have felt that she did not want to confront the student therapist's issues, but at least she could have gained by confronting her own and the changes in them from therapy.

More generally, of course, we can raise questions about the responsibilities of anyone in a subordinate position to raise questions that may threaten a supervisor or other superior. There is no particular gain in advocating martyrdom. Neither student status nor client status is a good position from which to challenge entrenched authority. Supervisors should be open to learning about emerging student concerns, especially around ethnic validity issues; it is distressing that at times they are not. Nevertheless, it does make sense for the student to pursue the alternative of trying to seek enough convergence with such a supervisor to work out some of the conflicts and uncertainties that arise.

For the student, those issues may be ones of trying to sort out personal confusions, trying to sort out issues with the professional community and its values and constraints, and trying to chart a course that seems compatible with one's own ethnic validity as well as with one's professional career goals. Sorting out those issues is a painful process, particularly since the issues of ethnic validity are not fully accepted as basic to our psychological natures. We are in an unprecedented era of exploration of their nature and relevance. We are far from believing or advocating that we have answers to those questions. What we are advocating is that it is of value to confront them. It is of value as a student therapist to raise them with a supervisor in a way that can seek convergence, control conflict, and evolve areas of divergence. We would go even further to emphasize the importance of divergence. A major buffer in all human interactions is the defining of a shared acceptance of divergence.

It is exceedingly valuable to establish a means for any two of us to accept that in some ways we will be different and that those differences are not only alright, they are desirable. Unless we can define a domain of difference we must be either totally alike or be in conflict. No such pattern is tolerable in the long run.

With those thoughts in mind we come back to the position that it is of value to all of us to try to understand the other person's perspective as well as our own. It is important to seek areas of convergence and divergence and work out constructive ways to handle conflict. It may be that an area of conflict that a student cannot work out with a particular supervisor is that of the relevance and relationship of racial or ethnic issues to therapy. It makes sense to find out in as professional a manner as possible whether that area is taboo. It then makes sense to keep that conflict in perspective as effectively as possible. Resolving the conflict may involve seeking another supervisor, or it may involve limiting the ways of interacting with an existing one. It is not in a student's interest to let that conflict become so destructive that it interferes with the student's development or with the client's well-being. If such an eventuality occurs, it becomes important for the student to explore the issues involved with others in the agency, with an advisor, or with a confidant. We would like to think that there are not prejudiced and unreasonable supervisors or students. Unfortunately, there are some of each. Fortunately, they are outnumbered by those who are relatively open and reasonable and have a commitment to these broader values. Look for those people, give them a chance to help, and work with them.

Student–Student Interactions

One of the most important and powerful aspects of the educational experience of each of us is the part provided by peers. We learn immense amounts from them. That is true while we are student therapists as well as in other student roles. Those interactions also confront us with ethnic validity issues. In some of the earlier sections we talked about a context in which student therapists are grouped together to form a heterogeneous class to enhance their opportunity to learn about ethnic validity issues. Even in that kind of context the task of coming to understand and manage one's own biases and frustrations is difficult, and it does not go smoothly. It would seem to follow that such explorations are likely to be even more difficult in contexts that are not organized to facilitate that kind of learning. We come back to the basis from which we began. We think that ethnic validity issues are vital, although we are aware that they aren't the only issues involved in relationships. To us it makes sense to encourage student therapists to explore those perspectives with their peers. In doing so it is important to seek convergences and to respect divergences. It is through those efforts that we begin to build trust. Those efforts also provide a climate for beginning to manage conflict. After all, we do have different perceptions about ethnic/racial issues, and they do involve us in ways that affect our sense of our own humanity and our sense of social justice as well as our ways of conducting therapy.

We will, inevitably, encounter peers with whom we cannot find common cause. We need to learn how to examine ourselves for our contribution to those issues without becoming consumed with self-condemnation. We need also to learn how to learn from those misunderstandings. Unfortunately, the burden in developing constructive interactions between students often falls disproportionately on NCDG students. It does not necessarily fall on them because CDG students are personally prejudiced. To some extent the burden falls on NCDG group students because CDG students have ordinarily not had similar experiences of being an outsider so are less aware of their enculturated ethnocentrism. We are quite aware that everyone has been an outsider at one time or another, but those experiences just are not comparable. Culture-defining group students have not had to contend with and become aware of an organized societal context and group that systematically devalues them and discriminates against them. Nor, on the other hand, have they had to contend with the patronizing manner of some from the culture-defining group.

The fact that we have all been treated as outsiders and we have all been patronized is an important reference point. We want to emphasize that those personal experiences provide a basis for beginning to understand the ethnic ecosystem of non-culture-defining groups and individuals from such backgrounds. Yet those individual experiences in and of themselves are lacking in the pervasiveness and inescapability of permanent status as marked by one's color or accent or official racial designation.

Students from the culture-defining group have their own ethnicity, and it has positive characteristics as well as limitations. In the United States, with its Anglo heritage, many students from that heritage do have constructive prosocial orientations. For them it is difficult to be labeled as oppressors and to have their efforts to seek convergence dismissed automatically. It is difficult to have their efforts to work on the injustices and inequities within the dominant culture dismissed as simply self-serving.

We come back to emphasizing the importance of working to seek bases for convergence across these barriers. To us that work begins with establishing informal and often nonverbal convergences of empathy, caring, and support. Student status is inherently threatening, and learning to become a therapist confronts us all with our own unspoken and unresolved conflicts. Learning to become therapists is a very demanding undertaking. It does not make our learning easier to revert to our own self-protective shells. In fact, the task we confront is the same one we ask of our clients. That is, we say we know that you are under stress and that your problems look overwhelming, but you can not solve them by staying within your shell. We will support you and help you sort out alternative courses of action, but you are going to have to take steps on your own behalf. That is what we are saying to students who work with each other. Take the same ethnic validity approach with each other that you take with your clients. It will give you a basis for your own development and for contributing to that of others as well.

TRAINING CONTEXT: WORKING IN SOMEONE ELSE'S WORLD

Choosing a Context

Often, psychotherapy training begins in a university counseling center or clinic setting. We will use that hypothetical situation as a reference point. Although our general ideas apply to any setting, there are a number of advantages to a university setting. One such advantage is the rhythm of the beginnings and endings of semesters. Beginnings and endings are an important part of life and, consequently, of therapy. Their occurrences at frequent intervals in a college setting provide excellent opportunities for working with those issues. Another advantage is the availability of diverse students and clients. And further, because those settings are organized as educational settings, they expect to provide for such training and often have specialized facilities for that purpose.

For example, for educational purposes it is ideal if we can observe each other at work. The availability of an observation suite enables teachers and students to observe each other conducting therapy. It is ideal if we can sit down and talk with others (who are also learning and teaching) about what we are doing. It is ideal if we have resource materials available.

A pattern that one of the authors has used is to select as a class four students who make up a diverse group on the basis of ethnicity, race, and gender. Arrangements are then made so that the students and the teacher can work in an observational suite, which permits them to observe each other. Such an approach helps the participants to become aware of their humanity and to observe the therapeutic approaches others use. It creates a context in which everyone can see their own and one another's strengths as well as limitations. Such observations help to demythologize the process of therapy and the mythic aura of therapists. They also help to provide a much wider range of direct and vicarious experiential learning than can be obtained otherwise. (This arrangement need not and should not violate any basic agreements of confidentiality with the agency or the clients. Its use can and should be made explicit. Years of experience have suggested that most clients are quite agreeable to such an approach. Those who are not can be provided other therapeutic arrangements.)

This arrangement also provides a context in which trainees can learn to serve as supervisors as well as supervisees. One possibility is to have the students arrange a round-robin in which they participate in supervising each other in the observational suite. Each student can also be provided with at least one client to see separately from this general forum under the supervision of a classmate. The faculty supervisor can serve as a backup supervisor as issues arise. If we are successful in creating an open and supportive climate, then such an arrangement facilitates the development of therapeutic perspectives and skills on the part of the students. It also helps them to learn about consulting others when issues seem unclear or troublesome or outside of their capabilities at the moment. Feedback from peers can be more insightful than that of the teacher and at times it can be more easily accepted. Other potential advantages include the possibility that peer supervision will be presented from a different generational as well as other racial perspective, particularly if the group is diverse. One more potential benefit is that a student is more likely to question or challenge a faculty supervisor if there is peer support available.

Status as Guests

Particularly in a situation of working with new psychotherapy trainees, it is important to impress on those trainees that they have role responsibilities to the agency in which they are working as well as to their clients. Agencies have many responsibilities and they have more than enough work to do. It is important for a supervisor and for students to learn the agency's rules and follow them. That task often requires substantial involvement and oversight on the part of the faculty supervisor, but it is essential in teaching students to be responsible therapists (of course, the teaching and the learning go more smoothly if the faculty supervisor serves as a responsible role model). At least one assumption we make is that therapists who are insensitive to others in an agency are going to find that conduct counterproductive. Insensitivity often gets passed on in the manner in which the staff treat clients and in what the staff conveys explicitly and implicitly to clients about the therapist.

Teaching Formats

There are a multitude of formats that can be used for teaching psychotherapy. It would be presumptuous to suggest that any one is the best. However, another teaching format that can contribute is one of having training workshops at the beginning, in the middle, and at the end of a semester or school year. Focus can be placed, respectively, on forming a relationship, sustaining and utilizing it, and terminating it. Those are the activities in sequence that are characteristic foci in therapy at those points in the year.

Finally, it is important to involve everyone in reading about therapy and talking about what they are reading. It seems more important that they read, than that they read anything in particular. The point is to bring into the ongoing dialogue as many perspectives as possible. After all, we have been suggesting all along that there is no one way of living that is the best for everyone in all situations. We are also suggesting that no one has all of the answers about therapy. If we can explore a variety of perspectives as we go along, then perhaps we can keep ourselves open as we learn and as we teach. Part of that exploration involves sharing with one another what we are reading and what values we see in it as well as what issues it raises that we cannot accept or incorporate. For that matter, providing a wide-ranging bibliography can be a valuable stimulus to learning. Such a bibliography can include historical material, biographies, novels, culturally pertinent materials, experimental and field studies, and of course materials on theories and techniques of therapy. No given student is likely to read the entire list, but having such a broad list makes the point that there are many sources that can contribute to our understanding of ourselves and others.

TEACHING CONTEXTS AND TECHNIQUES

The format we have outlined has involved a teacher–supervisor and a small heterogeneous group of students in a context in which the students are learning to become individual therapists. Nevertheless, we think the ethnic validity model has far more generality. These ideas can be taught in a wide variety of contexts and as bases for a range of intervention activities. Specifically, we have emphasized that we can use a few central ideas as a framework for understanding any of us. We have a sense of ourselves and a sense of the world, and from those we evolve ways of interpreting and negotiating the events in our lives. Our worlds contain both supports and threats, and they in turn shape how we think about ourselves and the world and how we interpret and negotiate events. Further, those facets of our existence are shaped by and integrated at any number of levels. We have emphasized the individual level and the ethnic/cultural/racial level. It is in that sense that we emphasize the importance of ethnic validity, of acknowledging that each of us has a sense of our own and our ethnic/racial/cultural group's validity as the framework of our existence. It is that person-in-context framework that we view as essential to understanding ourselves and others and to forming relationships, therapeutic and otherwise. In the following sections we cite a few such examples.

Workshops for Heterogeneous Groups of Therapists

We mentioned in an earlier discussion some of our experiences providing a workshop for a diverse group of therapists. They varied in level of sophistication, theoretical orientation, and racial/cultural/ethnic identity. The two of us who presented the workshop differed in race, gender, and age. We saw as our task exposing them to an ethnic validity framework in a fashion that would enable them to apply it to the specific context of the therapy they practice. We did not seek to challenge their particular theoretical orientations. Our emphasis was on accepting how they view themselves and their work. We wanted to ask them to look with us and with one another at the issue of ethnic validity as a way of enriching their work and their understanding of themselves in that work.

The central point of our effort was not to confront white–black issues *per se,* though that is a worthy point. One central point of our effort was to heighten their awareness that they bring their own racial/ethnic/cultural and gender background into the therapy context whether they think so or not. We were not trying to induce guilt about that reality. Rather, a central point of our effort was to help them to work out a way of accepting that neither we nor our clients can escape from our heritage, but that we can use our awareness of our heritage and of the heritage of our clients in a constructive way.

Another example involves a multidisciplinary team of which one of the authors has been a member. We were asked to provide a series of counseling workshops for the counselors employed at a social service outreach agency serving Latin American youth. The counselors' own heritages and identities spanned South and Central America, Africa, and the United States. Their background education ranged from high school to master's degrees in social work. Their responsibilities included helping clients to find homes, employment, medical care, reduce alcohol and drug use, understand the culture of the United States and learn to function effectively within it, and evolve or maintain a meaningful and constructive psychological adjustment for themselves.

These counselors were themselves struggling with these acculturation and adaptation issues, and sessions on crisis intervention, abuse, culture, and adolescent development readily captured their attention. Sessions on moving beyond advice giving and direct intervention to the more complicated and less explicit tasks of therapeutic counseling were more frustrating. Realistically, they saw themselves and their clients as faced with overwhelming problems, but with limited resources and options.

Latinos from different countries and backgrounds are socialized differently. Yet there are come common cultural patterns. Compared to United States norms, Latinos tend to rely more on personal relationships, on respect for authorities, on their entitlement to respect and obedience from their children, on authorities as problem solvers, and on the belief that their role is to endure conditions imposed on them by others and controlled by others. Our emphasis in the workshops was on helping the counselors to see that these characteristics have had value in the context in which they are learned. In contrast, in their present context they have significant limitations. We sought to emphasize an ethnic validity perspective that would facilitate the counselors' learning to view culturally effective approaches in the United States as useful in this context, not as superior or better than those of their home countries. In workshop sessions we encouraged the counselors to bring in their own vignettes and experiences. We worked with that material in role-playing groups to explore new ways of understanding the issues, the perspectives involved, and the patterns underlying their interactions with each client. We also explored with them ways of helping clients to develop alternatives.

We return to a point made much earlier in this book: You have to solve your own problem first; then you can help others with theirs. That was much the case in this context. The counselors were struggling in different ways with acculturation. They were all struggling with the social injustices with which they and their clients must contend. Those injustices have created a work situation for them that confronts them with deep human misery and suffering and with limited possibilities for alleviating it. For us an important part of the workshop series was to help them develop ways of understanding that reality and coping with it rather than becoming immobilized by their own frustrations or passing them on to their clients. Thus, we had to solve our problem of understanding their lives by learning from them about their perspectives and their context—personal, professional, and ethnic/racial/cultural.

We then tried to help them construct an ethnically valid framework that would enable them to cope more effectively and counsel their clients more effectively. To do so we sketched out two diagrams for our discussions and their use. The first diagram emphasized the general point that people live in a context of support and threats. We sketched out how in a counseling environment we can provide supports that help clients solve life problems as well as others that help them to develop more adequate ways of coping with their lives and better understandings of themselves and their worlds. We also outlined the kinds of threats with potentially destructive impacts on the client and the therapy itself that we as counselors can introduce.

The second diagram outlined the general nature of the coping process as we envision it and have described it throughout this book. The point is that we want to help clients learn to see an active planful approach as a generally productive one. We also want to model it and help them to acquire it as a way of negotiating the events in their lives. We thought that providing this approach as a visual guide could be useful to counselors as they explored their own approaches to life, to counseling, and to guiding counselees toward more constructive lifestyles.

In at least this one effort, we were only partially successful. The group's supervisor wanted a structured series of lectures about counseling topics. Some of the staff wanted specific counseling techniques and ways of applying them to specific problems and to different people from different Central American backgrounds. In essence, we faced conflicting pressures between a universalist supervisor and particularist participants. We bridged these differences more effectively around specific topic areas such as crisis intervention and physical or sexual abuse, which permitted more direct structuring. We were least successful and both we and the participants most frustrated around issues of general counseling that called for a more active structuring role on the participants' part and more responsiveness to individual and cultural differences among the clients.

Crisis Centers, Emergency Rooms, and Other Challenges

Emergency rooms or crisis centers are particularly salient contexts in which to emphasize the importance of and learn about the role of ethnic validity factors. Trainees as well as staff working in those contexts are faced with individuals who need immediate assistance. Trainees must learn to form a quick working relationship of some kind with a client quickly. Their effectiveness requires sensitivity to many informal cues and a knowledge of people's ethnic/racial/cultural ways of relating to illness and stress.

A professional colleague, director of a community mental health center, described an incident that illustrates this point. He was called because the crisis team was confronted with an elderly black woman who had locked herself in her apartment and would not admit them or anyone else. Out of his own heritage as a black person and his knowledge of that community, he asked immediately whether anyone had contacted the woman's pastor. They had not, so he did. The pastor came and in a relatively short time persuaded the woman to open her door. This community mental health director demonstrated an important sense of ethnic awareness that no amount of formal professional therapeutic education would, by itself, yield.

We seldom literally confront the question of how to get someone to open a locked door, yet we confront it figuratively in most crisis situations. We often do not even know what or where the person's doors are so that we can see whether they are unlocked. A combination of ethnic validity awareness and professional skill are not only desirable, they seem to us to be essential.

One of the authors has had the experience of supervising graduate psychology students in a mental hospital setting in which he had access to the hospital's staff and facilities plus the freedom to design a teaching program as he saw fit. His initial approach was to ask new trainees to spend time on the hospital grounds, rather than in the wards, to get acquainted with the people confined there for treatment as *people,* not as *patients.* That assignment proved very distressing for at least several of the students in each class. They wanted the structured role, the tasks, and the tools (e.g., a test kit) of their trade. As we explored their reactions further, it became clear that they were either afraid of patients or not interested in knowing them as people. The patients were from a different social class or racial/ethnic group. They were people whom these students would not ordinarily associate with or want to become acquainted with. To those students, the assignment was irrelevant or onerous or both. As individuals, they were approaching the assignment from either an ethnocentric universalist perspective (patients are exemplifications of universal pathology and that is what is to be understood), from an ethnocentric particularist perspective (people are different, we and they have nothing in common with or of interest to anyone other than our respective own reference groups), or from both an ethnocentric universalist and particularist perspective.

Our approach to teaching in crisis or other short-term interaction contexts is to focus on exploring ethnic validity issues. Those contexts are particularly well suited for teaching ethnic validity perspectives. Many NCDG group people have to learn to glean what they need from culture-defining gatekeeper personnel who are insensitive to and unsympathetic to them as individuals and to their world views. If they work with us over an extended period, they may have the personal resources and the commitment to explore beyond our limits and grow therapeutically from doing so. In a crisis or emergency, they do not have that time, and they do not have the personal resources. They are in a crisis or emergency situation precisely because the events in their lives have overwhelmed or incapacitated them. They need ethnically/racially and personally sensitive professional competence.

In some situations, we can ask trainees to leave their professional role and explore the lives and situation of hospitalized individuals as people. In workshops such as the one we described earlier, we can simulate situations that require people to explore their own ethnic/racial perspectives by manipulating the ethnic/racial characteristics of therapist–client pairs. We can create hypothetical crises or emergencies and explore how they are likely to be different as the context is different. In our experience, for example, the issue of physical and sexual abuse raises quite different issues and produces quite different reactions in males than they do in females, and in Latina than in Anglo women.

Presenting to Large Groups

Presenting an ethnic validity approach to a large audience limits the possibilities for hands-on interactions. Nevertheless, it is still possible to involve an audience in considering that perspective. We all have personal as well as professional experiences. What we often lack is a context in which to place them and redefine them. That is our emphasis and our goal, to help people appeal to their own resources and experiences in a somewhat different way. Ironically, it is often particularly difficult to get CDG individuals and NCDG individuals to grasp that majority individuals also represent an ethnic validity perspective. Culture-defining groups tend to be enculturated to see themselves as the universal standard, as representing what is natural. Non-culture-defining groups tend to see culture-defining group members as oppressors or even at times as the *natural* model to be imitated. They are less likely to see them as reflecting an ethnic tradition just as they themselves do. To convey an ethnic validity perspective effectively to a large heterogeneous audience, it is important to provide vignettes of the strengths and limitations of each of them while highlighting their ethnic nature. For example, the white middle-class emphasis on long-range planning represents a strength in the context of their world that provides them a predictable future, at least moderately benign institutional supports, and opportunities to obtain greater future rewards as a consequence of short-term sacrifices. That same emphasis has led to a diminution of the capabilities of white middle-class people to enjoy themselves on a day-to-day basis. At times they even seem unable to enjoy their long-term rewards when they are finally in a position to do so.

The focus of the rural and urban poor (black, white, Latin, etc.) on short-term gratification rests on their experience in an environment in which resources and options are limited and their world is both unpredictable and malign. It does limit their potential for benefitting from long-term goal opportunities if they arise, but it helps them to survive a harsh life situation. It also leads them to find joy in day-to-day activities, an often blunted capability in middle-class-oriented individuals. Unfortunately, these choices of short-term goals and day-to-day satisfactions are often cited as evidence of ethnic/cultural/racial inferiority. They can more legitimately be attributed to patterns of enculturation in harsh and unpredictable contexts.

There are other ethnic/racial/cultural variations that are more legitimately a function of long-enduring patterns that have been shaped historically by diverse societies. Cultural studies have indeed documented substantial stylistic differences among the Chinese, Japanese, Indians, Arabs, Jews, Russians, West Europeans, South Europeans, English, Africans, and immigrant populations of the Americas. Those variations include convergences, divergences, and conflicts in understanding our external and internal realities as well as convergences, divergences, and conflicts in how to negotiate life's events. Our task in exploring these ideas is to involve our audience in seeing those factors as relevant to their own lives and as vital to understanding or conducting therapeutic activities.

Multiple Models of Therapy

There are many models of therapy. They include cognitive, behavioral, cognitive-behavioral, humanistic, dynamic, social learning, and a growing number of others. We three authors have our own preferred models and styles, and they are not the same for the three of us. They have common elements, but they also have divergences, and even conflicts. Do we argue? Of course. Do we always come to convergence? Of course not. We continue to work on containing our conflicts and broadening our understanding of ourselves, each other, and our ethnic/racial/cultural and gender differences.

Perhaps a similar approach can be suggested as a way of relating ethnic validity concepts to various models of and approaches to therapy. For example, we can involve students in considering whether and why dynamically oriented therapists are more likely to emphasize internal processes and feedback mechanisms. We can ask them to consider whether there are ethnic validity considerations in the orientation of behaviorally oriented therapies. Another set of issues concerns whether it is an accident of history that dynamic therapies originated in Europe and behavioral therapies have originated in the United States. We are inclined to speculate that the cultural contexts that have nourished those differing approaches are to some extent enculturated in their advocates and in the people who benefit from them or resist them. We are inclined to suggest that neither school has a true fix on the ultimate nature of humanity, and that each may have some important contributions to make to our understanding of ways that people can function meaningfully.

Primary Health Care

People's interactions with their bodies' capacities, limits, and functions involve their enculturated and socialized psychological natures. We are both products of our experiences and interpreters and shapers of our lives. Thus when we are negotiating any particular interaction with our bodies we do so in the fashion we have acquired for doing so. If we are to work as professional helpers with those types of problems, it would seem to follow that our work will be more effective if we can understand and attend to the individual in whose life (and body) the problem exists. We would suggest that that individual has an ethnically valid way of relating to himself or herself. That ethnicity involves, for example, a concept of an appropriate body image and appropriate ways for a body to function. It also includes a conception of the meaning of dysfunctions or impairments and of how to respond to them. It is in these senses at a bare minimum that an ethnic validity perspective is relevant to a variety of helping disciplines.

For example, medicine, as practiced in the United States, is undergoing revisions. These changes have led to a rethinking of the way in which medicine is taught and practiced. Under particular scrutiny are the nontechnological aspects of medicine. For example, more attention is being paid to the role of psychological and behavioral factors in disease onset and treatment. Further, there is greater concern for the quality of the physician–patient relationship and its role in illness management. That relationship, after all, is the primary medicine through which illnesses are managed.

At this time, there is a substantial movement to rehumanize treatment in the field of primary care. An explicit distinction is being drawn between disease and dis-ease. The latter perspective takes as its focus a person, an individual, a knower (of self, world, his or her perceived disease and personal dysfunction, and coping possibilities) who is suffering from and contending with a disease. There is an implication that the physician has a responsibility to learn about and to learn to know patients in the full context of their humanity as well as about disease processes, human anatomy and physiology, medical and pharmacological possibilities and consequences. Further, that context includes their cultural/racial/ethnic, class, community, family, gender, developmental status, and genetic validity. It also includes their individual ways of organizing and implementing their own senses of self, of the world, and of how to negotiate the events in their lives.

We believe that the ethnic validity model can provide a useful framework for understanding many of these issues. In the EVM, emphasis is placed on sharing power, sharing decision-making, and forming a new collective paradigm that the parties bring to bear on the particular problem at hand. In this regard, the EVM is a resource collaborator model. From that perspective, each of us is seen as both knower and known. A person as patient in the medical context has personal paradigms about his or her body functioning, about the causes of his or her illness, and about ways to get well. These paradigms, also based on self-knowledge and life experiences, are legitimate foci as resources in the process of patient care. The ethnic validity model orients physicians to explore their patients' complaints and ways of coping with them outside of a pathology framework as well as within it. It orients them to explore each patient's conception of the nature, implications, and potential treatments and consequences of pathology. This approach is in itself helpful in its basic humanness. Beyond that it has been demonstrated to be of value in contributing improved physician–patient relationships.

Some of the issues surrounding the physician–patient relationship concern the degree to which patients are respected as "knowers" as well as the degree to which they actively participate in the physician–patient interaction. Traditionally, the role of the patient has been passive and unassertive. Power is not shared, nor is decision-making collaborative. The impact of these dynamics is varied. For example, patient satisfaction and treatment adherence are directly tied to the interpersonal ecology of the physician–patent interaction (Meichenbaum, 1989). When patients feel devalued and mistreated they become dissatisfied, do not adhere to treatment recommendations, and are more likely to pursue legal recourse for any perceived doctor error in the course of being treated.

Recent research suggests that *activating* patients and engaging them in a resource collaborative style of interaction improves patient care on several dimensions. When patients are treated more as allies, they show more remission of their symptoms; request more information (Greenfield, Kaplan, & Ware, 1985); gain more control over their blood pressures; improve in self-efficacy; take more responsibility for their health (Schulman, 1979); return for follow-up visits; and share more relevant personal information (Roter, 1977).

The EVM model is particularly relevant in primary care settings in which many of the illnesses seen are caused by maladaptive lifestyles. Patients are far more familiar with the nuances of their lifestyles than anyone else. They are more knowledgeable about which aspects of their ways of being are more amenable to change and which are relatively resistant to it. Therefore, recommendations for lifestyle changes are best made jointly with the patient—the one who ultimately translates these plans into action.

Recommendations for changes in dietary habits, for example, clearly must be done within the framework of the patient's existing eating habits as well as within his or her definition of obesity. Also, weight has cultural, ethnic, class, and gender implications. Incorporating an ethnic validity perspective can contribute substantially to our efficacy as professionals seeking to help others achieve an enhanced quality of life.

Through collaboration, patients also share their ethnically and culturally defined ways of expressing distress. In some communities a problem with "nerves" does not mean an ostensible dysfunction of the nervous system or signal the need for an extensive neurological workup, but rather it is a metaphor for psychological and emotional distress. If a physician learns to know the individual in his or her context, that physician may come to see such complaints as culturally formed expressions of stress reactions. A physician who hears these paradigms and takes them seriously can make quicker and more accurate assessments of the patient's problems and treat them more efficiently. Does such a perspective mean that a physician can ignore individual differences among members of a particular group? By no means; we are advocating sensitivity to ethnic differences, not stereotyping on the basis of ethnic characteristics. Does such a perspective mean that the physician should ignore basic medical diagnostic procedures? No, but it does mean that the physician can avoid resorting to elaborate, and often costly, tests and procedures that can have iatrogenic effects.

In summary, the ethnic validity model is a potentially useful theoretical framework from which to begin thinking about some of the nontechnological issues in primary health care delivery. Providers who recognize their patients as knowers and their patients' knowledge as valid can help to reduce unnecessary costs, improve efficiency, and also forestall iatrogenic harm and prolonged harmful suffering. Ultimately, they can help to rehumanize medicine.

11

Research Questions and Directions

In the preceding chapters we have advanced a number of relatively nontraditional thoughts about existing approaches to understanding and practicing psychotherapy. We have questioned their adequacy and their appropriateness as frameworks for providing people a better understanding of important aspects of their lives and problems. In doing so we have ventured beyond existing bodies of therapeutic literature. In part we have done so because we believe existing therapeutic approaches and the research about them have for the most part ignored some of the issues that we consider to be central to understanding, conducting, and gaining from psychotherapy.

There is very little research that bears directly on much of what we have proposed. Further, what research there is has not been integrated into mainstream analyses of the state of knowledge about psychotherapy or recommended directions for research or utilization of existing knowledge. For example, in three recent reviews of the psychotherapy literature, these ethnic and ecosystem issues receive practically no mention. In 1986, complementary special issues of the *Journal of Consulting and Clinical Psychology* (JCCP) and of the *American Psychologist* (AP) were published. The JCCP article was "designed to bring together different types of articles, including discussion and review articles as well as empirical investigations, to address theoretical and methodological issues, to convey current thinking in substantive areas, and to outline further directions" (Kazdin, 1986, p. 3). The AP article "was designed to address topics of psychotherapy research that interface with broadly defined 'public' utilization of such knowledge" (Vandenbos, 1986, p. 112). In 1989, a special issue of the *Clinical Psychology Review* was devoted to reviews of "in-therapy behavior and experiences and their relationship to outcome" to recognize and provide some impetus to the development of such "key process and process/outcome phenomena, and to promoting innovative research programs" (Russell, 1989, p. 411).

The articles in these three special issues are scholarly, well-documented, and thoughtfully written. They include reference to psychotherapy as a learning process and as an interpersonal process (Strupp, 1986). There is also a reference to social meanings (Greenberg, 1986) and a figure that includes *society* as an input variable (Orlinsky, 1989). There is attention to the contributions of individual therapists to psychotherapy with reference to demographic, personality, adjustment, attitude, value, training, theoretical orientation, experience, and process variables. Even so, these variables are discussed primarily as individual difference variables, not as ecosystem or psychosocial variables (Lambert, 1989). There is consideration given to gender issues (Cooke & Kipnis, 1986) and to sexual attraction between cross-sex therapist–client pairs (Pope, Keith-Spiegel, & Tabachnick, 1986). There is one reference to an article by Szapocznik, Lasaga, Perry, and Solomon (1979) that identifies its sample in terms of its ethnicity. That article is referred to in a paper on generalizability of findings (Krupnick, Shea, & Elkin, 1986). There is one reference to an article that mentions race (E. E. Jones, 1978) in a paper on client experiences (Elliott & James, 1989). Even so, ethnicity and race are not identified as the relevant or significant factors in these studies. In sum, the articles are written as though the issues addressed in psychotherapy and by its participants (therapists and clients) are not influenced by nor do they bear upon race, ethnicity, or other ecosystem considerations.

It is as though there is an underlying assumption of the following kind. "It does not matter whether you are black, white, Latin, Asian; Buddhist, Christian, Muslim, Jew; South or North American; European or African; psychotherapy is psychotherapy." The psychosocial content, meaning, and significance of lives—with the possible exception of gender issues—and of the ecosystems in which they are lived are not seen as important to study or understand in their own right. To the extent that they are seen as relevant it is largely for purposes of identifying individual characteristics of participants in therapeutic interchanges. These special issues tell us much about how psychotherapy is viewed in the field of psychology. Further, the research questions considered important for advancing our understanding and practice of psychotherapy are framed in this life context- and content-free fashion.

We are more than happy to endorse the directions pointed out and the approaches to research advances that are detailed in these special issues as invaluable for anyone with an interest in psychotherapy research. Nevertheless, we want to argue that there are other equally, if not more, important considerations that also require our attention. These other considerations must be integrated into our formulation of theories, practices, and research approaches. Only then will we be able to answer how the issues of ecology and ethnic validity and the mainstream issues of psychotherapy research and practice are interrelated.

We believe that there are grounds for what we are advocating. In Chapter 2 we emphasized that there has been relatively little attention to questions about the impact of the therapist's ethnic/racial background or to what the therapist may need to learn from the client about the therapist's or the client's ethnic/racial perspectives or blinders. Rather, even transcendist-oriented research has tended to focus primarily on the potential of sensitive individual therapists overcoming ethnic barriers through experience and sensitivity to the different needs of clients with different backgrounds. There has also been emphasis on the capacity of the therapist to find convergence with the ethnically different client, at least at the level of individual issues.

We have cited evidence in support of our views from a variety of sources. Those sources include our own experiences, which, admittedly, are as subject to self-deception as anyone else's. We can only claim that we have, however, subjected those experiences to one another's scrutiny, with our disparate backgrounds and identities. We have also subjected them to the scrutiny of our students, our clients, and a range of professional audiences. In addition, we have cited indirect evidence such as Ezekiel's (1984) report of his experiences, insofar as we could locate it and bring it to bear on the questions that concern us here. Now we want to outline some thoughts about the kinds of questions that need to be investigated and about some of the issues that arise in conducting those investigations. We hope that doing so will serve to direct our efforts as well as those of our readers to challenging what we have set forth in the most rigorous ways possible.

We have organized this chapter into three major sections with the full realization that doing so is arbitrary and does some violence to what we have been saying. The material we have been presenting is integrated; it is, so to speak, "whole cloth." Nevertheless, we need to cut it up to work with it and to investigate its utility. In the following sections we have sketched out a framework as a guide to its further investigation. First, we will try to outline the broad general hypotheses that provide the defining structure of our approach. In some sense, they are metahypotheses and rightly so. They articulate the general challenges we feel need to be made to our conceptions of psychotherapy. Second, we will explore to some extent the methodological hurdles and issues that need to be considered in formulating research studies to test these ideas and to test the model more generally. Third, we will outline some "first" questions that need investigation as part of any serious efforts to establish the validity of the model we have proposed.

THE METAHYPOTHESES OF THE MODEL

We start with the assumption that human experience and conduct are a function of *destiny* (nature as humans, gender, the life cycle and one's position in it, and the era in which one lives), *history* (collective and individual), *context* (personal, family, community, ethnic, cultural), and *autonomy* (discretionary aspects of our functioning as we have formed and utilized ourselves as individuals). At a most inclusive level, knowledge of all of these factors is relevant to our understanding of ourselves and others. What we call our metahypotheses are statements that identify the factors that interact to influence who we are and how we experience and live our lives. At more specific levels we consider some of these factors to contribute more directly than others to particular activities and choices. As we are outlining hypotheses, we will try to identify those nested configurations that we consider to be of more central significance in understanding and managing our lives.

In the preceding paragraph, we have presented four groups of characteristics in an ascending order from least mutable (destiny) to most mutable (autonomy). We are in part going to reverse that order in focusing on the metahypotheses and hypotheses of the model. The reason for doing so is that, by the very nature of the psychotherapy process, we focus on the capacity of humans to effect change. In psychotherapy, we concentrate on people changing themselves, their environment, their relationships with their realities, and their understanding and interpretation of the meaning of those realities, be they internal or external.

In some general sense, what we have called our autonomy is our potential for changing those factors. What is central in psychotherapy is changing those factors that we define as relevant to ourselves as persons. Thus, one of our metahypotheses is the following: *People have empirically identifiable potentials for changing their personal perceptions of themselves as persons. They also have identifiable potentials for changing their relationships with their internal and external realities as well as their understandings and interpretations of the meaning of those realities, be they internal or external.* The origin, nature, and influence of those factors, which we have grouped under the term *autonomy,* are subject to empirical investigation and need study and specification.

However, we want to emphasize that the word *autonomy* is not equated here with the Western stereotypes of self-contained individualism. To be autonomous involves being an agent in one's own life, and it involves what we usually call voluntary action. However, it can be as voluntary (as autonomous) to form a friendship or a marriage relationship as it is to remain unattached to others. It can be as voluntary (as autonomous) to join with others in a shared commitment to a group's well-being as it is to go one's own solitary way. The core of *autonomy* is willing voluntary involvement, not unwilling involuntary constraint.

Destiny, history, and context are relevant because they shape the ecosystem we contend with in the task of living, and they are crucial factors in the forming of our sense of autonomy. They have shaped us by the time we turn to psychotherapy as a vehicle for attaining understanding about and change of ourselves. They also shape, expand, or constrict the possibilities of change, the domains in which change is possible, and the potential gains and limits from different types of change. Our research task involves understanding those factors and how they interact with our autonomy.

For example, at the level of genetic endowment, a core issue in a number of theories of therapy is whether there are genetically based (destiny) qualities that predispose distinct racial/ethnic and gender groups to experience reality in unique ways. Are blacks destined to experience reality differently from whites? For example, is the Afrocentric "we-ness" attributed to blacks genetically determined to some extent so that whites can never experience it in the same way or to the same degree? Are men destined to experience reality differently from women? Is the concept of maternal love somewhat a product of genetic endowment such that men can never experience it in the same way or to the same degree? To answer these questions we must study them. To study them, we must free ourselves and others who share our own historical time and our own cultural/ethnic/racial and gender contexts from our own biases. In proceeding we must confront the intermingling and confounding that arises from the presence of these external (historical and contextual) and internal (genetic and personal experience) factors in all of us, researchers and subjects as well. Those who study these questions half a century from now will do so in a different historical time and in a different ecological context. As individuals they too will combine confounding genetic and personal experience factors in their observations. Over generations we can potentially achieve a clearer understanding of the ways in which these factors do shape our possibilities and limits. However, we can do so only if we acknowledge their relevance and at the very least document their presence in our studies and in the generalizations we draw from them. That is, studies of the characteristics of black people conducted by black investigators for purposes of demonstrating the uniqueness of blacks as individuals and as a race are subject to these kinds of biases, and their findings need to be interpreted accordingly. Studies of whites by white investigators for purposes of demonstrating the uniqueness of whites as individuals and as a race are also subject to such biases, and their findings need to be interpreted accordingly. In most of the literature we have cited, the studies by and about blacks and about women have been considered to be subject to bias and/or special pleading. The studies by and about whites and men have not been. Studies conducted in earlier eras have been considered to be limited by the narrower visions of those times. Studies conducted now are not considered to be limited by the legacy of those earlier eras or by the limits of our current vision. It is these kinds of discrepancies that need to be addressed.

Specifically, a black female college student in the United States in the 1990s may not be different from a black female college student in the United States in the 1940s in her gender and racial nature (genetic endowment). However, she lives at a quite different time in the history of the world and has had a quite different personal history, even if she has experienced a similar personal family history. Further, the racial, community, and college contexts are quite different for those two women. The woman in the 1940s lived in a more segregated world that offered far fewer possibilities of defining herself; far fewer possibilities for relating to other students and to professors; far fewer possibilities for socializing and forming a family; and far fewer career choices and life options in general.

It seems almost banal to say it, but the consequences of the differences just noted are immense. Unfortunately, we have paid relatively little attention to those differences and to those consequences. A general metahypothesis of our approach is that those consequences need to be investigated, and this increased understanding needs to be incorporated into our theories of psychotherapy and into our conduct. Thus we would formulate the following metahypothesis: *Distal as well as proximal historical as well as personal events and experiences of racial, ethnic, and sex discrimination and oppression impact on individuals and are relevant to therapeutic issues for the therapist and for the client.* For example, white therapists who have had a long history of family continuity and stability may favor their clients' defining their lives in terms of the historic continuity of those families. Black therapists and black clients who know of the history of white oppression, with its accompanying vulnerability of black women (including their mothers and grandmothers) to unwanted sexual access by white men and of black men to physical as well as psychological degradation (including lynching), may want to define their lives in terms of future possibilities, of future continuity. Whether therapists and clients explore the past and the future together or separately, their divergent histories seem likely to lead therapists and clients to experience those explorations in divergent and conflicting, as well as convergent, ways.

As we have noted, gender enters as a consideration. Whether there are gender differences in how men and women experience reality is a question that is unanswered in any definitive sense. Yet people, including therapists, have differing views as to the answer to that question. Those differing views have consequences for our research as well as for our therapeutic practices. In a broader sense, our questions about gender are accompanied by analogous questions about race and even, possibly, life stage. Those questions can be formulated in the following metahypothesis: *The nature, form, and extent to which presumably genetically determined factors such as gender and race influence the nature of human experience and the range of human possibilities is empirically investigable, but requires (1) study over a substantial period of time, (2) study of a broad context of possibilities and outcomes, and (3) investigators with representative identities to ensure a sufficient sample of findings to approximate a nonbiased domain of possibilities and limits.* Our current reference perspectives, or baselines, have been influenced in indeterminate ways and can hardly be considered to be unbiased.

The world of therapy as well as the broader world of people's lives, includes many examples of the confounding effect of beliefs and their impact on the ways in which such factors as gender shape peoples' lives, individually and collectively. For example, women who accept a so-called traditional role as appropriate define themselves and the issues of their lives in relation to that set of expectations. Therapists who view the reality of women in the same way define the task of therapy as helping women to make the most of that reality. Such a woman and such a therapist can potentially be effective in resolving the client's therapeutic issues insofar as they can be resolved in that paradigmatic view. If there are issues that require a different paradigm to permit their more effective resolution, then those two cannot resolve them. They may concur in viewing them as unresolvable. That convergence may reduce the client's subjective frustration but not other effects. For example, if they both share the view that a woman's fulfillment rests only in being as prolific as possible during her childbearing years, they may help her adapt to that lifestyle. They may be less successful in helping her to accomplish the goal of a long life, since she may succumb to the stresses or multiple pregnancies and of rearing a large number of children. They will be quite unsuccessful in examining whether their paradigmatic view is empirically substantiated. Further, if they serve as research subjects, the effects of those beliefs on their lives and on their reports of their experiences need to be taken into consideration by investigators.

As we focus on our model, and want to offer ways to explore its utility, we then focus on such issues. That is, we focus on such questions as those human possibilities and these definitions of "good lives" and life possibilities. We have noted in our presentations of the psychosocial competence model and the ethnic validity model that to some extent people define themselves (and are defined by themselves and others) in relation to the nature of their psychosocial milieus, individually and contextually. Thus, another of our metahypotheses is the following: *People's psychosocial milieus, including their histories as well as their time in history, have an empirically measurable impact on the psychosocial reality of their internal and external lives.* We need to investigate how they impact that reality and what kind of impact it is.

We have also argued that people need not constrain their lives by other people's definitions of who they are and what their possibilities are. Thus, the woman who wants to develop her life beyond her presumed genetic commitment to a maternal or relational role is entitled to an empirical answer about the extent and the limits of those possibilities for herself, as well as about their potential costs and benefits. We have a personal and professional responsibility to challenge the belief systems that constrain her and those that seem to offer her limitless possibilities. We have a comparable responsibility to explore the utilization of therapeutic knowledge and techniques to help her achieve the extent of those possibilities as well as accommodate to their limitations. We also have a responsibility to challenge the belief systems that constrain us and to explore the potentials of collaborating with her as we and she learn about the struggles and the rewards as well as the costs of pursuing those possibilities.

Do the above suggestions lead to the conclusion that we, as therapists, need to be guided exclusively by any and all wishes of clients to change as they see fit? No, that is not the logical conclusion of our argument. We bear additional responsibilities to ourselves and others, as well as to our clients. Those responsibilities include our responsibility to assess the potential limits as well as the potential possibilities of change and to inform society, our clients, and ourselves of those limits. We have a responsibility to honor our own value systems, heritages, and knowledge bases. In essence, the responsibility we bear is to accord the same status to our own and others' individual, psychosocial, and ethnic/racial/cultural realities. Beyond that we have a special responsibility to our scientific and professional standards. We are vested by society with such special responsibilities. For example, we are not to support or countenance individuals harming themselves or others. We are not to support or countenance unfounded beliefs, prejudices, and practices. We have a responsibility to ask for evidence about what constitutes harm of self and others. We have a responsibility to seek evidence about the consequences of beliefs, prejudices, and practices. Finally, we have a responsibility to act in accordance with our findings.

We are also not to countenance society harming its members, individually or collectively, although this responsibility is less clearly identified and acted upon. These are responsibilities we should bear wisely. We must be careful not to presume to define those standards and make those judgments without careful study of these background considerations. In short, particularly in these domains, we have a responsibility to investigate and question the bases and the consequences of the beliefs, standards, and practices that we espouse and follow.

Finally, we should be particularly attuned to the responsibility of investigating the relationship between those beliefs that provide us with privileged status and protection from challenge and the manner in which we relate to society and to our clients. In short, another of our metahypotheses is the following: *Therapists and investigators are also members of the human community. Their perspectives are subject to all of the factors that influence their clients and are thus influenced by those factors in ways that are subject to empirical investigation.* Our privileged status gives us a special responsibility to investigate all of these issues—ecosystem variables as well as individual variables and the ecological, historical, and personal context of the therapist as well as that of the client. They require us to pay particular attention to scrutinizing our roles as therapists and investigators because of the disproportionate power of our status and our potential for self-justification. They also obligate us to report those findings to our clients, the public, and our colleagues and to assume responsibilities for modifying our theories and practices as indicated by those findings.

Methodological Hurdles and Issues to Consider in Researching the Model

There already exists an extensive body of literature about psychotherapy research. Its character as well as its methodological strengths and limitations have been described, and that material is readily accessible and quite useful. Earlier in this chapter we referred to three recent articles summarizing the import of that work. We wish again to recommend that individuals wishing to conduct psychotherapy and/or psychotherapy research familiarize themselves with that material. In this section we call attention to issues that arise more particularly from ethnic validity and resource collaborator perspectives.

A resource collaborative model emphasizes that both therapist and client are involved as active participants as well as products of their own heritage and nature; more traditional models tend to view therapists as active participants and clients as products of their own heritage and nature. Resource collaborative approaches emphasize that both therapist and client contribute to their interaction and that, for both, that interaction has costs as well as benefits. More traditional approaches tend to emphasize that the interaction is unidirectional; the influence and benefits flow from the therapist to the client. (An example of a resource collaborative group counseling project is that of Tyler and Gatz, 1977, discussed in Chapter 2.)

We suggest that the psychotherapy research literature has been dominated by a culture-defining group perspective that is not resource collaborative oriented. Most of it has been based on a few paradigms (psychodynamic, humanistic, behavioral) that assume there is a universal psychological life process. They also assume that there is a universal psychotherapeutic process that therapists can direct and that can change clients. If we follow the psychodynamic or humanistic theories, we assume that those processes are primarily not amenable to rational understanding and correction. If we follow the behavioral tradition, we assume that those processes in the client are subject to direct cue-reinforcement manipulations and that the client has no, or very limited, autonomy. Recent elaborations of these approaches offer more complexity but tend to be basically unchanged in their underlying assumptions. The recent reviews of psychotherapy research cited earlier in this chapter seem to confirm this orientation. Actually, they seem even to strengthen it by their neglect of the growing body of research that documents the relevance of racial sensitivity, feminist perspectives, and even life span changes.

Particularist models have tended to rest on comparable beliefs of universality but have restricted their views to the assertion that there is universality within each diverse gender or race/ethnic/cultural group. For example, particularists with regard to cross-racial therapy involving blacks and whites in the United States may assume that there is a distinctive psychodynamic process for blacks and a distinctive, but different, one for whites. However, such particularists also assume there are no trans-racial/ethnic commonalities in the domains of experience and conduct which psychotherapy addresses. They may also assume that the psychotherapeutic processes for these different racial/ethnic/cultural groups are not commensurable. Understanding one is of no help in understanding the other.

We are proposing a perspective that endorses the position that people are involved in constructing their own realities. People converge, diverge, and conflict in how they form their lives and how they have been formed by their lives. Those convergences, divergences, and conflicts exist at all levels of destiny, history, context, and autonomy. We communicate and understand each other because of overlaps (convergences), but creating a conceptual understanding of the nature and role of those convergences is a complex task. To us it is one that requires that we create that broader framework by incorporating and assigning equal status to a range of perspectives. In other words, basing our conceptual understanding on an explicit or implicit culture-defining group perspective is unacceptably flawed. Basing it on a unilateral therapist defined model of interaction and of research rather than a resource collaborator approach is also unacceptably flawed. Unfortunately, most available research has been built on such a perspective. That is, most communities of therapists and therapy investigators have consisted of small groups of homogeneous people living and working in a common context and having experienced similar individual histories and educations. Further, their work has tended to assume that clients are objects of study, not participating members in an ongoing dialogue.

What we are proposing is that we focus on the methodological issues that arise if we start from the assumption that our research must meet the requirements of a broader multifaceted perspective. To do so we must focus on considering the many factors that may potentially contribute to a comprehensive understanding of what goes on in forming, maintaining, and changing the people we are. It is these factors that we need to understand and address in therapy. We must also explore how to inform our theories of therapy so that they incorporate that matrix of factors. In summary, what we are emphasizing is that we need to look at psychotherapy in, and as part of, the ecology (the contextual matrix) of the ordinary nature of lives in which it is enmeshed. As an aid to that process, we have listed in Table 1 those parameters whose contributions must be specified in conducting research within an ethnic validity framework. These parameters are what we consider to be important and are an outgrowth of our perspectives on psychosocial competence and on the influence of the ecology on human expression and interaction.

TABLE 1 *Research Matrix*

Parameters	Variables
World view	Autonomy, continuity, history, destiny
Sociocultural attributes	Culture, race, ethnicity, gender
Ecological context	CDG status, NCDG status, family, community, therapy, group, dyad
Psychosocial dimensions	Self, self–world, coping, supports, threats, experiences, behaviors
Type of measure	Holistic/analytic; qualitative/quantitative; investigator constructed/respondent constructed; jointly constructed
Form of knowing	Knowledge/value, fact/belief, enduring/temporary; state/process
Respondent	Therapist, client, other
Therapist–client relationship	Convergent/divergent/conflict
Time of measurement	Before therapy, during therapy, after therapy, life stage

Defining Domains of Questions

Our basic premise is that any information we obtain is context dependent. To establish how and in what ways any information that can be gathered is shaped by its context, the matrix in Table 1 or another one like it is needed. That is, we can identify the influences that contribute to information only to the extent that we identify potential influences and account for, or control for, their effect. Table 1 specifies nine broadly defined parameters. They are:

1. *World view,* which pertains to the researcher or participants' perspective on agency and on the factors that influence it;
2. *Sociocultural attributes,* which pertain to the sociological level at which the researcher or participant targets as important in defining him- or herself or others;
3. *Ecological context,* which identifies the ecosystem and ecological variables within which world view and sociocultural attributes are expressed, translated, and reformulated;
4. *Psychosocial dimensions,* which are those variables that define the domains of human relatedness and functioning and the behaviors that accompany them;
5. *Type of measure,* which pertains to the way information is collected and assembled;

6. *Form of knowing,* which pertains to the characteristics and nature of the information assessed;
7. *Respondent,* which pertains to the participants of the research;
8. *Therapist–client relationship,* which refers to the process or aspect of the relationship being investigated; and
9. *Time of measurement,* which is related to ecological context since both context and time of measurement inform our understanding of ways humans construct meaning from their experiences.

For example (see Table 1), we may be interested in studying the relationship between the nature of the self and sense of autonomy as manifested in individual therapy. In our study, we may choose to study the nature and role of autonomy as it is manifest in the sense of self as expressed in individual therapy by the members of the culture-defining group. We may further decide to focus on the self as an enduring belief system as exhibited during therapy in a period of therapist–client conflict between a therapist and client who are both members of the culture-defining group. We may use an investigator-constructed qualitative measure based on therapist ratings. We do not ordinarily specify all of these factors when we undertake a research project, nor when we interpret its findings. Characteristically, we do not repeat such a study using client ratings, client-constructed measures, periods of convergence, or non-culture-defining clients. We ordinarily attend to these parameters only in an asystematic fashion.

It is true that we can study only a limited set of these factors at any given time. Nevertheless, we cannot assume that they do not influence our results without identifying them and investigating them systematically. Nor can we assume that the significant meanings of our findings are relevant to the therapy process itself without accounting for the contribution of these many factors. That is, the form and nature of the therapeutic interchanges and of the characteristics exhibited by the parties involved in such a study may be a function of their shared cultural backgrounds, not the therapeutic aspects of their interaction. Their findings may reflect how a client from that cultural milieu interacts with an authority figure from that milieu and have little to do with the presumably therapeutic aspects of their relationship.

We can perhaps highlight this point further if we consider how the resulting interactions and data might be different in the United States if the therapist was from a non-culture-defining group (e.g., black) and the client was from a culture-defining group (e.g., white). We can also consider what differences might result in the United States if, in addition, the therapist was female (i.e., a black woman) and the client was male (i.e., a white man).

We can add another domain of considerations if we shift from studying autonomy to studying continuity. In modal cultural views in the United States, emphasis is placed on differentiation of the self from peers, from previous and succeeding generations, and from one's community and/or ethnic group. In some non-culture-defining groups (e.g., blacks, Latins, Asians), much more emphasis is placed on interrelatedness of the self with others. For example, Afrocentric-oriented black psychologists emphasize the *we self-referent* as more central than the *I self-referent*. Gilligan (1982) emphasizes that even culture-defining group women in the United States are more relational oriented than men. Their autonomy, their sense of self, is developed more by defining autonomy as encompassing relatedness than as an alternative to it, which is more the case for culture-defining group men.

Are we to conclude that these differences are relatively inconsequential, are simply manifestations of the content of people's lives but not central to their psychological conflicts, or are reflections of the deficiencies or aberrations in women and non-culture-defining group individuals? If these differences in the nature of the self, or autonomy, or the like, are not trivial, then we must conclude that understanding them is central to our understanding of people in therapy as well as out of therapy.

If we are to understand the many contextual parameters that can potentially be identified within a matrix such as the one we have outlined, we must begin to create an ecologically and ethnically grounded understanding of psychotherapeutic processes, therapeutic effects, and the appropriateness of therapeutic goals. We must study them as a source of the meaning in therapeutic and other human exchanges. We cannot continue to treat them as extraneous variables to be ignored or controlled for experimentally or statistically. We must document and report on these factors in all of our studies. We must establish systematically interrelated research programs that inform one another about the relevance and import of these factors. In this chapter we can only hope to point out a few of the considerations that are important in directing our research efforts more effectively toward those goals.

To illustrate the issues involved, we have chosen as another example the oft-researched question of the extent to which people are externally or internally oriented. We have included issues of using qualitative in contrast to quantitative measures, holistic in contrast to analytic approaches, black in contrast to white respondents, and investigator-constructed in contrast to respondent-constructed definitions of internal–external orientation. We could select other variables or combinations of variables to make our point. Any choice is to some extent arbitrary. In the long run, of course, we need to conduct a systematically designed set of studies across overlapping contextual domains until we understand more fully how these variables do contribute to who we are and how we live our lives.

We can and often do ask whether blacks are more externally oriented than whites (race/ethnicity). We do not ask what an external orientation (self and self–world belief) means in the context of or to the members of either group. The context of being black or white in the United States (non-culture-defining versus culture-defining status) can be described and/or explained in holistic terms, and changes in it can be identified and documented without using numbers. We can extend that description by defining our categories or variables in a quantifiable fashion and establishing numerical or statistical differences.

We can also reverse that sequence. That is, we can begin with quantifiable variables such as internality–externality and study the quantitative differences between blacks and whites in the United States. We can then extend beyond those quantitative differences to make holistic statements about the nature of blacks and whites in the United States, about the nature of the ecological contexts in which they live, and about their convergences, divergences, and conflicts. Those two approaches will lead to overlapping outcomes, but not to exactly the same outcome. We can take an additional step and construct a descriptive and explanatory framework that incorporates the descriptions and explanations obtained from those two perspectives—analytic and holistic.

This process is potentially endless. At some point we must exercise our judgments as to the relative benefits and costs of gaining more encompassing perspectives rather than taking action on the basis of the perspectives we have obtained. Nevertheless, our emphasis at this point is on how we can enrich and extend the currently available and, in our judgment, limited perspectives on the ethnic validity issues in psychotherapy.

The internality–externality variable has been originally conceptualized out of an analytic stimulus–response framework. We can ask and extend our understanding of that variable and concept by having it defined by respondents or jointly by investigators and respondents. We can have it defined by black populations and by white populations with our only beginning point being a shared minimal convergence on what that dimension of internality–externality means. We can also extend our understanding by starting at a holistic level and trying to develop a descriptive and quantitative sense of the internality–externality dimension from that beginning point. That is, we can begin by formulating descriptive or comparative statements including an overall holistic sense of what each group's context and life is like and of how those lives differ in an overall sense with regard to internality–externality.

A central question about holistic attributes is that of how we can quantify those characteristics we consider to be holistically measurable and not lose the significance of the overall contextual meaning on which we also want to focus. The answer to that question rests on our conceptual skill in attending to how we use numbers as well as holistic terms. In this instance, even if we say that blacks are more external than whites, we need to state the contextual meaning of that statement. For example, about what are they more external? Are they more external about those domains of their lives that are unique to their ethnic/racial reality? Are they just more external about those domains of their lives that are shaped by the culture-defining whites? In either case, asking and seeking to explore these questions in an ethnic validity context can lead us to a fuller understanding of both qualitative and quantitative representations and their interrelationships. Asking these questions can also lead us to a fuller understanding of the nature and implications of ethnic validity characteristics. Most importantly, they can lead us to a contextually richer and fuller understanding of people, black and white, and of how to use psychotherapy to help them resolve problems and enrich their lives.

There is a rich tradition of approaching the study of psychotherapy from a holistic, phenomenological, or at least qualitative, perspective. That tradition has been accompanied by an ongoing debate over the commensurability of qualitative and quantitative methods, measures, and criteria. Introducing an ethnic validity perspective does not solve, complicate, or change the underlying issues in that debate. It simply points to the importance of considering other questions such as that of the role of ecosystem perspectives on forming the nature of interpersonal relationships. For example, later in this section we ask a number of questions about the meaning of *rapport,* and whether its meaning for culture-defining group members and non-culture-defining group members is equivalent. From our point of view, questions about therapeutic concepts such as rapport, or more generally about our understanding of and practice of psychotherapy, are likely to be more fully answered by studies combining qualitative and quantitative approaches.

Another kind of example we can identify in the research matrix (Table 1) will serve to make a different kind of point about research approaches. Specifically, how do we assess convergence, divergence, and conflict? This question is somewhat unique; the methodology for answering it is not. We measure convergence, divergence, and conflict by studying processes and outcomes. Primarily, it is necessary to gather data independently from therapists and clients. We may do so directly or use a procedure such as having them keep diaries or otherwise record their ongoing impressions. We may use audiotape or videotape records, then have reviewers listen to or look at them independently or edit them so that raters hear or see only one of the participants' perspectives. With judgments thus made independently, we have a basis for studying their convergences, divergences, and conflicts, plus the correlates of those patterns.

What is crucial in enriching our understanding of ethnic validity considerations is that we begin to formulate questions, approaches, and answers from the perspectives of clients as well as therapists. Further, it is imperative that we formulate and ask our questions with an explicit awareness of and effort to answer ethnic validity-relevant questions such as the commonality of meaning that words have across groups. For example, we need to know whether blacks and whites in the United States mean the same thing when they say that they have *rapport* or that they agree on something or understand each other. By *mean the same thing* we mean Does that agreement (convergence) have equivalent ecological, psychosocial, and environmental antecedents, correlates, and consequences? To put it another way, we speak often of empathy and rapport in the psychotherapy literature. Is my sense of empathy ethnic validity based and limited to those with similar ethnic histories and identities? Is rapport between a black therapist and client comparable to that between a white therapist and client? At present we do not know. We are going to learn only by asking these kinds of questions and trying to answer them.

Defining the Nature of Psychotherapy

Life is an extended segmental process, and psychotherapy takes place as an extended segment of living. Psychotherapy is not a totally artificial and isolated event in our lives. We must look at pre–post issues as well as process issues in a program development and program evaluation context. We need to examine the beginning point of psychotherapy, the process itself, the changes involved in it, the endpoint or outcome of psychotherapy, and the longer-term follow-up consequences. And we need to look at those components in relation to each other.

Another issue that needs scrutiny is that of the relationship for clients between traditional psychotherapeutic topics and activities and the ongoing events in their lives. There are widespread beliefs that ongoing events must be put aside from the domain of therapy and that one's therapist should be someone with whom there is no ongoing life ties. These beliefs are a product of a dominant cultural, class, gender, and intellectual tradition, that of western Europe and of the twentieth-century United States. They may simply be a luxury of that group to have the time and leisure for detached intrapsychic contemplation. They may be a preferred style of a culture-defining group. That style may have its roots in cultural or religious traditions that emphasize the value of sanctuary as a means of understanding and resolving conflict, facilitating growth (the attaining of maturity, self-actualization, or whatever generally equivalent objective is indicated), or otherwise contributing to the quality of an individual's life. The idea of sanctuary, of seeking a safe, protected setting or relationship as a relief from overburdening life issues and as a setting in which to engage in contemplation, review issues and past actions and understandings, and consult with a trusted figure (real or spiritual) is by no means new or exclusive to the field of psychotherapy. There is abundant documentation of the benefits of such approaches. Nevertheless, it is by no means a universal human characteristic to approach problem solving by first focusing on internal feelings and assuming that doing so will lead to more satisfactory ways of living. Nor, for that matter, is it clear that the use of a sanctuary approach is without limitations, or even beneficial in all contexts and for all presumably psychological problems and conflicts.

In contrast, there may be benefits to focusing more directly on working out problems in a regular life context and expecting internal states to reflect the gains from that approach. There may be advantages to working our problems with a professional who is part of a client's community and who knows the client and his or her context and is in turn known by the client. This latter pattern seems to be a preferred one among, for example, Latin populations (Zwerling *et al.*, 1976). Our point is that we need to inform our theories and practices in the psychotherapy field by asking and answering these kinds of ethnic validity-relevant questions.

We must also consider and explore the possibility that there is a program development character to psychotherapy. That is, the processes involved may generate interactive changes that modify the context and nature of therapy as it proceeds. Therapists do think of the client as resisting the psychotherapeutic process and regimen. That perception could be seen as the therapist's view of the client's efforts to define the interaction in a different way, that is, as the client viewing the interaction from within another paradigm. From the traditional therapeutic perspective, that resistance indicates the client's pathology. We are suggesting that it may, at least in part, not indicate pathology (deviance or dysfunction in terms of the therapist's paradigm) but rather indicate another paradigm, a different ethnic validity way of being human. We need not reject the client's assertion that he or she has life-based problems within that different world view. We can begin by accepting the validity of that world view and then work collaboratively with the client to form a new paradigm of interaction between therapist and client. If that new paradigm is formed interactively, then neither therapist nor client can know at the beginning of their therapeutic interactions what the form of that process is going to be. Such interactive processes need specification, and we have much to gain from exploring them and their consequences. How do we trace such change processes? What are their antecedents, correlates, and consequences? How do we trace an ecosystem? Again, the methodologies involved are not unique. These questions may be. We can answer them by applying the usual methodologies to them. We trace an ecosystem or a change process within it by measuring it at different points in time, identifying its changes, and relating them to intervening events. We may also modify those intervening events and thereby develop quasi-experimental design studies.

Defining and Measuring Outcomes

We face several issues in conceptualizing the nature of outcomes and their desirability. First, the traditional criterion of symptom reduction is woefully limited. For example, do we consider it a desirable outcome when we have reduced anxiety, outrage, or depression by influencing people to believe that those feelings have come from intrapsychic inadequacy so that they now focus on organizing their resources to contain those feelings rather than focusing on changing certifiably unjust circumstances? Symptom reduction is also limited in that it presumes a universalist definition of what is a "symptom."

We need to define our criteria so that they also include quality of life indicators, such as manifestations of satisfactions, resources, strengths, and other indicators of well-being. We need, as well, to measure dissatisfactions, including what are usually called symptoms. We suggest that they should possibly be more appropriately labeled as indicators of dysfunctions.

A second issue arises around the question of whether any set of universal (cultural-defining group) criteria is appropriate in and of itself for any group. Thus we would suggest that the ethnic (and other contextual) base of any set of criteria be specified, particularly until we have developed independent sets of contextually based criteria for definable ethnic/racial/cultural and gender groups. Further, we need at least to consider defining different ecologically and ethnically syntonic criteria of human well-being in relation to the ethos of those distinctive ethnic validities. Finally, we would emphasize the importance of defining any set of criteria in such a way that the definitions acknowledge and allow for the heterogeneity of human groups and the divergent ways in which individuals define themselves in any context.

To attain these sets of criteria, it seems important to define the form of adequate sets of criteria. At this point in time, we can look to the work of black, Hispanic, and Asian psychologists and to the work of feminists as guides. They have begun to establish guidelines for developing ethnically valid judgments. Our concern can be expressed as defining criteria—for instance, "of black people, by black people, and for black people" or "of women, by women, and for women." Yet, even as we articulate such an aim that ethnically valid judgments about a group must be defined and at least include their own definition of themselves, we must also keep in mind that blacks and women have been defined primarily by white men. Their first approximations at defining themselves are going to be influenced by that history and their own socialization within it (including at times a reaction against the view of themselves as lesser humans). That history of necessity provides powerful external and internal pressures on how they define themselves. Further, self-definition is always an interactive process that incorporates others' views as well as one's own. Nevertheless, establishing a beginning point is essential. After we have defined these indigenous or non-culture-defining group sets of criteria, we will have ahead of us the task of defining overarching sets of criteria. Both distinctive and overarching criteria are essential for somewhat disparate groups who live in the same world to interact with and understand each other.

We then need to explore the short- and long-term characteristics of life as lived within those contextually defined sets of characteristics. We said much earlier that there is more than one way to be human. The research mentioned earlier of street children illustrates dramatically the ways even children can find to deal with harsh realities and still build a strong prosocial sense of their own humanity. Yet our criteria of well-being, therapeutic benefit, and the like, have not acknowledged the pluralism and diversity inherent in that statement. It will only be as we have studied alternative life conceptions that we will be in a position to assess their relative value or to assess the costs and benefits of combining different life conceptions.

Further, we must consider whether, at the beginning point of their interactions, either therapist or client should specify completely what the end point of psychotherapy should look like. In some sense we are arguing that both will undergo a type of paradigm shift as a function of their interaction. That is why they should not (and cannot) specify in advance what makes sense in general or in particular as an ending point. Consequently, we are arguing that formation of criteria for favorableness of outcomes cannot be fully specified in advance.

We do believe that making an initial statement of desired final end points is important. We just do not believe that it is a sufficient criterion on which to base final evaluations. We also need reference points about how to evolve new understandings and criteria along the way and about how to include them as part of our criteria as to the desirability of outcomes. We think that we must include both original criteria and modified ones, and with appropriate rationales for any changes from our initial criteria. Since it is an ongoing process, we need to check out in future studies whether such changes and rationales provide more general benefits for clients or just serve to provide rationales for our self-deceptions. For example, do we find that clients' changing conceptions of their own future well-being include more divergence from our views of their possibilities, not just more convergence with what we consider desirable for them.

MAJOR FIRST AREAS IN RESEARCHING THE MODEL

A useful reference framework for identifying a comprehensive set of research questions about any model is Kuhn's (1970) suggested categories of research that are important in developing and testing a paradigm. They are, namely, (1) direct tests of the theory, (2) tests of matters directly relevant to articulating and extending the theory, and (3) tests of significant practical applications of the theory. In a broad sense, any research on the relationships between ecological considerations and individual functioning qualify as pertinent to evaluations of the ethnic validity model. In this context, our goal is to be substantially more restrictive than those possibilities suggest and to point out a few potential areas of research that seem to bear on all three of these considerations and seem particularly central to determining whether the conception of an ethnic validity perspective is of substantial relevance or represents an essentially secondary or trivial set of considerations.

The Ecology of Therapy and Therapists

Some of our first questions deal with getting a good grasp on the ecology of therapy and of therapists. After all, unless we can demonstrate that there are substantially different ethnic validities and that they are related in substantial, not trivial, ways to people's psychosocial well-being, then there is no empirical basis for a theory of ethnic validity. We have suggested that there is evidence (see Chapters 2 and 3) to support our view. Even so, that evidence is sketchy indeed. Therapists, clients, and society are in need of a more substantive documentation of the nature of identifiable ethnic ecologies and the potential constructive as well as destructive life patterns they foster.

We must establish the "beginning point" for therapists as well as for clients. We cannot assume that either begins at a specified position of understanding of self or others. We cannot assume that either has a universally legitimate reference point. Rather, we need to develop a matrix of perspectives. For example, in our ethnic validity article (Tyler, Sussewell, & Williams-McCoy, 1985) we developed the four patterns of interrelations that exist in the possible pairings between white and black clients and therapists. We also suggested in that article that each of those pairings has its own ecology. We need to explore empirically what each of those ecologies is—not in reference to the others, but in and of itself.

We think that the task of defining a coherent picture of each such subgroup or pairing is important as a first step into this domain of questions. After all, the various pairings with all of the diversity they imply are and will continue to be elements within a pluralistic world. We need to know more about what each is like, what it contributes, and what it lacks. We can then ask how to make the most of its possibilities and how to shore up its limitations.

We also need to ask what are the advantages and disadvantages of the different pairings in relation to what individuals, purposes, problems, and contexts. Which shall we choose when we have a choice? How shall we make the most of the possibilities when our choices are limited?

Therapists also have different beliefs and expectations with regard to the ecosystems of different clients. Will exploring therapists' perspectives help us get at these issues? One question that needs asking is whether these therapist-defined expectations for different individuals provide insights about the different ecologies that characterize different ethnic/racial groups? In other words, are the ways in which therapists define the context of therapy for individually distinctive but culturally homogeneous clients, in contrast to those from different ethnic/racial ecologies, indicative of the significant character of these different ethnic validities? Are they indicative of the individual or ethnic biases and stereotypes of the therapists from different ethnic heritages? It is our suggestion that research investigations are needed to answer these questions.

There are in existence a number of studies and models for studying the expectations of teachers and their impacts on students and of investigators and their impact on subjects. Those models can serve as a springboard for investigations in the therapeutic area. We need to ask, for example, what NCDG therapists' expectations are in regard to interactions with and outcomes for their clients from the same NCDG. We need to ask whether and how their expectations are different for other NCDG clients. We need to ask whether and how their expectations are different for CDG clients. We need to ask similar questions about CDG therapists. And on and on we need to explore until we have in-depth pictures of these patterns.

Presumably, among the first questions that follow the identification of distinctive ethnic ecologies and life patterns are those about whether the different kinds of matches and biases we speak of make any difference. That is, are there different interactions among the different pairings? We agree that those questions are important, indeed essential, to ask and answer. That is, we need to know the consequences of these divergent and, perhaps, conflicting patterns for therapists, clients, and for society.

As we ask about the consequences of these differences among the various pairings, we encounter other important questions that need attention: Are NCDG members (as compared with CDG members) more concerned with indications of personal caring than of formal credentials and criteria? (Gibbs, 1980, suggests that possibility.) Do NCDG members achieve the levels of trust that characterize CDG members; or higher levels among themselves and lower levels with CDG members; or the converse? As we noted earlier, whatever rapport is, it may be different within the context of different psychosocial ecosystems.

We also need to investigate what outcome configurations are more characteristic, optimal, or dysfunctional for CDG members and NCDG members. Are there identifiable outcome configurations that are more characteristic, optimal, or dysfunctional for CDG members and NCDG members in their own ecosystem contexts; in contexts in which they are the majority; in contexts in which they are the minority?

Finally, are there a variety of identifiable ways of living within each ethnic validity tradition that have characteristic strengths as well as limitations, offer characteristic joys as well as sorrows, and thus provide different ways of being human and of imagining and creating lifestyles and solutions? Or, is each tradition characterized by a unitary way of judging the psychosocial integrity of its members and others? Does each tradition thus force the diversity of humanity to conform to some Procrustean bed (as defined by any group) or psychological fit? We can only begin to answer these questions by beginning with the assumption that they are legitimate and then trying to answer them. It is that process of exploration that we consider to be long overdue.

Convergence and Psychotherapy

We also encounter important first areas of questions when we look at the necessary conditions for constructive interactions between any two people, or for that matter when we look at the interactions we have with ourselves. That is, we either converge on a reference point, diverge about it (we are of two minds about it), or conflict over it. We apparently assume, at least implicitly, that by its nature, diversity is undesirable and conflict is intolerable. We assume that we must resolve conflict or shut down interacting. We raise the question of whether we can meaningfully interact across the presence of divergences and conflicts by assuming that we cannot, even at the level of differences between individuals. We say that we cannot work with someone because they are too warm, too cold, too combative, too sensitive, too insensitive, too affectionate, too anything.

Investigating the question of the possibilities of people interacting constructively in the absence of convergence merits our attention at the most general possible level. Nevertheless, we want to focus primarily on a select few particular aspects or manifestations of that question. Namely, do people continue with interactions even if they see the other person as ethnically/racially in conflict with them? Do they continue if one of them sees the other as not psychosocially competent to help with some of the issues that are central to that person? If they do continue such interactions, what are the consequences? Should they try to interact in spite of, or even because of, those differences?

We do not really know what the differing correlates of convergences, divergences, and conflicts in psychotherapy are, at least not in any systematic way. We do not know very much about those issues for individual therapist–client pairings except for very extreme instances. We know even less about them when we focus on cross-racial/ethnic pairings. We do not even know how to sort out the impact of individual stylistic characteristics in contrast to ethnic/racial stylistic characteristics because we have not attended to that issue in any depth. For example, there are ethnically/racially characteristic ways of viewing ourselves and presenting ourselves. There are individual differences within those patterns. When a therapist and client from different ethnic/racial groups interact, we need to know whether they are typical or atypical of their own heritage, and whether they are interacting with each other and interpreting those interactions as individual or group characteristics. We also need to know what the different correlates are of the two kinds of interpretations. For example, it is important to study what difference it makes to a therapist to approach that role as a black therapist rather than as a therapist who is black, and as a white therapist rather than as a therapist who is white. Further, what additional difference does it make in relation to clients who are of a similar rather than a different ethnic heritage; to clients with a similar rather than a different view of the role of that ethnic heritage and identity? Maybe it makes no difference, but let us at least ask and find out.

In this section so far we have been asking questions about the exploration of ethnic/racial issues. We want to note also that we are advocating a resource collaborator model of psychotherapy, not a unidirectional model of change. It is important to focus also on the question of whether users of a resource collaborator model will interact differently, be perceived differently, and/or have different impacts from others like themselves who approach psychotherapy in a more traditional fashion. Also, will they come to think of clients more as people and less as diagnostic categories? How does the model shape the socialization of the therapist? How does it shape the socialization of the client? More broadly, what difference does it make, if any, and in what ways? Unless it makes some differences, then our approach is of no consequence, theoretically or practically. If it does make a difference, then we face a long overdue reconceptualization of our theories of psychotherapy and of psychological well-being and dysfunction. We also face important new directions in research in these areas.

Process Questions

Throughout our discussion so far, we have stressed that psychotherapy involves a process. We need to explore the nature of that process, or of those processes, to assess whether there are the kinds of differences and gains and losses we speak of as related to ethnic validity issues. Models for asking and answering those questions exist with regard to theories and techniques of therapy. They have not been explored in a systematic and definitive sense with regard to ethnic validity issues. It seems to us that there would be great benefit in doing so. For example, how do therapists' and clients' ethnic/racial attitudes about clients, therapy, ethnicity, and the like, create realities and changes that shape therapeutic processes? How do they shape approaches to change as those approaches relate to gains and losses; as they relate to the ways people change their competence configuration functioning, their related lifestyles, and their satisfaction or dissatisfaction with their lives? We have noted in another context that there are therapists who seem unable to work with anyone other than people like themselves. We have not said and do not know what is involved in those negative interactions or how to change them. At one level it is important for therapists to understand their deficiencies and change them. At another level it is important for clients to know how to make the most of the therapeutic possibilities available to them and understand which limitations are in their therapists, not in them.

Training

A literature review in the *Psychological Bulletin* (Garb, 1989) ended with the conclusion that experience does not improve clinical judgment, but that training may. That statement is both depressing and encouraging. It is depressing because the psychotherapy field relies heavily on experience as a means of training and uses it as a justification for many therapeutic theories, judgments, and practices. It is encouraging because it supports the belief that it is possible to educate and train people and thereby improve their clinical judgment. Now it leads us to ask what training helps, and how does it do so? Further, how can we introduce ethnic validity issues into that training in a fashion that will improve clinical judgments and, more generally, psychotherapy?

There are many such questions to ask. We want to focus on only a few as particularly important and as instructive examples. As they seek to become therapists, students are confronted with many issues and questions about themselves, their clients, their chosen profession, and, for that matter, their world. Generally, training focuses on individual characteristics, not ethnic validity ones. We want to ask about training to deal with institutional as well as individual racism and related ethnic validity attitudes and attributes such as racial identity. We want to ask about students' level of comfort with diversity (does it last; how is it kept alive; how generalizable is it to other areas of their lives?). We want to ask how to include these issues in training therapists in ways that have more benign than malign effects. We also want to ask comparable questions about how to train clients to gain the most from their investment in psychotherapy. We can answer those questions only by carefully exploring alternative possibilities within and between culture-defining and non-culture-defining groups.

SUMMARY

There are an infinite number of research questions to be asked in the domain of ethnic validity and psychotherapy. We have suggested only a few. Central to our focus is the task of bringing destiny, history, and context into the forefront of our research. Possibly less highlighted, but equally important, has been our stress on the view that autonomy is psychosocial, even as destiny, history, and context are. Autonomy is a function of individual experience, but it is also a function of ethnic, racial, and cultural, experience. Each of us defines self, the world, and choice in relation to many levels of nested existence. Thus to some extent, freedom and understanding are a matter of degree in relation to particular areas and choices as well as domains. We may be quite free and feel we have much control over our options in our personal existence, in our family, and in our ethnically homogeneous work and community, but not in our cross-ethnic interactions. Thus understanding our ethnicity as an anchor in defining ourselves is crucial for us, for those we relate to, for our therapists (when we are clients), and for our clients (when we are therapists). We can enrich that understanding only to the extent that we see those factors as parts of ourselves and of our ecology. What we are suggesting is that we can begin to view our theories and therapeutic approaches as more meaningful to the extent that we begin to see them as embedded in and also reflective of the history, destiny, context, and autonomy of their creators and practitioners. They are not content-free sets of principles nor value-free sets of universal goods and bads, rights and wrongs, insights and defenses. They are imbedded in us and we in them. It is important that we begin to inform ourselves and others of the imbeddedness of culture-defining group perspectives as well as those of non-culture-defining group perspectives. This chapter has been intended to point out some of the ways that we can go about that task. We hope that it can serve for our readers as a beginning point, not as an end.

IN CLOSING

We have presented the ethnic validity model as one we have found to be of value for learning to be a therapist and teaching others who would be therapists as well as for conducting psychotherapy. We have elaborated on its possibilities at some length and are not inclined to say more at this point. What we do want to say is that we have tried to provide a model that can serve as a framework for developing what we have called psychosocial competence. It is a model for thinking about ourselves and the process of living. We have included an extensive account of what we see as important ethnic validity issues. We see them as significant components of our social environments, our psychological makeups, and our ways of interacting with the world. We include in that latter category our ways of conducting and experiencing therapy as therapists and our ways of conducting and experiencing therapy as clients.

We have elaborated on the long-term aspects of therapeutic relationships. Conducting psychotherapy involves three phases, forming a relationship, maintaining and using it to accomplish therapeutic purposes, and terminating it. We have elaborated on those same phases as the parts of a single interview. An interview has a beginning (exploring our status and organizing our goals), a working through (implementing our intentions), and a termination (culminating, concluding, and redefining). We have also pointed out that working through an issue has the same elements in it.

We have also pointed out the importance of learning about ourselves and seeing ourselves as part of what is going on in a therapeutic interaction. We have discussed the importance of viewing therapy as a reciprocal interaction process. We have indicated that there is asymmetry in such processes but that it does not negate their reciprocal nature. As therapists our objective is to be helpful; that does not elevate us or inoculate us from our human limitations. As clients our objective is to get help; that does not diminish us or take away our capabilities and our humanness.

In sum then, what we have tried to provide is some perspectives for readers to build on. We leave you with our firm conviction that your greatest asset is your own humanness, personal and ethnic/racial/cultural. There is much to learn from your own research and experiences and from the research and experiences of others. That learning can be facilitated by incorporating it in a model such as the one we have tried to describe. Some of us will be more abstract and intellectual, some of us will be more concrete and emotional. These styles and the many others we can imagine all have their utilities and their limitations. Each of us can build most effectively on our own unique way of living by acknowledging it as our base and moving on from there. That is what the process of learning to be a therapist and the process of teaching someone else to be a therapist seem to be about. Finally, it is our hope that exploring these ideas and approaches is as enriching for you as outlining our views has been for us.

References

Abramowitz, S. I., & Murray J. (1983). Race effect in psychotherapy. In J. Murray & P. R. Abrams (Eds.), *Bias in psychotherapy* (pp. 215–255). New York: Praeger.

Acosta, F. X. (1979). Preferences and self-disclosure in relation to psychotherapist professional and ethnic identification. *Journal of Psychology, 103,* 129–134.

Acosta, F. X. (1980). Self-described reasons for premature termination of psychotherapy by Mexican American, Black American, and Anglo-American patients. *Psychological Reports, 47*(2), 435–443.

Acosta, F. X., & Sheehan, T. G. (1976). Preferences toward Mexican-American and Anglo-American psychotherapists. *Journal of Consulting and Clinical Psychology, 44,* 272–279.

Acosta, F. X., & Sheenan, J. (1978). Self-disclosure in relation to psychotherapist expertise and ethnicity. *American Journal of Community Psychology, 6*(6), 541–553.

Acosta, F. X., Yamamoto, J., & Evans, L. A. (1982). *Effective psychotherapy for low income and minority patients.* New York: Plenum.

Alston, L. (1974). Minority students and the college mental health clinic. *Journal of American College Health Association, 23,* 22–29.

Anderson, C. R. (1977). Locus of control, coping behaviors, and performance in a stress setting: A longitudinal study. *Journal of Applied Psychology, 62,* 446–451.

Argyris, C. (1968). Some unintended consequences of rigorous research. *Psychological Bulletin, 70,* 185–197.

Argyris, C. (1975). Dangers in applying results from experimental social psychology. *American Psychologist, 30,* 469–485.

Atkinson, D. R. (1983). Ethnic similarity in counseling psychology: A review of the research. *Counseling Psychologist, 11*(3), 79–92.

Atkinson, D. R. (1985). A meta-review of research on cross-cultural counseling psychology. *Journal of Multicultural Counseling and Development, 13*(4), 138–153.

Bahnson, C. B. (1980). Stress and cancer: The state of the art—I. *Psychosomatics, 21,* 975–981.

Bahnson, C. B. (1981). Stress and cancer: The state of the art—II. *Psychosomatics, 22,* 207–220.

Bandura, A. (1982). Self efficacy mechanisms in human agency. *American Psychologist, 37,* 122–147.

Banks, W. M. (1972). The differential effects of race and social class in helping. *Journal of Clinical Psychology, 28,* 90–92.

Barron, F. (1963). *Creativity and psychological health.* Princeton, NJ: Van Nostrand.

Baum, O. E., Felzer, S. B., D'zmura, T. L., & Shumaker, E. (1966). Psychotherapy dropouts and lower socioeconomic patients. *American Journal of Orthopsychiatry, 36,* 629–325.

Beale, A. V. (1986). A cross cultural therapeutic encounter. *Journal of Multicultural Counseling and Development, 14*(2), 73–76.

Benesch, K. F., & Ponterotto, J. (1989). East and west: Transpersonal psychology and cross-cultural counseling. *Counseling and Values, 33*(2), 121–131.

Bennett, L. (1964). *Before the Mayflower: A history of the Negro in America*. Baltimore, Penguin.

Bergin, A. E., & Lambert, M. J. (1978). The evaluation of therapeutic outcomes. In S. L. Garfield & A. E. Bergin (Eds.), *Handbook of psychotherapy and behavior change: An empirical analysis* (2nd ed., pp. 139–190). New York: Wiley.

Berkman, L. F., & Syme, L. (1979). Social networks, host resistance, and mortality: A nine-year follow up study of Alameda county residents. *American Journal of Epidemiology, 109*(2), 186–204.

Bernal, G., & Flores, O. (1982). Latino families in therapy: Engagement and evaluation. *Journal of Marriage and Family, 8*(3), 357–365.

Billingsley, A. (1968). *Black families in white America*. Englewood Cliffs, NJ: Prentice-Hall.

Blassingame, J. W. (1979). *The slave community: Plantation life in the Antebellum South*. New York: Oxford University Press.

Borus, J. F., Anastasia, M., Casoni, R., Russo, R. D., DiMascio, L., Fusco, L., Rubenstein, J., & Snyder, M. (1979). Psychotherapy in the goldfish bowl: The role of the indigenous therapist. *Archives of General Psychiatry, 236*, 187–190.

Breeden, J. (1980). *Advice among masters: The ideal in slave management in the old south*. Westport, CT: Greenwood Press.

Brown, L. S. (1986). Gender-role analysis: A neglected component of psychological assessment. *Psychotherapy, 23*(2), 243–248.

Bryson, S., & Bardo, H. (1975). Race and the counseling process: An overview. *Journal of Non-White Concerns, 4*(1), 5–15.

Bugaighis, M. A., Schumm, W. R., Bollman, S. R., & Jurich, A. P. (1983). Locus of control and marital satisfaction. *Journal of Psychology, 114*(2), 275–279.

Bulhan, H. (1985). *Frantz Fanon and the psychology of oppression*. New York: Plenum.

Burke, L. (1986). *Women, feminism, and biology: The feminist challenge*. Sussex Brighton: Harvester Press.

Butler, R. O. (1975). Psychotherapy: Implications of a black process model. *Psychotherapy: Theory, Practice, and Research, 12*, 407–411.

Byrne, P. (1984). Psychiatric morbidity in a gynecology clinic: An epidemiological survey. *British Journal of Psychiatry, 144*, 28–34.

Carkhuff, R. R., & Pierce, R. (1967). Differential effects of therapist race and social class upon rate and depth of self-exploration in the initial clinical interview. *Journal of Consulting Psychology, 31*, 632–634.

Carter R. T. (1990). Cultural value differences between African Americans and white Americans. *Journal of College Student Development, 31*(1), 71–79.

Charlesworth, E. A., & Nathan, R. G. (1982). *Stress management: a comprehensive guide to wellness*. Houston, TX: Biobehavioral Publishers and Distributors.

Cimbolic, P. (1972). Counselor race and experience effects on black clients. *Journal of Consulting and Clinical Psychology, 39*, 328–332.

Cobb, S. (1976). Social support as a moderator of life stress. *Psychosomatic Medicine, 38*, 300–314.

Coelho, G. V., Hamburg, D. A., & Murphey, E. B. (1963). Coping strategies in a new learning environment. *Archives of General Psychiatry, 9*, 433–443.

Comas-Diaz, L. (1981). Puerto Rican espiritismo and psychotherapy. *American Journal of Orthopsychiatry, 51*(4), 636–645.

Comas-Diaz, L., & Jacobsen, F. M. (1987). Ethnocultural identification in psychotherapy. *Psychiatry, 50*(3), 232–241.

Connolly, J. (1976). Life events before myocardial infarction. *Journal of Human Stress, 2*(4), 3–17.

Cooke, M., & Kipnis, D. (1986). Influence tactics in psychotherapy. *Journal of Consulting and Clinical Psychology, 54,* 22–26.

Cortese, M. (1979). Intervention research with Hispanic Americans: A review. *Hispanic Journal of Behavioral Sciences, 1*(1), 4–20.

Crisson, J. E., & Keefe, F. J. (1988). The relationship of locus of control to pain, coping strategies, and psychological distress in chronic pain patients. *Pain, 35*(2), 147–154.

Cross, W. E. (1980). Models of psychological nigrescence: A literature review. In R. L. Jones (Ed.), *Black psychology* (2nd ed., pp. 81–98). New York: Harper & Row.

Dana, R. H. (1986). Personality-assessment and Native Americans. *Journal of Personality Assessment, 50*(3), 480–500.

Davidson, L. (1987). The cross-cultural therapeutic dyad. *Contemporary Psychoanalysis, 23*(4), 659–675.

DeCharms, R. (1968). *Personal causation.* New York: Academic Press.

DeLongis, A., Folkman, S., & Lazarus, R. S. (1988). The impact of daily stress on health and mood: Psychological and social resources as mediators. *Journal of Personality and Social Psychology, 54*(3), 486–495.

Dillard, J. L. (1972). *Black English.* New York: Random House.

Dyal, J. (1984). Cross cultural research with the locus of control construct. In H. M. Lefcourt (Ed.), *Research with the locus of control construct: Extensions and limitations* (Vol. 3, pp. 209–306). New York: Academic Press.

Elkins, S. M. (1968). *Slavery* (2nd ed.). Chicago: University of Chicago Press.

Elliott, R., & James, E. (1989). Varieties of client experience in psychotherapy: An analysis of the literature. *Clinical Psychology Review, 9,* 443–469.

Evans, D., & Tyler, F. B. (1976). Is work competence enhancing for the poor? *American Journal of Community Psychology, 4,* 25–33.

Ewing, T. (1974). Racial similarity of client, and counselor satisfaction with therapy. *Journal of Counseling Psychotherapy, 21,* 446–447.

Ezekiel, R. S. (1968). The personal future and Peace Corps competence. *Journal of Personality and Social Psychology Monograph Supplement, 8*(2, Pt. 2).

Ezekiel, R. S. (1984). *Voices from the corner: poverty and racism in the inner city.* Philadelphia: Temple University Press.

Fanon, F. (1967). *Black skin, white masks.* New York: Grove Press.

Fleishman, J. A. (1984). Personality characteristics and coping patterns. *Journal of Health and Social Behavior, 25,* 229–244.

Ford, R. C. (1987). Cultural awareness and cross-cultural counseling. *International Journal for the Advancement of Counseling, 10*(1), 71–78.

Frank, J. (1947). Adjustment problems of selected Negro soldiers. *Journal of Nervous and Mental Disease, 105,* 647–650.

Freire, P. (1971). *Pedagogy of the oppressed.* New York: Herder and Herder.

Garb, H. N. (1989). Clinical judgment, clinical training and professional experience. *Psychological Bulletin, 105*(3), 387–396.

Garfield, S. L. (1978). Research on client variables in psychotherapy. In S. L. Garfield & A. E. Bergin (Eds.), *Handbook of psychotherapy and behavior change* (2nd ed., pp. 191–232). New York: Wiley.

Garmezy, N. (1983). Stressors of childhood. In N. Garmezy & M. Rutter (Eds.), *Stress, coping, and development in children* (pp. 43–84). New York: McGraw-Hill.

Gary, L. E. (1978). *Mental health: A challenge to the black community.* Philadelphia: Dorrane.

Gatz, M., Barbarin, O., Tyler, F. B., Mitchell, R., Moran, J., Wirzbicki, P., Crawford, J., & Engleman, A. (1982a). Enhancement of individual and community competence: The older adult as community worker. *American Journal of Community Psychology, 10,* 203–219.

Gatz, M., Gease, E. I., Tyler, F. B., & Moran, J. (1982b). Psychosocial competence characteristics of black and white women: The constraining effects of "triple jeopardy." *The Black Scholar, 13*, 5–12.

Gibbs, J. T. (1980). The interpersonal orientation in mental health consultation: Toward a model of ethnic variations in consultation. *Journal of Community Psychology, 8*, 195–207.

Gilligan, C. (1982). *In a different voice*. Cambridge, MA: Harvard University Press.

Goldfried, M., & D'Zurilla, T. (1969). A behavioral-analytic model for assessing competence. In C. Spielberger (Ed.), *Current topics in clinical and community psychology* (pp. 151–196). New York: Academic Press.

Gordon, M., & Grantham, R. J. (1979). Helper preference in disadvantaged students. *Journal of Counseling Psychology, 26*, 337–343.

Gossett, T. (1963). *Race: The history of an idea in America*. Dallas: Southern Methodist University Press.

Gould, S. J. (1981). *The mismeasure of man*. New York: W. W. Norton.

Grace, G. D., & Schill, T. (1986). Expectancy of personal control and seeking social support in coping style. *Psychological Reports, 58*(3), 757–758.

Greenberg, L. S. (1986). Change process research. *Journal of Consulting and Clinical Psychology, 54*, 22–26.

Greenfield, S., Kaplan, S., & Ware, J. E. (1985). Expanding patient involvement in care: Effects on patient outcomes. *Annals of Internal Medicine, 102*, 520–528.

Griffith, M. S. (1977). The influence of race on psychotherapeutic relationship. *Psychiatry, 40*, 27–40.

Griffith, M., & Jones, E. (1979). Race and psychotherapy: Changing perspectives. In J. Masserman (Ed.), *Current psychiatric therapies* (Vol. 18, pp. 225–235). New York: Grune & Stratton.

Grinker, R., Sr., Grinker, R., Jr., & Timberlake, J. (1962). "Mentally healthy" young males (homoclites). *Archives of General Psychiatry, 6*, 405–453.

Handy, W. S. (1978). *Traditional and ethnic perspective on black health*. Paper presented at the Eleventh Annual National Convention of the Association of Black Psychologists, St. Louis, MO.

Harrison, D. (1975). Race as a counselor–client variable in counseling and psychotherapy: A review of the research. *Counseling Psychologist, 5*, 124–133.

Hartmann, H. (1958). *Ego psychology and the problem of adaptation*. New York: International University Press.

Heath, D. (1977). *Maturity and competence*. New York: Gardner Press.

Hector, M. A., & Fray, J. S. (1987). The counseling process, client expectations, and cultural influences: A review. *International Journal for the Advancement of Counseling, 10*(4), 237–247.

Heine, R. W. (1950). The Negro patient in psychotherapy. *Journal of Clinical Psychology, 6*, 373–376.

Helms, J. E. (1985). Toward a theoretical explanation of the effects of race on counseling: A black and white model. *Counseling Psychologist, 12*(3), 153–164.

Helms, J. E. (1990). *Black and white racial identity: Theory, research and practice*. New York: Greenwood Press.

Hendricks, L. E., & Fullilove, R. E. (1983). Locus of control and the use of contraception among unmarried black adolescent fathers and their controls: A preliminary report. *Journal of Youth and Adolescence, 12*(3), 225–233.

Herskovits, M. J. (1956). *Man and his works*. New York: Knopf.

Hilliard, A. (1984). IQ testing as the emperor's new clothes: A critique of Jensen's bias in mental testing. In C. Reynolds (Ed.), *Perspectives on bias in mental tests* (pp. 139–170). New York: Plenum.

Hines, P. M., & Boyd-Franklin, N. (1982). Black families. In M. McGoldrick, J. Pearce, & J. Giordano (Eds.), *Ethnicity and family therapy* (pp. 84–107). New York: Guilford.
Holahan, C. J., & Moos, R. H. (1981). Social support and psychological distress: A longitudinal analysis. *Journal of Abnormal Psychology, 90,* 365–370.
Holahan, C. J., & Moos, R. H. (1985). Life stress and health: Personality, coping, and family support in stress resistance. *Journal of Personality and Social Psychology, 49*(3), 739–747.
Holahan, C. J., & Moos, R. H. (1986). Personality, coping, and family resources in stress resistance: A longitudinal analysis. *Journal of Personality and Social Psychology, 51*(2), 389–395.
Ibrahim, F. A. (1985). Effective cross-cultural counseling and psychotherapy. *Psychotherapy, 22*(2), 321–323.
Jackson, G. (1976). Cultural seedbeds of the black backlash in mental health. *Journal of Afro-American Issues, 4,* 70–91.
Jackson, G. (1979). The roots of backlash theory in mental health, *Journal of Black Psychology, 6*(1), 17–45.
Jackson, G. G., & Kirschner, S. A. (1973). Racial self-designation and preference for a counselor. *Journal of Counseling Psychology, 20,* 560–564.
Jahoda, M. (1958). *Current concepts of positive mental health.* New York: Basic Books.
James, W. H., Woodruff, A. B., & Werner, W. (1965). Effect of internal and external control upon changes in smoking behavior. *Journal of Consulting Psychology, 29,* 184–186.
Jones, E. E. (1978). Effects of race on psychotherapy process and outcome: An exploratory investigation. *Psychotherapy: Theory, Research and Practice, 15,* 226–236.
Jones, E. E. (1982). Psychotherapists impression of treatment outcome as a function of race. *Journal of Clinical Psychology, 38*(4), 722–731.
Jones, F. (1976). *White racism and Africanity in the development of Afro-American communities.* Paper presented at Annual Clinical Community Workshop, University of Maryland, College Park.
Jones, J. M. (1972). *Racism and prejudice.* Reading, MA: Addison-Wellesley.
Jordan, W. D. (1968). *White over black.* Chapel Hill: University of North Carolina Press.
Kaduchin, A. (1972). The racial factor in the interview. *Social Work, 17,* 88–98.
Kazdin, A. E. (1986). Editor's introduction to the special issue [Special issue]. *Journal of Consulting and Clinical Psychology, 54,* 3.
Kobasa, S. C. (1979). Stressful life events, personality, and health: An inquiry into hardiness. *Journal of Personality and Social Psychology, 37,* 1–11.
Korchin, S. (1980). Clinical psychology and minority problems. *American Psychologist, 35,* 262–269.
Kovel, J. (1970). *White racism: A psychohistory.* New York: Vintage Books.
Krupnick, J., Shea, T., & Elkin, E. (1986). Generalizability of treatment studies utilizing solicited patients. *Journal of Consulting and Clinical Psychology, 54,* 68–78.
Kuhn, T. (1970). *The structure of scientific revolutions.* Chicago: University of Chicago Press.
Lambert, M. J. (1989). The individual therapist's contribution to psychotherapy process and outcome. *Clinical Psychology Review, 9,* 469–486.
Lazarus, R. (1966). *Psychological stress and the coping process.* New York: McGraw-Hill.
Lefcourt, H. M. (Ed.). (1984). *Research with the locus of control construct: Vol. 3. Extensions and limitations.* New York: Academic Press.
Leong, F. T. L. (1986). Counseling and psychotherapy with Asian-Americans—Review of the literature. *Journal of Counseling Psychology, 33*(2), 196–206.
Lerner, S. (1972). *Therapy in the ghetto: Political impotence and personal disintegration.* Baltimore: Johns Hopkins University Press.
Li, R. D. (1980). Cultural influences on clinical perception: A comparison between Cauca-

sian and Chinese-American therapists. *Journal of Cross Cultural Psychology, 11*(3), 327–342.

Lin, K. M., Inui, T. S., Kleinman, A. M., & Womack, W. M. (1982). Sociocultural determinants of the help-seeking behavior of patients with mental illness. *Journal of Nervous and Mental Diseases, 170*(2), 78–85.

Loevinger, J. (1976). *Ego development: Conceptions and theory.* San Francisco: Josey Bass.

Lundy, J. R. (1972). Some personality correlates of contraceptive use among married female college students. *Journal of Psychology, 80,* 9–14.

Maish, K. A. (1977). *Black political orientation, political activism, and positive mental health.* Unpublished doctoral dissertation, University of Maryland, College Park.

McGoldrick, M. (1982). Ethnicity and family therapy: An overview. In M. McGoldrick, J. Pearce, & J. Giordano (Eds.), *Ethnicity and family therapy* (pp. 3–30). New York: Guilford.

McIntosh, P. (1988). *White privilege and male privilege: A personal account of coming to see correspondences through work in women's studies.* Working paper, Center for Research on Women, Wellesley College, Wellesley, MA.

Meichenbaum, D. (1989). Noncompliance. *Feelings and Their Medical Significance, 31,* 5–8.

Meier, A., & Rudwick, E. (1969). *The making of black America: Essays in Negro life & history, Vol. I.* New York: Atheneum.

Meyer, R. J., & Haggerty, R. J. (1962). Streptococcal infection in families: Factors altering individual susceptibility. *Pediatrics, 29,* 539–549.

Mitchell, K. M., & Atkinson, M. B. (1983). The relationship between therapist and client social class and participation in psychotherapy. *Professional Psychology, Research and Practice, 14*(3), 310–316.

Moffic, H. S. (1983). Sociocultural guidelines for clinicians in multicultural settings. *Psychiatric Quarterly, 55*(1), 47–54.

Mondell, S., & Tyler, F. B. (1981). Child psychosocial competence and its measurement. *Journal of Pediatric Psychology, 6,* 145–154.

Mondell, S., Tyler, F. B., & Freeman, R. W. (1981). Evaluating a psychotherapeutic day camp with psychosocial competence and goal attainment measures. *Journal of Clinical Child Psychology, 10,* 180–184.

Nobles, W. (1976). Extended self: Rethinking the so-called Negro self-concept. *Journal of Black Psychology, 2,* 15–24.

Nobles, W. W. (1980). African philosophy: Foundations for black psychology. In R. Jones (Ed.), *Black psychology* (2nd ed., pp. 99–105). New York: Harper & Row.

Nobles, W. (1990, February). *Culturally informed, group esteem enhancing prevention: The Afrocentric model.* Invited address given at the Office for Substance Abuse Prevention, Third National Learning Community Conference, Washington, DC.

Oakes, J. (1982). *The ruling race: A history of American slaveholders.* New York: Vintage Books.

Orlinsky, D. E. (1989). Researchers' images of psychotherapy: Their origins and influence on research. *Clinical Psychology Review, 9,* 469–486.

Otero, R. (1982). *The handling of stressful psychosocial life events as a function of a hierarchical pattern of competence.* Unpublished doctoral dissertation, University of Maryland, College Park.

Otero, R., Tyler, F. B., & Labarta, M. (1986). A cross-cultural comparison of behavioral attributes of psychosocial competence using a Spanish translation of the Tyler Behavioral Attributes of Psychosocial Competence. *Intramerican Journal of Psychology, 20,* 45–58.

Pargament, K. I., Steele, R. E., & Tyler, F. B. (1979). Religious participation, religious motivation, and psychosocial competence. *Journal for the Scientific Study of Religion, 18,* 412–419.

Parham, T., & Helms, J. E. (1981). The influence of black students' racial identity attitudes on preferences for counselor's race. *Journal of Counseling Psychology, 28,* 3, 250–257.

Parkes, K. R. (1984). Locus of control, cognitive appraisal, and coping in stressful situation. *Journal of Personality and Social Psychology, 46,* 655–668.

Parloff, M. B., Waskow, W. E., & Wolfe, B. E. (1978). Research on therapist variables in relation to process and outcome: In S. L. Garfield & A. E. Bergin (Eds.), *Handbook of psychotherapy and behavior change: An empirical analysis* (2nd ed., pp. 233–282). New York: Wiley.

Pedersen, P. (1987). Ten frequent assumptions of cultural bias in Counseling. *Journal of Multicultural Counseling and Development, 15*(1), 16–24.

Phares, E. J. (1976). *Locus of control in personality.* Morristown, NJ: General Learning Press.

Phillips, W. B. (1960). Section D: Counseling Negro pupils: An educational dilemma. *Journal of Negro Education, 28,* 504–507.

Pinderhughes, C. (1973). Racism and psychotherapy. In C. V. Willie, B. M. Kramer, & B. S. Brown (Eds.), *Racism and mental health* (pp. 61–122). Pittsburgh: University of Pittsburgh Press.

Pinderhughes, E. (1989). *Understanding race, ethnicity and power: The key to efficacy in clinical practice.* New York: Free Press.

Poe, C. A. (1973). Development of a psychological effectiveness scale. *Journal of Psychology, 85,* 81–85.

Ponterotto, J., & Casas, J. J. (1987). In search of multicultural competence within counselor education programs. *Journal of Counseling and Development, 65*(8), 430–434.

President's Commission on Mental Health. (1978). *Task panel of special populations.* Washington, DC: U.S. Government Printing Office.

Rahe, R. H., & Lind, E. (1971). Psychosocial factors and sudden cardiac death: A pilot study. *Journal of Psychosomatic Research, 15,* 19–24.

Ridley, C. R. (1984). Clinical treatment of the nondisclosing black client: A therapeutic paradox. *American Psychologist, 39*(11), 1234–1244.

Roll, S., Millen, L., & Martinez, R. (1980). Common errors in psychotherapy with Chicanos: Extrapolations from research and clinical experience. *Psychotherapy: Theory, Research and Practice, 17,* 158–168.

Roter, D. L. (1977). Patient participation in the patient–provider interaction: The effects of patient question asking on the quality of interaction, satisfaction and compliance. *Health Education Monographs,* (Winter), 281–315.

Rotter, J. (1966). Generalized expectancies for internal versus external control of reinforcement. *Psychological Monographs, 80*(609), 1–23.

Rotter, J. (1967). A new scale for the measurement of interpersonal trust. *Journal of Personality and Social Psychology, 35*(4), 651–665.

Rotter, J. (1975). Some problems and misconceptions related to the construct of internal versus external control of the new environment. *Journal of Consulting and Clinical Psychology, 43,* 56–67.

Rotter, J. B. (1980). Interpersonal trust, trustworthiness, and gullibility. *American Psychologist, 35*(1), 1–7.

Russell, R. L. (1989). Preface [Special issue]. *Clinical Psychology Review, 9,* 411.

St. Claire, H. (1951). Psychiatric interview experience with Negroes. *American Journal of Psychiatry, 108,* 113–119.

Sanchez, A. R., & Atkinson, D. R. (1983). Mexican-American cultural commitment, preference for counselor ethnicity, and willingness to utilize counseling. *Journal of Counseling Psychology, 30,* 215–220.

Sattler, J. M. (1970). Racial "experimenter effects" in the psychotherapy of Negro patient. *Psychiatric Quarterly, 34,* 9–27.

Sattler, J. M. (1977). The effects of therapist–client similarities. In A. S. Gurman & A. M. Razin (Eds.), *Effective psychotherapy: A handbook of research* (pp. 252–290). New York: Pergamon.

Schulman, B. A. (1979). Active patient orientation on and outcomes in hypertensive treatment: Application of a socio-organizational perspective. *Medical Care,* 267–280.

Seeman, J. (1959). Toward a concept of personality integration. *American Psychologist, 14,* 633–637.

Seeman, J. (1966). Personality integration in college women. *Journal of Personality and Social Psychology, 4,* 91–93.

Seeman, M., & Evans, J. W. (1962). Alienation and learning in a hospital setting. *American Sociological Review, 27,* 772–783.

Shane, M. (1960). Some subcultural considerations in the psychotherapy of a Negro patient. *Psychiatric Quarterly, 34,* 9–27.

Silber, E., Hamburg, D. A., Coelho, G. V., Murphey, E. B., Rosenberg, M., & Pearlin, L. I. (1961). Adaptive behavior in competent adolescents: Coping with the anticipation of college. *Archives of General Psychiatry, 5,* 354.

Smith, E. M. J. (1985). Ethnic minority: Life stress, social support, and mental health issues. *Counseling Psychologist, 13,* 537–579.

Smith, M. B. (1965). Explorations in competence: A study of Peace Corps teachers in Ghana. *American Psychologist, 21,* 555–566.

Smith, M. B. (1968). Competence and socialization. In J. Clausen (Ed.), *Socialization and society* (pp. 270–320). Boston: Little, Brown.

Spivack, G., & Shure, M. B. (1974). *Social adjustment of young children.* San Francisco: Jossey-Bass.

Stevens, M. (1945). Meeting the needs of dependent Negro children. *The Family, 2,* 176–181.

Stipek, D. (1980). A causal analysis of the relation between locus of control and academic achievement. *Contemporary Educational Psychology, 5*(1), 90–99.

Strupp, H. H. (1986). Psychotherapy: Research, practice, and public policy (How to avoid dead ends). *American Psychologist, 42,* 120–130.

Sue, D. W. (1978). Elementary cultural oppression in counseling: Toward a general theory. *Journal of Counseling Psychology, 25,* 419–428.

Sue, S. (1988). Psychotherapeutic services for ethnic-minorities—Two decades of research findings. *American Psychologist, 43*(4), 301–308.

Sue, S., & Zane, N. (1987). The role of culture and cultural techniques in therapy: A critique and reformulation. *American Psychologist, 42*(1), 37–45.

Sussewell, D. R. (1981). *Cross-racial study of double consciousness.* Unpublished doctoral dissertation, University of Maryland, College Park.

Szapocznik, J., Lasaga, J., Perry, P., & Solomon, J. R. (1979). Outreach in the delivery of mental health services to Hispanic elders. *Hispanic Journal of Behavioral Sciences, 1,* 21–40.

Terestman, N., Miller, D., & Weber, J. (1974). Blue collar workers at the psychoanalytic clinic. *American Journal of Psychiatry, 131,* 261–266.

Theorell, T., Lind, E., & Floderus, B. (1975). The relationship of disturbing life changes and emotions to the early development of myocardial infarctions and other serious illnesses. *International Journal of Epidemiology, 4,* 281–293.

Thomas, A. P., & Sillen, S. (1972). *Racism and psychiatry.* New York: Brunner/Mazel.

Tinloy, M. (1978). Counseling Asian-Americans: A contrast in values. *Journal of Non-White Concerns in Personnel and Guidance, 6*(2), 71–77.

Toupin, E. (1980). Counseling Asians: Psychotherapy in the context of racism and Asian-American history. *American Journal of Orthopsychiatry, 50*(1), 76–86.

Triandis, H., & Lambert, W. W. (1980). *Handbook of clinical and community psychology perspectives* (Vol. 1). Boston: Allyn & Bacon.

Turner, S., & Armstrong, S. (1981). Cross racial psychotherapy: What the therapists say. *Psychotherapy: Theory, Research and Practice, 18,* 375–378.

Tyler, F. B. (1978). Individual psychosocial competence: A personality configuration. *Education and Psychological Measurements, 38,* 309–323.

Tyler, F. B. (1979). Psychological competence differences among adolescents on entering group counseling. *Psychological Reports, 44,* 811–822.

Tyler, F. B. (1986). Ecology, ethnic validity, and psychotherapy. Paper presented at the Conference on Ethnic Minority Perspectives in Human Development and Clinical Psychology, University of Massachusetts/Boston, Boston, MA.

Tyler, F. B., Dhawan, N., & Sinha, Y. (1988). Adaptation patterns of Indian and American adolescents. *Journal of Social Psychology, 128,* 633–645.

Tyler, F. B., Dhawan, N., & Sinha, Y. (1989). Cultural contributions to constructing locus of control attributions. *Genetic, Social and General Psychology Monographs, 115*(2), 205–220.

Tyler, F. B., & Gatz, M. (1977). Development of individual psychosocial competence in a high school setting. *Journal of Consulting and Clinical Psychology, 45,* 441–449.

Tyler, F. B., Gatz, M., & Keenan, K. (1979). A constructivist analysis of the Rotter I-E scale. *Journal of Personality and Social Psychology, 47,* 11–35.

Tyler, F. B., Labarta, M., & Otero, R. (1986). Attributions of locus of control in a Puerto Rican sample. *InterAmerican Journal of Psychology, 20,* 23–44.

Tyler, F. B., Moran, J. A., Gatz, M., & Gease, E. I. (1982). Individual psychosocial competence and aging. *Academic Psychology Bulletin, 4,* 503–514.

Tyler, F. B., & Pargament, K. I. (1981). Racial and personal factors and the complexities of competence-oriented changes in a high school group counseling program. *American Journal of Community Psychology, 9,* 697–714.

Tyler, F. B., & Pargament, K. I. (1982). *The behavioral attributes of psychosocial competence.* Unpublished manuscript.

Tyler, F. B., Pargament, K. I., & Gatz, M. A. (1983). The resource collaborator role: A model for interaction between change agents and community members. *American Psychologist, 38,* 388–398.

Tyler, F. B., Sussewell, D., & Williams-McCoy, J. (1985). Ethnic validity in psychotherapy: A psychosocial competence perspective. *Psychotherapy, 22,* 311–320.

Tyler, F. B., Tyler, S. L., Echeverry, J. J. (1985). Psychosocial characteristics of Bogota gamins. *Cuadernos de Psicologia, 7,* 121–148.

Tyler, F. B., & Varma, M. (1988). Help-seeking and helping behavior in children as a function of psychological competence. *Journal of Applied Developmental Psychology, 9,* 219–231.

Vandenbos, G. (1986). Psychotherapy research: A special issue [Special issue]. *American Psychologist, 42,* 111–112.

Weiss, S. L., & Dlugokinski, E. (1974). Parental expectations of psychotherapy. *Journal of Psychology, 86,* 71–80.

Werner, E. E., Bierman, J. M., & French, F. E. (1971). *The children of Kauai: A longitudinal study from the prenatal period to age ten.* Honolulu: University of Hawaii Press.

Werner, E. E., & Smith, R. S. (1982). *Vulnerable but invincible: A study of resilient children.* New York: McGraw-Hill.

White, J. L. (1970). Guidelines for black psychologists. *Black Scholar, 21,* 522–525.

White, R. W. (1959). Motivational reconsidered: The concept of competence. *Psychological Review, 66,* 297–333.

Williams-McCoy, J., & Tyler, F. B. (1985). Selected psychosocial characteristics of black unwed adolescent fathers. *Journal of Adolescent Health Care, 6,* 12–16.

Willie, C. V., Kramer, B. M., & Brown, B. S. (1973). *Racism and Mental Health.* Pittsburgh: University of Pittsburgh Press.

Wolman, B. (1973). *Dictionary of behavioral science.* New York: Van Nostrand.

Wood, N. (1979). *Weusi suspiciousness.* Unpublished master's thesis, University of Maryland, College Park.

Wright, T. L., & Kirmani, A. (1977). Interpersonal trust, trustworthiness and shoplifting in high school. *Psychological Reports, 41,* 1165–1166.

Yamamoto, J., James, Q., Bloombaum, M., & Hattem, J. (1967). Racial factors in patient selection. *American Journal of Psychiatry, 5,* 630–636.

Young, K. A. (1975). *The relationship among black power orientation, self-concept, and behavioral competence in black adolescents.* Unpublished master's thesis, University of Maryland, College Park.

Zwerling, I., Batson, R., Carr, A., Parks, P., Peck, H., Sherrington, W., & Tyler, F. B. (1976). *Professionalism, elitism, and racism: Barriers to community of mental health.* New York: Jason Aronson.

Author Index

Subject Index